T0348402

2013
YEAR BOOK OF
CRITICAL CARE
MEDICINE®

The 2013 Year Book Series

Year Book of Critical Care Medicine®: Drs Dries, Zanotti-Cavazzoni, Latenser, Martinez, Rincon, and Zwank

Year Book of Emergency Medicine®: Drs Hamilton, Bruno, Handly, Minczak, Quintana, and Ramoska

Year Book of Endocrinology®: Drs Schott, Apovian, Clarke, Eugster, Meikle, Oetgen, Ovalle, Schteingart, and Toth

Year Book of Hand and Upper Limb Surgery®: Drs Yao, Adams, Isaacs, Lee, and Rizzo

Year Book of Medicine®: Drs Barker, Garrick, Gersh, Khardori, LeRoith, Panush, Talley, and Thigpen

Year Book of Neonatal and Perinatal Medicine®: Drs Fanaroff, Benitz, Donn, Neu, Papile, and Van Marter

Year Book of Neurology and Neurosurgery®: Drs Klimo, Minagar, Gandhi, House, Kevill, Liu, Mazia, Panagariya, Ragel, Riesenburger, Robottom, Schwendimann, Shafazand, Uhm, and Yang

Year Book of Obstetrics, Gynecology, and Women's Health®: Drs Dungan and Shulman

Year Book of Oncology®: Drs Arceci, Bauer, Chiorean, Gordon, Lawton, Murphy, Thigpen, and Tsao

Year Book of Ophthalmology®: Drs Rapuano, Cohen, Flanders, Hammersmith, Milman, Myers, Nagra, Nelson, Penne, Pyfer, Sergott, Shields, Talekar, and Vander

Year Book of Orthopedics®: Drs Morrey, Huddleston, Rose, Swiontkowski, and Trigg

Year Book of Otolaryngology-Head and Neck Surgery®: Drs Sindwani, Balough, Franco, Gapany, and Mitchell

Year Book of Pathology and Laboratory Medicine®: Drs Raab and Bissell

Year Book of Pediatrics®: Dr Stockman

Year Book of Plastic and Aesthetic Surgery™: Drs Miller, Boehmler, Gosman, Gutowski, Ruberg, Salisbury, and Smith

Year Book of Psychiatry and Applied Mental Health®: Drs Talbott, Ballenger, Buckley, Frances, Krupnick, and Mack

Year Book of Pulmonary Disease®: Drs Barker, Jones, Maurer, Spradley, Tanoue, and Willsie

Year Book of Sports Medicine®: Drs Shephard, Cantu, Feldman, Galea, Jankowski, Janssen, Lebrun, and Nieman

Year Book of Surgery®: Drs Copeland, Behrns, Daly, Eberlein, Fahey, Huber, Klodell, Mozingo, and Pruett

Year Book of Urology®: Drs Andriole and Coplen

Year Book of Vascular Surgery®: Drs Moneta, Gillespie, Starnes, and Watkins

2013

The Year Book of
CRITICAL CARE
MEDICINE®

Editors-in-Chief

David J. Dries, MSE, MD

John F. Perry, Jr. Chair of Trauma Surgery, Professor of Anesthesiology, Adjunct Professor of Clinical Emergency Medicine, University of Minnesota; Assistant Medical Director for Surgical Care, HealthPartners Medical Group, Minneapolis, Minnesota; Director of Critical Care Services and Director of Academic Programs, Department of Surgery, Regions Hospital, St. Paul, Minnesota

Sergio L. Zanotti-Cavazzoni, MD

Assistant Professor of Medicine, Cooper Medical School of Rowan University; Adjunct Professor, Robert Wood Johnson Medical School, University of Medicine and Dentistry of New Jersey; Program Director, Critical Care Medicine Fellowship, Division of Critical Care Medicine, Cooper University Hospital, Camden, New Jersey

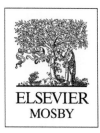

ELSEVIER
MOSBY

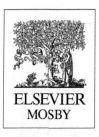

ELSEVIER
MOSBY

Vice President, Continuity: Kimberly Murphy
Developmental Editor: Patrick Manley
Production Supervisor, Electronic Year Books: Donna M. Skelton
Electronic Article Manager: Mike Sheets
Illustrations and Permissions Coordinator: Dawn Vohsen

2013 EDITION
Copyright 2013, Mosby, Inc. All rights reserved.

No part of this publication may be reproduced, stored in a retrieval system, or transmitted, in any form or by any means, electronic, mechanical, photocopying, recording, or otherwise, without prior written permission from the publisher.

Permission to photocopy or reproduce solely for internal or personal use is permitted for libraries or other users registered with the Copyright Clearance Center, provided that the base fee of $35.00 per chapter is paid directly to the Copyright Clearance Center, 21 Congress Street, Salem, MA 01970. This consent does not extend to other kinds of copying, such as copying for general distribution, for advertising or promotional purposes, for creating new collected works, or for resale.

Composition by TNQ Books and Journals Pvt Ltd, India

Printed and bound by CPI Group (UK) Ltd, Croydon, CR0 4YY

Transferred to digital print 2012

Editorial Office:
Elsevier
Suite 1800
1600 John F. Kennedy Blvd.
Philadelphia, PA 19103-2899

International Standard Serial Number: 0734-3299
International Standard Book Number: 978-1-4557-7273-5

Associate Editors

Barbara A. Latenser, MD
Professor of Surgery, Division of Acute Care Surgery, Department of Surgery, University of Iowa, Iowa City, Iowa

Elizabeth A. Martinez, MD, MHS
Associate Professor of Anesthesia, Critical Care and Pain Medicine, Massachusetts General Hospital, Harvard University, Boston, Massachusetts

Fred Rincon, MD, MSc, FACP
Assistant Professor of Neurology and Neurological Surgery, Department of Neurological Surgery, Thomas Jefferson University and Jefferson College of Medicine; Staff Neurointensivist, Division of Critical Care and Neurotrauma, Jefferson Hospital for Neurosciences, Philadelphia, Pennsylvania

Michael D. Zwank, MD, RDMS, FACEP
Assistant Professor, Department of Emergency Medicine, University of Minnesota Medical School, Minneapolis, Minnesota; Staff Physician, Emergency Department, Regions Hospital, St. Paul, Minnesota

Guest Editors

Guest Editor for Transfusion in the Critically Ill
David R. Gerber, DO
Associate Professor of Medicine, Cooper Medical School of Rowan University; Adjunct Professor, Robert Wood Johnson Medical School, University of Medicine and Dentistry of New Jersey; Associate Director, Medical/Surgical Intensive Care Unit, Cooper University Hospital, Camden, New Jersey

Guest Editor for Infection
Anand Kumar, MD
Associate Professor of Medicine, Cooper Medical School of Rowan University; Adjunct Professor, Robert Wood Johnson Medical School, University of Medicine and Dentistry of New Jersey; Division of Critical Care Medicine and Division of Infectious Diseases, Cooper University Hospital, Camden, New Jersey; Associate Professor of Medicine, Sections of Critical Care Medicine and Infectious Disease, University of Manitoba, Winnipeg, Canada

Guest Editor for Cardiology
Steven W. Werns, MD
Professor of Medicine, Cooper Medical School of Rowan University; Adjunct Professor, Robert Wood Johnson Medical School, University of Medicine and Dentistry of New Jersey; Director, Invasive Cardiovascular Services, Cooper University Hospital, Camden, New Jersey

Guest Editor for Ethics
Vijay Rajput, MD, FACP, SFHM
Professor of Medicine, Head, Division of Medical Education, Department of Medicine, Assistant Dean for Curriculum, Cooper Medical School of Rowan University, Camden, New Jersey

Contributing Editors

M. Kamran Athar, MD
Division of Neurocritical Care, Hospital of the University of Pennsylvania, Philadelphia, Pennsylvania

Duane Funk, MD
Assistant Professor of Anesthesia, University of Manitoba; Department of Anesthesia and Section of Critical Care Medicine, Winnipeg Health Sciences Center, Winnipeg, Manitoba, Canada

Zoulficar Kobeissi, MD
Assistant Professor of Clinical Medicine, Weill-Cornell School of Medicine, New York, New York; Intensivist, Division of Critical Care Medicine, The Methodist Hospital, Houston, Texas

Jocelyn Mitchell-Williams, MD, PhD
Associate Dean for Multicultural and Community Affairs, Cooper Medical School of Rowan University; Adjunct Professor, Robert Wood Johnson Medical School, University of Medicine and Dentistry of New Jersey; Department of Obstetrics and Gynecology, Cooper University Hospital, Camden, New Jersey

Nitin Puri, MD
Medical Intensivist, Inova Fairfax Hospital, Falls Church, Virginia

Collaborative Reviewers

J. Baker, MS
4th Year Medical Student, Class of 2013, Thomas Jefferson University, Philadelphia, Pennsylvania

Ryan T. Bourdon, MD
Emergency Medicine Resident, Regions Hospital, Saint Paul, Minnesota

T. Clark, MD
Internal Medicine Resident, Philadelphia College of Osteopathic Medicine Consortium, Philadelphia, Pennsylvania

Saugat Dey, MBBS
Clinical Observer and Research Volunteer, Neurological Surgery, Thomas Jefferson University, Philadelphia, Pennsylvania

M. Gardecki, MD
Neurocritical Care Fellow, Department of Neurology, Thomas Jefferson University, Philadelphia, Pennsylvania

Sayantani Ghosh, MBBS
Clinical Observer and Research Volunteer, Neurological Surgery, Thomas Jefferson University, Philadelphia, Pennsylvania

Shravan Kethireddy, MD
Associate Physician in the Departments of Critical Care and Infectious Diseases at Geisinger Medical Center, Danville, Pennsylvania

Lauren Ng, MD, MPH
Neurocritical Care Fellow, Department of Neurology, Thomas Jefferson University, Philadelphia, Pennsylvania

S. Siow, MD
4th Year Medical Student, Class of 2013, Thomas Jefferson University, Philadelphia, Pennsylvania

K .Vakharia, MD
4th Year Medical Student, Class of 2013, Thomas Jefferson University, Philadelphia, Pennsylvania

David Yaron, MD
4th Year Medical Student, Class of 2013, Thomas Jefferson University, Philadelphia, Pennsylvania

Joshua Weinstock, BS
1st Year Medical Student, Cooper Medical School of Rowan University, Camden, New Jersey

William Rafelson, MBA
4th Year Medical Student, Robert Wood Johnson Medical School at Camden, New Jersey

Krysta Contino, BS
4th Year Medical Student, Robert Wood Johnson Medical School at Camden, New Jersey

Phil Wilse, DO
3rd Medicine Resident, Cooper University Hospital, Cooper Medical School of Rowan University

Rajani Sharma, BS
Fourth Year Medical Student, Robert Wood Johnson Medical School at Camden, NJ

Paul McMackin, MD
Attending, Hospitalist, Cooper University Hospital, Camden, NJ

Emily Damuth, MD
Chief Fellow, Division of Critical Care Medicine, Cooper University Hospital, Cooper Medical School of Rowan University, Camden, NJ

Ben Goodgame, MD
Chief Fellow, Division of Critical Care Medicine, Cooper University Hospital, Cooper Medical School of Rowan University, Camden, NJ

Zoulficar Kobeissi, MD
Assistant Professor of Clinical Medicine, Weill-Cornel School of Medicine, New York, NY; Intensivist, Division of Critical Care Medicine, The Methodist Hospital, Houston, TX

Carleen Cho, MD
Resident, Department of Surgery, Cooper University Hospital, Cooper Medical School of Rowan University, Camden, NJ

Anthony F. Miller, MD
Resident, Department of Radiology, Hahnemann University Hospital, Philadelphia, Pennsylvania

Mithil Gajera, MD
Intensivist, Division of Critical Care Medicine, Christiana Healthcare System, Newark, Delaware

Table of Contents

JOURNALS REPRESENTED   xvii

PREFACE   xix

1. Airways/Lungs   1
   Acute Lung Injury/Acute Respiratory Distress Syndrome . .   1
   Airway   4
   Other   7
2. Cardiovascular   13
   Cardiac Arrest   13
   Cardiopulmonary Resuscitation/Other.   16
   Myocardial Infarction/Cardiogenic Shocks   20
   Pulmonary Embolism/Pulmonary Artery   48
3. Hemodynamics and Monitoring.   55
4. Infectious Disease   63
   Nosocomial/Ventilator-Acquired Pneumonia   63
   Other   64
5. Postoperative Management.   99
   Cardiovascular Surgery   99
   Miscellaneous.   120
   Other   128
6. Sepsis/Septic Shock.   135
7. Metabolism/Gastrointestinal/Nutrition/Hematology-Oncology   177
8. Neurologic: Traumatic and Non-traumatic   191
9. Renal   223
10. Trauma and Overdose   229
11. Ethics/Socioeconomic/Administrative Issues.   291
   Other   291
   Quality of Life/End of Life/Outcome Prediction   299
12. Pharmacology/Sedation-Analgesia   339

ARTICLE INDEX   349

AUTHOR INDEX   359

Journals Represented

Journals represented in this YEAR BOOK are listed below.
Academic Emergency Medicine
Alimentary Pharmacology & Therapeutics
American Journal of Medicine
American Journal of Respiratory and Critical Care Medicine
American Journal of Surgery
American Surgeon
Anaesthesia
Anesthesiology Clinics
Annals of Emergency Medicine
Annals of Internal Medicine
Annals of Surgery
Annals of Thoracic Surgery
Antimicrobial Agents and Chemotherapy
Archives of Internal Medicine
Archives of Physical Medicine and Rehabilitation
Archives of Surgery
British Journal of Surgery
Burns
Chest
Circulation
Circulation Cardiovascular Interventions
Circulation Cardiovascular Quality and Outcomes
Clinical Infectious Diseases
Critical Care Medicine
European Journal Cardio-Thoracic Surgery
European Journal of Obstetrics & Gynecology and Reproductive Biology
Heart
Injury
Intensive Care Medicine
Interactive Cardiovascular and Thoracic Surgery
Journal of Burn Care & Research
Journal of Cardiothoracic and Vascular Anesthesia
Journal of Critical Care
Journal of Electrocardiology
Journal of Emergency Medicine
Journal of Medical Ethics
Journal of Pain and Symptom Management
Journal of Surgical Research
Journal of the American College of Cardiology
Journal of the American College of Surgeons
Journal of the American Medical Association
Journal of the American Society of Nephrology
Journal of Thoracic and Cardiovascular Surgery
Journal of Trauma
Journal of Trauma and Acute Care Surgery
Journal of Vascular and Interventional Radiology
Lancet

Lancet Infectious Diseases
Mayo Clinic Proceedings
Medicine, Health Care and Philosophy
Neurosurgery
New England Journal of Medicine
Obstetrics & Gynecology
Otolaryngology-Head and Neck Surgery
Public Library of Science One
Resuscitation
Shock
Stroke
Surgery
Transfusion

STANDARD ABBREVIATIONS

The following terms are abbreviated in this edition: acquired immunodeficiency syndrome (AIDS), cardiopulmonary resuscitation (CPR), central nervous system (CNS), cerebrospinal fluid (CSF), computed tomography (CT), deoxyribonucleic acid (DNA), electrocardiography (ECG), health maintenance organization (HMO), human immunodeficiency virus (HIV), intensive care unit (ICU), intramuscular (IM), intravenous (IV), magnetic resonance (MR) imaging (MRI), and ribonucleic acid (RNA).

NOTE

The YEAR BOOK OF CRITICAL CARE MEDICINE® is a literature survey service providing abstracts of articles published in the professional literature. Every effort is made to assure the accuracy of the information presented in these pages. Neither the editors nor the publisher of the YEAR BOOK OF CRITICAL CARE MEDICINE® can be responsible for errors in the original materials. The editors' comments are their own opinions. Mention of specific products within this publication does not constitute endorsement.

To facilitate the use of the YEAR BOOK OF CRITICAL CARE MEDICINE® as a reference tool, all illustrations and tables included in this publication are now identified as they appear in the original article. This change is meant to help the reader recognize that any illustration or table appearing in the YEAR BOOK OF CRITICAL CARE MEDICINE® may be only one of many in the original article. For this reason, figure and table numbers will often appear to be out of sequence within the YEAR BOOK OF CRITICAL CARE MEDICINE®.

Preface

Welcome to the YEAR BOOK OF CRITICAL CARE MEDICINE for 2013!

Dr David J. Dries from Surgery at Regions Hospital and the University of Minnesota along with Dr Sergio L. Zanotti-Cavazzoni from the Cooper Medical School of Rowan University and Cooper University Hospital have placed greater emphasis on the ongoing submission of abstracts for the YEAR BOOK during the past year. If you follow YEAR BOOK abstracts online in Critical Care Medicine, you will see that approximately half of the abstracts were submitted prior to the close of the publishing year. This way, we hope to keep the most current information before our readers.

We again thank the other senior members of the editorial team. Dr Barbara Latenser from the University of Iowa continues to provide abstract review in burn care. Dr Elizabeth Martinez from the Massachusetts General Hospital reviews in perioperative care and anesthesiology, while Dr Michael Zwank of the University of Minnesota and Regions Hospital reviews emergency medicine management for a variety of problems. Dr Fred Rincon of Thomas Jefferson University adds the dimension of neurologic critical care.

As always, editors and associate editors receive invaluable input from other authorities serving as guest editors for this edition.

In addition, there are several key individuals participating in facilitating our editorial work. Ms Toni Piper at Cooper University Hospital continues as a key editorial resource for the YEAR BOOK OF CRITICAL CARE MEDICINE. Mrs Sherry Willett at Regions Hospital in St. Paul, Minnesota has joined her and is doing a large part of the essential editing. Mr Patrick Manley and the editorial team at Elsevier provide the link between editorial offices at Regions Hospital and Cooper University Medical Center.

Thank you for joining us! Enjoy this issue of the YEAR BOOK OF CRITICAL CARE MEDICINE.

Respectfully,

David J. Dries, MSE, MD
Sergio L. Zanotti-Cavazzoni, MD

1 Airways/Lungs

Acute Lung Injury/Acute Respiratory Distress Syndrome

Early alveolar and systemic mediator release in patients at different risks for ARDS after multiple trauma
Raymondos K, Martin MU, Schmudlach T, et al (Med School Hannover, Germany; Justus-Liebig-Univ, Giessen, Germany)
Injury 43:189-195, 2012

Alveolar IL-8 has been reported to early identify patients at-risk to develop ARDS. However, it remains unknown how alveolar IL-8 is related to pulmonary and systemic inflammation in patients predisposed for ARDS. We studied 24 patients 2–6 h after multiple trauma. Patients with IL-8 > 200 pg/ml in bronchoalveolar lavage (BAL) were assigned to the group at high risk for ARDS (H, $n = 8$) and patients with BAL IL-8 < 200 pg/ml to the group at low risk for ARDS (L, $n = 16$). ARDS developed within 24 h after trauma in 5 patients at high and at least after 1 week in 2 patients at low risk for ARDS ($p = 0.003$). High-risk patients had also increased BAL IL-6, TNF-α, IL-1β, IL-10 and IL-1ra levels ($p < 0.05$). BAL neutrophil counts did not differ between patient groups (H vs. L, 12% (3–73%) vs. 6% (2–32%), $p = 0.1$) but correlated significantly with BAL IL-8, IL-6 and IL-1ra. High-risk patients had increased plasma levels of pro- but not anti-inflammatory mediators. The enhanced alveolar and systemic inflammation associated with alveolar IL-8 release should be considered to identify high-risk patients for pulmonary complications after multiple trauma to adjust surgical and other treatment strategies to the individual risk profile.

▶ These authors demonstrate that alveolar and intravascular levels of interleukin (IL)-8 may be predictive of early adult respiratory distress syndrome development after blunt injury. I note that other contributing factors are not well-characterized. For example, patient use of blood products is reported, but the distribution of the use of these materials is not clearly specified.[1] In addition, chest x-ray was used to screen for pulmonary contusion. Computed tomography imaging would be a much better indicator.[2] All but 1 patient survived. There was no incremental change in mortality. One remarkable finding in all patients was the predominant proinflammatory pattern of cytokines identified.

We will need far more data to confirm the value of IL-8 as a predictor of pulmonary dysfunction after injury.[3] At this point, I cannot recommend IL-8 blockade or other anti-inflammatory cytokine strategies. I have 2 reasons for this suggestion. First, this system is highly redundant and blockade of 1 factor is unlikely to have a consistent outcome benefit. Second, a proinflammatory response may be associated with survival advantage compared with a situation where this response has been reduced.

D. J. Dries, MSE, MD

References

1. Dries DJ. The contemporary role of blood products and components used in trauma resuscitation. *Scand J Trauma Resusc Emerg Med.* 2010;18:63.
2. Miller PR, Croce MA, Bee TK, et al. ARDS after pulmonary contusion: accurate measurement of contusion volume identifies high-risk patients. *J Trauma.* 2001; 51:223-230.
3. Dicker RA, Morabito DJ, Pittet JF, Campbell AR, Mackersie RC. Acute respiratory distress syndrome criteria in trauma patients: why the definitions do not work. *J Trauma.* 2004;57:526-528.

Association Between Use of Lung-Protective Ventilation With Lower Tidal Volumes and Clinical Outcomes Among Patients Without Acute Respiratory Distress Syndrome: A Meta-analysis
Serpa Neto A, Cardoso SO, Manetta JA, et al (ABC Med School, Santo André, São Paulo, Brazil; et al)
JAMA 308:1651-1659, 2012

Context.—Lung-protective mechanical ventilation with the use of lower tidal volumes has been found to improve outcomes of patients with acute respiratory distress syndrome (ARDS). It has been suggested that use of lower tidal volumes also benefits patients who do not have ARDS.

Objective.—To determine whether use of lower tidal volumes is associated with improved outcomes of patients receiving ventilation who do not have ARDS.

Data Sources.—MEDLINE, CINAHL, Web of Science, and Cochrane Central Register of Controlled Trials up to August 2012.

Study Selection.—Eligible studies evaluated use of lower vs higher tidal volumes in patients without ARDS at onset of mechanical ventilation and reported lung injury development, overall mortality, pulmonary infection, atelectasis, and biochemical alterations.

Data Extraction.—Three reviewers extracted data on study characteristics, methods, and outcomes. Disagreement was resolved by consensus.

Data Synthesis.—Twenty articles (2822 participants) were included. Meta-analysis using a fixed-effects model showed a decrease in lung injury development (risk ratio [RR], 0.33; 95% CI, 0.23 to 0.47; I^2, 0%; number needed to treat [NNT], 11), and mortality (RR, 0.64; 95% CI, 0.46 to 0.89; I^2, 0%; NNT, 23) in patients receiving ventilation with lower tidal volumes. The results of lung injury development were similar when stratified by the type of study (randomized vs nonrandomized) and were significant only in randomized trials for pulmonary infection and only in nonrandomized trials for mortality. Meta-analysis using a random-effects model showed, in protective ventilation groups, a lower incidence of pulmonary infection (RR, 0.45; 95% CI, 0.22 to 0.92; I^2, 32%; NNT, 26), lower mean (SD) hospital length of stay (6.91 [2.36] vs 8.87 [2.93] days, respectively; standardized mean difference [SMD], 0.51; 95% CI, 0.20 to 0.82; I^2, 75%), higher mean (SD) $PaCO_2$ levels (41.05 [3.79] vs 37.90 [4.19] mm Hg, respectively; SMD, -0.51; 95% CI, -0.70 to -0.32; I^2, 54%), and lower mean (SD) pH values (7.37 [0.03] vs 7.40 [0.04], respectively; SMD, 1.16; 95% CI, 0.31 to 2.02; I^2, 96%) but similar mean (SD) ratios of PaO_2 to fraction of inspired oxygen (304.40 [65.7] vs 312.97 [68.13], respectively; SMD, 0.11; 95% CI, -0.06 to 0.27; I^2, 60%). Tidal volume gradients between the 2 groups did not influence significantly the final results.

Conclusions.—Among patients without ARDS, protective ventilation with lower tidal volumes was associated with better clinical outcomes. Some of the limitations of the meta-analysis were the mixed setting of mechanical ventilation (intensive care unit or operating room) and the duration of mechanical ventilation.

▶ This meta-analysis examines the balance of literature favoring lower tidal volumes even in patients without adult respiratory distress syndrome or acute lung injury.[1] With a number of reservations, as listed below, a low tidal volume strategy appears to be applicable across most patients.

Several important limitations in this work have been acknowledged by the authors and must be mentioned. First, many of the key observations and events recorded do not come from randomized trials. Second, duration of mechanical ventilation in these patients was brief in many of the studies included. Thus, a time-dependent treatment effect could be masked. Third, it appears that these authors included ventilation both in the operating room and in the critical care unit. Application of mechanical ventilation in these 2 settings is frequently quite different, and again, a treatment effect could be reduced with the inclusion of operating room data. Finally, it is important to note that many of the phenomena assessed are difficult to quantify. For example, definitions of pneumonia versus atelectasis associated with mechanical ventilation continue to be controversial (Fig 2 in the original article). Therefore, infection data proposed here could be seriously flawed. Definitions of various forms of lung injury also continue to evolve. The most recent Berlin definition is cited among the references in this trial.[2,3]

Within the context of physiologic stability, low tidal volumes can be supported in patients placed on critical care ventilation. However, additional study is needed to determine a mechanism of benefit.[4]

D. J. Dries, MSE, MD

References

1. Plötz FB, Slutsky AS, van Vught AJ, Heijnen CJ. Ventilator-induced lung injury and multiple system organ failure: a critical review of facts and hypotheses. *Intensive Care Med.* 2004;30:1865-1872.

2. The ARDS Definition Task Force, Ranieri VM, Rubenfeld GD, Thompson BT, et al. Acute respiratory distress syndrome: the Berlin Definition. *JAMA*. 2012; 307:2526-2533.
3. Bernard GR, Artigas A, Brigham KL, et al. The American-European Consensus Conference on ARDS. Definitions, mechanisms, relevant outcomes, and clinical trial coordination. *Am J Respir Crit Care Med*. 1994;149:818-824.
4. Gajic O, Dara SI, Mendez JL, et al. Ventilator-associated lung injury in patients without acute lung injury at the onset of mechanical ventilation. *Crit Care Med*. 2004;32:1817-1824.

Airway

Measurement of forces applied during Macintosh direct laryngoscopy compared with GlideScope® videolaryngoscopy

Russell T, Khan S, Elman J, et al (Univ of Toronto, Canada)
Anaesthesia 67:626-631, 2012

Summary Laryngoscopy can induce stress responses that may be harmful in susceptible patients. We directly measured the force applied to the base of the tongue as a surrogate for the stress response. Force measurements were obtained using three FlexiForce Sensors® (Tekscan Inc, Boston, MA, USA) attached along the concave surface of each laryngoscope blade. Twenty-four 24 adult patients of ASA physical status 1−2 were studied. After induction of anaesthesia and neuromuscular blockade, laryngoscopy and tracheal intubation was performed using either a Macintosh or a GlideScope® (Verathon, Bothell, WA, USA) laryngoscope. Complete data were available for 23 patients. Compared with the Macintosh, we observed lower median (IQR [range]) peak force (9 (5−13 [3−25]) N vs 20 (14-28 [4−41]) N; $p = 0.0001$), average force (5 (3−7 [2−19]) N vs 11 (6−16 [1−24]) N; $p = 0.0003$) and impulse force (98 (42−151 [26−444]) Ns vs 150 (93−207 [17−509]) Ns; $p = 0.017$) with the GlideScope. Our study shows that the peak lifting force on the base of the tongue during laryngoscopy is less with the GlideScope videolaryngoscope compared with the Macintosh laryngoscope.

▶ This article examined the forces applied to the laryngoscope/patient during intubation using a standard Macintosh (Mac) blade and using a GlideScope (Verathon, Bothell, WA, USA). Experienced anesthesiologists performed laryngoscopy on 24 healthy patients with normal anatomy. Both devices were used in random order on each patient and forces were measured with multiple sensors attached to the blades. The GlideScope required less peak, average, and impulse force (integral force over time) during the intubation. There was large variability in the forces used by various providers during the intubation and it appeared that this variation was greatest using the Mac blade. Incidentally, when using the Mac blade, 3 patients needed more than one attempt and 8 needed external laryngeal manipulation. The authors of this study discuss possible affects of the force on the patients (cervical spine movement, local tissue trauma). In contrast, I think this study takes the first step at examining effects on the provider. Laryngoscopy is hard work, and I have witnessed more than 1 example of a provider not having enough strength/force to obtain an adequate view of a patient's airway. This article would support the notion that if you have limited might in your arm or if the patient has a lot of mass to lift, consider using the GlideScope.

M. D. Zwank, MD

Difficult airway management in the emergency department: GlideScope videolaryngoscopy compared to direct laryngoscopy
Mosier JM, Stolz U, Chiu S, et al (Univ of Arizona College of Medicine, Tucson)
J Emerg Med 42:629-634, 2012

Background.—Videolaryngoscopy has become a popular method of intubation in the Emergency Department (ED), however, little research has compared this technique with direct laryngoscopy (DL).

Objective.—To compare the success rates of GlideScope (Verathon Inc., Bothell, WA) videolaryngoscopy (GVL) and DL in emergent airways with known difficult airway predictors (DAPs).

Methods.—We evaluated 772 consecutive ED intubations over a 23-month period. After each intubation, the physician completed a data collection form that included: demographics, DAPs, Cormack-Lehane view, optical clarity, lens contamination, and complications. DAPs included: cervical immobility, obesity, small mandible, large tongue, short neck, blood or vomit in the airway, tracheal edema, secretions, and facial or neck trauma. Primary outcome was first-attempt success rates. Multivariate logistic regression was performed to evaluate the odds of failure for DL compared to GVL.

Results.—First-attempt success rate with DL was 68%, GVL 78% (Fisher's exact test, $p = 0.001$). Adjusted odds of success of GVL compared to DL on first attempt equals 2.20 (odds ratio [OR] 2.2, 95% confidence interval [CI] 1.51−3.19). After statistically controlling for DAPs, GVL was more likely to succeed on first attempt than DL (OR 3.07, 95% CI 2.19−4.30). Logistic regression of DAPs showed that the presence of blood, small mandible, obesity, and a large tongue were statistically significant risk factors for decreasing the odds of success with DL and increasing the odds of success of GVL.

Conclusion.—For difficult airways with the presence of blood or small mandible, or a large tongue or obesity, GVL had a higher success rate at first attempt than DL.

▶ Tracheal intubation is front and center in the protocol of care for critically ill patients. Traditionally, this was accomplished with direct laryngoscopy by lifting the tongue and mandible with a suitable laryngoscope and placing an endotracheal tube into the trachea under direct visualization. Although the end goal remains the same, options for accomplishing the task have advanced over the past decade. This study retrospectively compared success rates among normal and difficult airways using traditional direct laryngoscopy (DL) with one of the more popular video laryngoscopes—the Glidescope. Not surprisingly, new school (Glidescope) outperformed old school (DL), especially among those airways deemed difficult. The odds ratio of first attempt success was 2.20 for all airways and 3.07 for difficult airways. This adds to prior literature supporting videolaryngoscope use in intubation. The study has limitations, including its retrospective nature and nonrandomized use of the techniques. However, given the plethora of literature already available, the results are consistent with previous studies. There are a number of videolaryngoscope products on the market and each has its strengths and weaknesses. In any case, in 2012, videolaryngoscopy should be available at least as a backup for all intubations, although ideally it should be used as first-line treatment, especially in airways deemed difficult.

M. D. Zwank, MD

A Comparison of the C-MAC Video Laryngoscope to the Macintosh Direct Laryngoscope for Intubation in the Emergency Department
Sakles JC, Mosier J, Chiu S, et al (Univ of Arizona, Tucson; Univ of Arizona College of Medicine, Tucson)
Ann Emerg Med 60:739-748, 2012

Study Objective.—We determine the proportion of successful intubations with the C-MAC video laryngoscope (C-MAC) compared with the direct laryngoscope in emergency department (ED) intubations.

Methods.—This was a retrospective analysis of prospectively collected data entered into a continuous quality improvement database during a 28-month period in an academic ED. After each intubation, the operator completed a standardized data form evaluating multiple aspects of the intubation, including patient demographics, indication for intubation, device(s) used, reason for device selection, difficult airway characteristics, number of attempts, and outcome of each attempt. Intubation was considered ultimately successful if the endotracheal tube was correctly inserted into the trachea with the initial device. An attempt was defined as insertion of the device into the mouth regardless of whether there was an attempt to pass the tube. The primary outcome measure was ultimate success. Secondary outcome measures were first-attempt success, Cormack-Lehane view, and esophageal intubation. Multivariate logistic regression analyses, with the inclusion of a propensity score, were performed for the outcome variables ultimate success and first-attempt success.

Results.—During the 28-month study period, 750 intubations were performed with either the C-MAC with a size 3 or 4 blade or a direct laryngoscope with a Macintosh size 3 or 4 blade. Of these, 255 were performed with the C-MAC as the initial device and 495 with a Macintosh direct laryngoscope as the initial device. The C-MAC resulted in successful intubation in 248 of 255 cases (97.3%; 95% confidence interval [CI] 94.4% to 98.9%). A direct laryngoscope resulted in successful intubation in 418 of 495 cases (84.4%; 95% CI 81.0% to 87.5%). In the multivariate regression model, with a propensity score included, the C-MAC was positively predictive of ultimate success (odds ratio 12.7; 95% CI 4.1 to 38.8) and first-attempt success (odds ratio 2.2; 95% CI 1.2 to 3.8). When the C-MAC was used as a video laryngoscope, a Cormack-Lehane grade I or II view (video) was obtained in 117 of 125 cases (93.6%; 95% CI 87.8% to 97.2%), whereas when a direct laryngoscope was used, a grade I or II view was obtained in 410 of 495 cases (82.8%; 95% CI 79.2% to 86.1%). The C-MAC was associated with immediately recognized esophageal intubation in 4 of 255 cases (1.6%; 95% CI 0.4% to 4.0%), whereas a direct laryngoscope was associated with immediately recognized esophageal intubation in 24 of 495 cases (4.8%; 95% CI 3.1% to 7.1%).

Conclusion.—When used for emergency intubations in the ED, the C-MAC was associated with a greater proportion of successful intubations and a greater proportion of Cormack-Lehane grade I or II views compared with a direct laryngoscope.

▶ Airway management lies at the very core of emergency medicine. Central to airway management is tracheal intubation. This retrospective cohort study evaluated a video laryngoscope (C-MAC; Karl Storz, Tuttlingen, Germany) in comparison with standard direct laryngoscopy in the emergency department. It was indeed the first study to make this comparison in this setting. This was a busy level I trauma center and most of the intubations were performed by emergency medicine residents. It comes as little surprise that the C-MAC outperformed direct laryngoscopy in nearly every aspect of intubation. Although one can break down the numbers in many different ways (eg, first pass attempt, predicted difficult airway), the question that matters most is: "When the dust had settled, was there an endotracheal tube in the trachea?" This key outcome occurred in 248/255 of the C-MAC attempts but only 418/495 of the direct laryngoscopy attempts. This is despite the fact that C-MAC was more likely to be chosen when an airway was expected to be difficult. Rescue devices included C-MAC, GlideScope, ILMA, and cricothyrotomy. The strengths of this article include the number of patients and the rigorous manner in which data was collected. This article adds to a growing body of literature supporting video laryngoscopy use during tracheal intubation. I am a big proponent of video laryngoscopy. If you have a video laryngoscope, you already know the benefits; if you don't have one, it is time to get one.

M. D. Zwank, MD

Other

Early Administration of Systemic Corticosteroids Reduces Hospital Admission Rates for Children With Moderate and Severe Asthma Exacerbation

Bhogal SK, McGillivray D, Bourbeau J, et al (McGill Univ, Montreal, Quebec, Canada; Montreal Children's Hosp of the McGill Univ Hosp Centre, Quebec, Canada)
Ann Emerg Med 60:84-91, 2012

Study Objective.—The variable effectiveness of clinical asthma pathways to reduce hospital admissions may be explained in part by the timing of systemic corticosteroid administration. We examine the effect of early (within 60 minutes [SD 15 minutes] of triage) versus delayed (>75 minutes) administration of systemic corticosteroids on health outcomes.

Methods.—We conducted a prospective observational cohort of children aged 2 to 17 years presenting to the emergency department with moderate or severe asthma, defined as a Pediatric Respiratory Assessment Measure (PRAM) score of 5 to 12. The outcomes were hospital admission, relapse, and length of active treatment; they were analyzed with multivariate logistic and linear regressions adjusted for covariates and potential confounders.

Results.—Among the 406 eligible children, 88% had moderate asthma; 22%, severe asthma. The median age was 4 years (interquartile range 3 to 8 years); 64% were male patients. Fifty percent of patients received systemic corticosteroids early; in 33%, it was delayed; 17% of children failed to receive any. Overall, 36% of patients were admitted to the hospital. Compared with delayed administration, early administration reduced the odds of admission by 0.4 (95% confidence interval 0.2 to 0.7) and the length of active treatment by 0.7 hours (95% confidence interval −1.3 to −0.8 hours), with no significant effect on relapse. Delayed administration was positively associated with triage priority and negatively with PRAM score.

Conclusion.—In this study of children with moderate or severe asthma, administration of systemic corticosteroids within 75 minutes of triage decreased hospital admission rate and length of active treatment, suggesting that early administration of systemic corticosteroids may allow for optimal effectiveness.

▶ It has already been shown that giving oral corticosteroids to emergency department (ED) patients with moderate to severe asthma can reduce hospitalizations. This Canadian study examined whether the timing of steroids given to children ages 2 to 17 with moderate to severe asthma affects hospitalization. In other words, if you give steroids early or late, does it make a difference? They showed that early steroid administration (defined as within 60 minutes of arrival) does lead to decreased hospitalization. In fact, for every 30-minute delay in giving steroids, there was an increased likelihood of admission of (odds ratio 1.23) and an increase in ED treatment time of 60 minutes. The strength of the study was that the hospital used an asthma treatment protocol that aimed to standardize care of these children. They also used a validated asthma score (Preschool Respiratory Assessment Measure) that helped grade asthma severity in an objective manner. This was a very well done study and shows that you should be giving steroids to any child with moderate or severe asthma and you should be giving them as early as possible. If you really want to make a difference, help your ED develop an asthma treatment protocol including triage evaluation to help standardize the treatment of these patients.

M. D. Zwank, MD

Burns, inhalation injury and ventilator-associated pneumonia: Value of routine surveillance cultures

Brusselaers N, Logie D, Vogelaers D, et al (Ghent Univ Hosp, Belgium; Ghent Univ, Belgium)
Burns 38:364-370, 2012

Purpose.—Burn patients with inhalation injury are at particular risk for ventilator-associated pneumonia (VAP). Routine endotracheal surveillance cultures may provide information about the causative pathogen in subsequent VAP, improving antibiotic therapy. Our objective was to assess the incidence of VAP in burn patients with inhalation injury, and the benefit of routine surveillance cultures to predict multidrug resistant (MDR) pathogens.

Procedures.—Historical cohort ($n = 53$) including all burn patients with inhalation injury requiring mechanical ventilation, admitted to the Ghent burn unit (2002—2010).

Main Findings.—Median (interquartile range) age and total burned surface area were 44y (39—55y) and 35% (19—50%). Overall, 70 episodes of VAP occurred in 46 patients (86.8%). Median mechanical ventilation days (MVD) prior to VAP onset were 7d (4—9d). The incidence was 55 episodes/1000 MVD. In 23 episodes (32.9%) at least one MDR causative pathogen was involved, mostly *Pseudomonas aeruginosa and Enterobacter* spp. The sensitivity and specificity of surveillance cultures to predict MDR etiology in subsequent VAP was respectively 83.0% and 96.2%. The positive and negative predictive value was 87.0% and 95.0%, respectively.

Conclusions.—The incidence of VAP in burn patients with inhalation injury is high. In this cohort routine surveillance cultures had excellent operating characteristics to predict MDR pathogen involvement.

▶ Like some of the other literature we are now seeing regarding burns, this work comes from a fairly small country (Belgium has a population of approximately 11 million) that has not traditionally published burn-related work in English-speaking journals. If you did not know better, you would be tempted to believe that we now know the incidence of ventilator-associated pneumonia (VAP) in patients with inhalation injury. Sadly, the authors seem unaware of the Consensus Conference on Burn Sepsis and Infection published in 2007,[1] wherein infections were clearly defined, including the criteria for pneumonia in the burn population. One of the main reasons for using uniform definitions for each infective process in any group of patients is to have cogent discussions about the same process, comparing apples to apples, if you will. The definitions of pneumonia must be uniform in order for the information regarding the use of routine surveillance cultures presented here to be meaningful and relevant. It would be interesting to know if the practitioners in this burn center adopted any of the VAP bundle strategies that have been effective in reducing the VAP incidence in the general intensive care unit population. Although it is not yet clear the exact impact of the VAP bundle on pneumonia prevention in the burn population, the early ambulation of the ventilated burn patient that has been in practice in some burn centers for decades is now finding favor in the nonburn critical care literature, an intervention that is long overdue.

B. A. Latenser, MD, FACS

Reference

1. Greenhalgh DG, Saffle JR, Holmes JH, et al; American Burn Association Consensus Conference on Burn Sepsis and Infection Group. American Burn Association consensus conference to define sepsis and infection in burns. *J Burn Care Res.* 2007;28:776-790.

Review of Burn Injuries Secondary to Home Oxygen
Murabit A, Tredget EE (Univ of Alberta, Edmonton, Canada)
J Burn Care Res 33:212-217, 2012

The use of long-term home oxygen therapy (HOT) has become increasingly common for treatment of chronic pulmonary diseases. Although illegal to smoke while on HOT, there is an increasing incidence of burn injuries in those patients who smoke while on HOT. The importance of recognition of the prevalence of this injury, the obstacles faced when treating these patients, and understanding the proposed algorithmic approach to be taken with patients on HOT, including prescription, reassessment, and prevention of burn injury are outlined in this review. Retrospective epidemiological data including circumstances, admission, treatment, and disposition were collected and reviewed on the patients treated from 1999 to 2008 with burns secondary to smoking while on HOT. Seventeen patients sustained injuries secondary to smoking on HOT over the 9-year period; 9 patients were female and 8 were male. All the patients were on HOT for chronic obstructive pulmonary disease. Mean patient age was 69.1 ± 2.5 years and mean TBSA 2.8 ± 0.4%; 11.8% (2/17) sustained inhalation injury requiring intubation and 23.5% (4/17) required wound debridement and skin grafting. Mean hospital stay was 42.8 ± 12.5 days; 10.3 ± 5.4 days in the burn intensive care unit and 32.5 ± 11.0 days in the ward. Before the burn injury, 23.5% (4/17) lived in long-term care facilities. On discharge from hospital, 47.1% (8/17) were transferred to extended care facilities or other acute care hospitals, and 11.8% (2/17) died during their hospitalization. After recovery, there was a 35.3% reduction in patients able to return home and/or live independently. A significant number of burn injuries secondary to smoking while on HOT was observed. These patients differ from standard burn patients because they are older in age, have higher rates of inhalation injury, and have much longer lengths of hospitalization, despite smaller TBSA injuries. Prevention of this injury would improve the safety of the patient and those around them as well as healthcare resource allocation. A proactive multidisciplinary algorithmic approach is presented which can be used to manage patients on HOT at risk for continued smoking

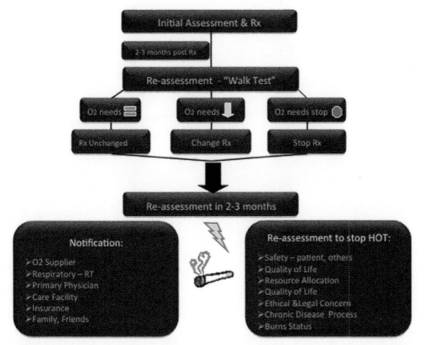

FIGURE 5.—Algorithm Overview consisting of initial assessment made with the prescription of oxygen, subsequent reassessment, and finally, the necessary repercussions if found to be smoking on home oxygen therapy (HOT). Rx, prescription; O₂, oxygen; RT, respiratory therapy. (Reprinted from Murabit A, Tredget EE. Review of burn injuries secondary to home oxygen. *J Burn Care Res.* 2012;33:212-217, with permission from the American Burn Association.)

to decrease the incidence and the impact of burn injuries in this patient population (Fig 5).

▶ The authors have done a great job illustrating how a very small problem affecting only a few patients is actually a serious public health hazard. That 17 patients with small body surface area burns cost the Canadian government more than $1.5 million Canadian dollars should grab the attention of health care providers everywhere. Burn care providers are not the physicians prescribing home oxygen therapy, but we care for patients when they misuse the therapy and continue to smoke while using home oxygen. It should not surprise us that the authors found that up to 50% of patients continue to smoke while using home oxygen. Education of the family and general health care providers must certainly be part of the process. Adding teeth to regulations whereby patients injured in a "smoking while on home oxygen therapy" event bear some financial responsibility for their injuries may be a reasonable step to consider. The authors present a very nice algorithm in Fig 5, to guide the practitioner through the process. Sadly, until there is a sudden outbreak of safety, these injuries will continue to be seen with their devastating consequences.

B. A. Latenser, MD, FACS

2 Cardiovascular

Cardiac Arrest

Hypothermia in Comatose Survivors From Out-of-Hospital Cardiac Arrest: Pilot Trial Comparing 2 Levels of Target Temperature
Lopez-de-Sa E, Rey JR, Armada E, et al (Hospital Universitario La Paz, Madrid, Spain; et al)
Circulation 126:2826-2833, 2012

Background.—It is recommended that comatose survivors of out-of-hospital cardiac arrest should be cooled to 32° to 34°C for 12 to 24 hours. However, the optimal level of cooling is unknown. The aim of this pilot study was to obtain initial data on the effect of different levels of hypothermia. We hypothesized that deeper temperatures will be associated with better survival and neurological outcome.

Methods and Results.—Patients were eligible if they had a witnessed out-of-hospital cardiac arrest from March 2008 to August 2011. Target temperature was randomly assigned to 32°C or 34°C. Enrollment was stratified on the basis of the initial rhythm as shockable or asystole. The target temperature was maintained during 24 hours followed by 12 to 24 hours of controlled rewarming. The primary outcome was survival free from severe dependence (Barthel Index score ≥ 60 points) at 6 months. Thirty-six patients were enrolled in the trial (26 shockable rhythm, 10 asystole), with 18 assigned to 34°C and 18 to 32°C. Eight of 18 patients in the 32°C group (44.4%) met the primary end point compared with 2 of 18 in the 34°C group (11.1%) (log-rank $P = 0.12$). All patients whose initial rhythm was asystole died before 6 months in both groups. Eight of 13 patients with initial shockable rhythm assigned to 32°C (61.5%) were alive free from severe dependence at 6 months compared with 2 of 13 (15.4%) assigned to 34°C (log-rank $P = 0.029$). The incidence of complications was similar in both groups except for the incidence of clinical seizures, which was lower (1 versus 11; $P = 0.0002$) in patients assigned to 32°C compared with 34°C. On the contrary, there was a trend toward a higher incidence of bradycardia (7 versus 2; $P = 0.054$) in patients assigned to 32°C. Although potassium levels decreased to a greater extent in patients assigned to 32°C, the incidence of hypokalemia was similar in both groups.

Conclusions.—The findings of this pilot trial suggest that a lower cooling level may be associated with a better outcome in patients surviving out-of-hospital cardiac arrest secondary to a shockable rhythm. The benefits observed here merit further investigation in a larger trial in out-of-hospital cardiac arrest patients with different presenting rhythms.

Clinical Trial Registration.—URL: http://www.clinicaltrials.gov. Unique identifier: NCT01155622.

▶ Therapeutic hypothermia (TH) is currently indicated for patients who achieve return of spontaneous circulation but do not follow commands immediately after cardiac arrest according to guidelines published by the American Heart Association (AHA). TH has been shown to improve neurologic outcomes and increase survival in this patient population, specifically with respect to patients who had a ventricular fibrillation or ventricular tachycardia dysrhythmia. The AHA currently recommends that these patients be cooled to 32°C from 34°C for 12 to 24 hours. This small (n = 32) single center clinical trial randomly assigned patients to cooling to 32°C versus 34°C for 24 hours. The protocol included the use of cold saline infusion and placement of a cooling catheter in the intravenous catheter. For patients with a shockable rhythm (n = 13 in both groups), 8 patients cooled to 32°C were alive and free from severe dependence at 6 months compared with only 2 patients who were cooled to 34°C. Although seizures were more frequent in the 34°C group, other adverse events were similar between the groups. All patients with asystole died within 6 months regardless of the treatment arm. Given the small numbers, no concrete conclusions can be drawn from this study, but it does take an important step in this research realm and strongly suggests that 32°C is superior to 34°C.

R. T. Bourdon, MD

High prevalence of corrected QT interval prolongation in acutely ill patients is associated with mortality: Results of the QT in Practice (QTIP) Study
Pickham D, Helfenbein E, Shinn JA, et al (Univ of California San Francisco; Advanced Algorithm Res Ctr, San Jose, CA; Stanford Univ Med Ctr, CA; et al)
Crit Care Med 40:394-399, 2012

Objective.—To test the potential value of more frequent QT interval measurement in hospitalized patients.

Design.—We performed a prospective, observational study.

Setting.—All adult intensive care unit and progressive care unit beds of a university medical center.

Patients.—All patients admitted to one of six critical care units over a 2-month period were included in analyses.

Interventions.—All critical care beds (n = 154) were upgraded to a continuous QT monitoring system (Philips Healthcare).

Measurements and Main Results.—QT data were extracted from the bedside monitors for offline analysis. A corrected QT interval >500 msecs was considered prolonged. Episodes of QT prolongation were manually over-read. Electrocardiogram data (67,648 hrs, mean 65 hrs/patient) were obtained. QT prolongation was present in 24%. There were 16 cardiac

TABLE 3.—Logistic Regression of the Predictors for QT Prolongation

Variables	Wald	Degrees of Freedom	p	Odds Ratio	95% Confidence Interval	
Age[a]	5.948	3	.114			
40–49 yrs	2.490	1	.115	1.869	0.859	4.064
50–64 yrs	5.827	1	.016	2.240	1.164	4.310
>65 yrs	4.393	1	.036	1.991	1.046	3.790
Female	8.111	1	.004	1.726	1.186	2.513
Cerebrovascular accident	8.005	1	.005	2.085	1.253	3.469
Hypothyroidism	4.327	1	.038	1.838	1.036	3.263
Hypocalcemia (<9 mg/dL)	5.984	1	.014	3.076	1.250	7.566
Hypokalemia (<3.5 mEq/L)	15.294	1	.000	2.155	1.467	3.167
High serum creatinine (>2.5 mg/dL)	8.655	1	.003	1.881	1.235	2.864
Hyperglycemia[b]	7.961	2	.019			
125–199 mg/dL vs. <124 mg/dL	2.913	1	.088	1.514	0.940	2.439
>200 mg/dL vs. <124 mg/dL	7.958	1	.005	2.259	1.282	3.980
Proarrhythmic drug administration[c]	21.491	4	.000			
1 drug	4.113	1	.043	1.588	1.016	2.482
2 drugs vs. 0 drugs	2.111	1	.146	1.503	0.867	2.606
3 drugs vs. 0 drug	12.253	1	.000	4.432	1.926	10.200
4 drugs vs. 0 drugs	12.848	1	.000	5.933	2.241	15.708

[a]Reference group: <39 yrs.
[b]Reference group: <124 mg/dL.
[c]Reference group: 0 drugs.

arrests, with one resulting from Torsade de Pointes (6%). Predictors of QT prolongation were female sex, QT-prolonging drugs, hypokalemia, hypocalcemia, hyperglycemia, high creatinine, history of stroke, and hypothyroidism. Patients with QT prolongation had longer hospitalization (276 hrs vs. 132 hrs, $p < .0005$) and had three times the odds for all-cause in-hospital mortality compared to patients without QT prolongation (odds ratio 2.99 95% confidence interval 1.1–8.1).

Conclusions.—We find QT prolongation to be common (24%), with Torsade de Pointes representing 6% of in-hospital cardiac arrests. Predictors of QT prolongation in the acutely ill population are similar to those previously identified in ambulatory populations. Acutely ill patients with QT prolongation have longer lengths of hospitalization and nearly three times the odds for mortality then those without QT prolongation (Table 3).

▶ This is intriguing data generated from a single academic medical center. Female gender, electrolyte and renal abnormalities, and administration of proarrhythmic drugs are associated with QT prolongation, torsades, and hospital mortality (Table 3).[1] We are given little other demographic information on these patients. Where demographic data are compared, patients with QT prolongation had a greater burden of organ dysfunction. Is QT prolongation a simple manifestation of acuity of illness?

Subsequent studies could better delineate patients at risk and identify risk reduction strategies, including tight control of electrolytes, particularly in patients with renal dysfunction. In addition, these data imply that the number, and possibly combination, of proarrhythmic drugs administered could affect QT prolongation and adverse outcomes. Will these results change with appropriate corrective action?

Torsades de pointes is noted to represent 6% of in-hospital cardiac arrests. Does QT prolongation predict other arrhythmias and non-torsades cardiac arrest as well? Should other hospitals obtain software sufficient to provide continuous QT interval measurement?[2]

D. J. Dries, MSE, MD

References

1. Drew BJ, Ackerman MJ, Funk M, et al. Prevention of torsade de pointes in hospital settings: a scientific statement from the American Heart Association and the American College of Cardiology Foundation. *J Am Coll Cardiol.* 2010; 55:934-947.
2. Helfenbein ED, Zhou SH, Lindauer JM, et al. An Algorithm for continuous real-time QT interval monitoring. *J Electrocardiol.* 2006;39:S123-S127.

Cardiopulmonary Resuscitation/Other

Effectiveness of the LUCAS device for mechanical chest compression after cardiac arrest: systematic review of experimental, observational and animal studies
Gates S, Smith JL, Ong GJ, et al (The Univ of Warwick, UK)
Heart 98:908-913, 2012

Context.—The LUCAS mechanical chest compression device may be better than manual chest compression during resuscitation attempts after cardiac arrest.

Objective.—To summarise the evidence about the effectiveness of LUCAS.

Data Sources.—Searches of 4 electronic databases, reference lists of included studies, review articles, clinical guidelines, and the manufacturer's web site. No language restrictions were applied. Date of last search: September 2011.

Study Selection.—All studies, of any design, comparing mechanical chest compression using LUCAS with manual chest compression, with human or animal subjects. Studies published only as abstracts were included. Manikin studies, and case reports or case series, were excluded.

Data Extraction.—Data were extracted on study methodology and outcomes, including return of spontaneous circulation, survival, injuries caused by resuscitation, and physiological parameters.

Results.—22 papers reporting 16 separate studies were included. There was one randomised trial, nine cohort studies, 2 before/after studies and 4 animal studies. No meta-analyses were performed because of high risk of bias and heterogeneity in the study designs. Animal studies suggested an advantage to LUCAS in terms of physiological parameters, but human studies did not suggest an advantage in ROSC or survival. Existing evidence is low quality because most studies were small and many were poorly reported.

Conclusions.—There is insufficient evidence to make any recommendations for clinical practice. Large scale, high quality randomised trials of LUCAS are needed. Studies that have so far been published only as abstracts should be reported fully.

▶ The LUCAS chest compression device is a tool aimed at improving the quality of chest compressions during cardiopulmonary resuscitation (CPR). It consists of a suction cup that attaches to a patient's chest and a solid frame that wraps around a patient's chest. The plunger compresses at a standard rate to a standard depth with a goal of providing both active compression and decompression. There has been a mix of literature supporting and refuting its benefit. This article provided a summary of all of the literature currently printed on the LUCAS. The authors found only 1 randomized trial and a small number of cohorts, before and after, and animal studies. Several of the animal studies showed good physiologic benefit. In regard to return of spontaneous circulation (ROSC), 2 prehospital human studies from the same "low-quality" article showed the benefit of the LUCAS with relative risk greater than 2. A number of other human and animal studies favored ROSC benefit though the relative risk ratio confidence intervals crossed 1, indicating that there was insufficient statistical power to prove benefit. Six studies evaluating survival benefit showed no benefit, whereas 1 study showed significant benefit though a very wide confidence interval because of small numbers. For those of us who have seen this device in use (we use it at our primary hospital), it seems that LUCAS should provide benefit. It makes sense both from a practical standpoint (it never gets tired) and from a physiologic standpoint (active decompression should increase blood return to the heart). However, this study shows that a large randomized, controlled trial is sorely needed before widespread recommendation or adoption.

M. D. Zwank, MD

Effects of fluid resuscitation with synthetic colloids or crystalloids alone on shock reversal, fluid balance, and patient outcomes in patients with severe sepsis: A prospective sequential analysis
Bayer O, Reinhart K, Kohl M, et al (Friedrich-Schiller-Univ Jena, Germany; Furtwangen Univ, Schwenningen, Germany; et al)
Crit Care Med 40:2543-2551, 2012

Objective.—To assess shock reversal and required fluid volumes in patients with septic shock.

Design.—Prospective before and after study comparing three different treatment periods.

Setting.—Fifty-bed single-center surgical intensive care unit.

Patients.—Consecutive patients with severe sepsis.

Interventions.—Fluid therapy directed at preset hemodynamic goals with hydroxyethyl starch (predominantly 6% hydroxyethyl starch 130/0.4) in the first period, 4% gelatin in the second period, and only crystalloids in the third period.

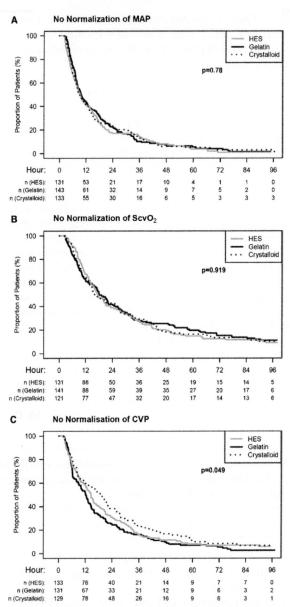

FIGURE 2.—Reaching of hemodynamic goals estimated by the Kaplan-Meier method. Time to normalization of preset hemodynamic goals, including mean arterial pressure (*MAP*) of ≥70 mm Hg, central venous pressure (*CVP*) of ≥8 mm Hg, central venous oxygenation saturation (*ScvO₂*) of ≥70%. Significance testing by log-rank tests. n denotes patients not having reached hemodynamic goals at the respective time. *HES*, hydroxyethyl starch. (Reprinted from Bayer O, Reinhart K, Kohl M, et al. Effects of fluid resuscitation with synthetic colloids or crystalloids alone on shock reversal, fluid balance, and patient outcomes in patients with severe sepsis: a prospective sequential analysis. *Crit Care Med.* 2012;40:2543-2551, with permission from the Society of Critical Care Medicine and Lippincott Williams & Wilkins.)

Measurements and Main Results.—Main outcome was time to shock reversal (serum lactate < 2.2 mmol/L and discontinuation of vasopressor use). Hemodynamic goals were mean arterial pressure > 70 mm Hg; $ScvO_2$ < 70%; central venous pressure > 8 mm Hg. Safety outcomes were acute kidney injury defined by Risk, Injury, Failure, Loss, and End-stage kidney disease criteria and new need for renal replacement therapy. Hemodynamic measures, serum lactate, and creatinine were comparable at baseline in all study periods (hydroxyethyl starch n = 360, gelatin n = 352, only crystalloids n = 334). Severity scores, hospital length of stay, and intensive care unit or hospital mortality did not differ significantly among groups. All groups showed similar time to shock reversal. More fluid was needed over the first 4 days in the crystalloid group (fluid ratios 1.4:1 [crystalloids to hydroxyethyl starch] and 1.1:1 [crystalloids to gelatin]). After day 5, fluid balance was more negative in the crystalloid group. Hydroxyethyl starch and gelatin were independent risk factors for acute kidney injury (odds ratio, 95% confidence interval 2.55, 1.76–3.69 and 1.85, 1.31–2.62, respectively). Patients receiving synthetic colloids received significantly more allogeneic blood products.

Conclusions.—Shock reversal was achieved equally fast with synthetic colloids or crystalloids. Use of colloids resulted in only marginally lower required volumes of resuscitation fluid. Both low molecular weight hydroxyethyl starch and gelatin may impair renal function (Fig 2).

▶ This is a carefully analyzed convenience study in which more than 300 patients were initially resuscitated from sepsis or septic shock with hetastarch, then by gelatin, and then by colloids as a matter of critical care unit policy over multiple years.[1] Data on resource consumption and resuscitation outcomes were carefully collected. There is no obvious difference in fluid requirements in the 3 groups (Fig 2). Fluid balance was higher in the crystalloid group in initial days but after day 5, fluid balance became more negative with crystalloid administration. Time on mechanical ventilation was increased in both synthetic colloid groups and a pattern of increasing renal injury was seen with colloid administration. Intensive care unit and hospital mortality were similar among all patients. Finally, the colloid groups received more blood products. The contribution of blood product administration to the organ injury seen is unclear.[2]

This study does not address the beneficial effect of albumin in sepsis or septic shock identified by the Saline versus Albumin Fluid Evaluation study investigators.[3] The value of other synthetic colloids in this setting must be questioned.

D. J. Dries, MSE, MD

References

1. Perel P, Roberts I. Colloids versus crystalloids for fluid resuscitation in critically ill patients. *Cochrane Database Syst Rev.* 2012;(6):CD000567.
2. Napolitano L. Cumulative risks of early red blood cell transfusion. *J Trauma.* 2006;60:S26-S34.
3. Finfer S, Bellomo R, Boyce N, et al; SAFE Study Investigators. A comparison of albumin and saline for fluid resuscitation in the intensive care unit. *N Engl J Med.* 2004;350:2247-2256.

Myocardial Infarction/Cardiogenic Shocks

2-Hour Accelerated Diagnostic Protocol to Assess Patients With Chest Pain Symptoms Using Contemporary Troponins as the Only Biomarker: The ADAPT Trial
Than M, Cullen L, Aldous S, et al (Christchurch Hosp, New Zealand; Royal Brisbane and Women's Hosp, Australia; et al)
J Am Coll Cardiol 59:2091-2098, 2012

Objectives.—The purpose of this study was to determine whether a new accelerated diagnostic protocol (ADP) for possible cardiac chest pain could identify low-risk patients suitable for early discharge (with follow-up shortly after discharge).

Background.—Patients presenting with possible acute coronary syndrome (ACS), who have a low short-term risk of adverse cardiac events may be suitable for early discharge and shorter hospital stays.

Methods.—This prospective observational study tested an ADP that included pre-test probability scoring by the Thrombolysis In Myocardial Infarction (TIMI) score, electrocardiography, and 0 + 2 h values of laboratory troponin I as the sole biomarker. Patients presenting with chest pain due to suspected ACS were included. The primary endpoint was major adverse cardiac event (MACE) within 30 days.

Results.—Of 1,975 patients, 302 (15.3%) had a MACE. The ADP classified 392 patients (20%) as low risk. One (0.25%) of these patients had a MACE, giving the ADP a sensitivity of 99.7% (95% confidence interval [CI]: 98.1% to 99.9%), negative predictive value of 99.7% (95% CI: 98.6% to 100.0%), specificity of 23.4% (95% CI: 21.4% to 25.4%), and positive predictive value of 19.0% (95% CI: 17.2% to 21.0%). Many ADP negative patients had further investigations (74.1%), and therapeutic (18.3%) or procedural (2.0%) interventions during the initial hospital attendance and/or 30-day follow-up.

Conclusions.—Using the ADP, a large group of patients was successfully identified as at low short-term risk of a MACE and therefore suitable for rapid discharge from the emergency department with early follow-up. This approach could decrease the observation period required for some patients with chest pain. (An observational study of the diagnostic utility of an accelerated diagnostic protocol using contemporary central laboratory cardiac troponin in the assessment of patients presenting to two Australasian hospitals with chest pain of possible cardiac origin; ACTRN12611001069943).

▶ Stable patients with chest pain notoriously cause angst among emergency physicians. A number of studies in the past have looked at 6-hour algorithms to effectively rule out acute coronary syndrome. In many emergency departments, 6 hours is an impractically long time to keep a patient prior to disposition. This study from New Zealand determined if a 2-hour "rapid rule-out" could accomplish the goal of determining if a patient's chest pain represents acute coronary syndrome. It was similar to another study published last year (ASPECT) and determined patients to be low risk if they had a TIMI score of 0, a normal or unchanged electrocardiogram, and a conventional troponin level that was normal at presentation and at 2 hours. Of the 1975 patients enrolled, 302 met these low-risk criteria. Of those, only 1 had an adverse event (non-ST-elevation myocardial infarction) within 30 days. No patients were lost to follow-up. This was a great study with a large patient population, thorough follow-up and use of a conventional (not highly sensitive, which is not universally available) troponin assay. With the results from this and the ASPECT study, you can feel comfortable using a 2-hour rule out. Be sure that you are only using it for patients with a TIMI score of 0 because this was a key part of the rule.

M. D. Zwank, MD

Ultrafiltration in Decompensated Heart Failure with Cardiorenal Syndrome
Bart BA, for the Heart Failure Clinical Research Network (Hennepin County Med Ctr, Minneapolis, MN; et al)
N Engl J Med 367:2296-2304, 2012

Background.—Ultrafiltration is an alternative strategy to diuretic therapy for the treatment of patients with acute decompensated heart failure. Little is known about the efficacy and safety of ultrafiltration in patients with acute decompensated heart failure complicated by persistent congestion and worsened renal function.

Methods.—We randomly assigned a total of 188 patients with acute decompensated heart failure, worsened renal function, and persistent congestion to a strategy of stepped pharmacologic therapy (94 patients) or ultrafiltration (94 patients). The primary end point was the bivariate change from baseline in the serum creatinine level and body weight, as assessed 96 hours after random assignment. Patients were followed for 60 days.

Results.—Ultrafiltration was inferior to pharmacologic therapy with respect to the bivariate end point of the change in the serum creatinine level and body weight 96 hours after enrollment ($P = 0.003$), owing primarily to an increase in the creatinine level in the ultrafiltration group. At 96 hours, the mean change in the creatinine level was -0.04 ± 0.53 mg per deciliter (-3.5 ± 46.9 µmol per liter) in the pharmacologictherapy group, as compared with $+0.23 \pm 0.70$ mg per deciliter (20.3 ± 61.9 µmol per liter) in the ultrafiltration group ($P = 0.003$). There was no significant difference in weight loss 96 hours after enrollment between patients in the pharmacologic-therapy group and those in the ultrafiltration group (a loss of 5.5 ± 5.1 kg [12.1 ± 11.3 lb] and 5.7 ± 3.9 kg [12.6 ± 8.5 lb], respectively; $P = 0.58$). A higher percentage of patients in the ultrafiltration group than in the pharmacologic-therapy group had a serious adverse event (72% vs. 57%, $P = 0.03$).

Conclusions.—In a randomized trial involving patients hospitalized for acute decompensated heart failure, worsened renal function, and persistent congestion, the use of a stepped pharmacologic-therapy algorithm was superior to a strategy of ultrafiltration for the preservation of renal function at 96 hours, with a similar amount of weight loss with the two approaches. Ultrafiltration was associated with a higher rate of adverse events. (Funded by the National Heart, Lung, and Blood Institute; ClinicalTrials.gov/ number, NCT00608491.)

▶ The 30-day readmission rate, which is used as an indicator of hospital quality and a benchmark for reimbursement, was 24.8% among 1 330 157 Medicare beneficiaries who were hospitalized for heart failure from 2007 through 2009.[1] Hospitals with high readmission rates after hospitalization for heart failure now face reductions in reimbursement from the Centers for Medicare and Medicaid Services.[1] Consequently, there is an increased financial incentive to reduce the rate of readmission after hospitalization for heart failure.

The most common reason for readmission after hospitalization for heart failure is recurrent heart failure, which accounts for 35% of readmissions.[2] One reason for readmission after hospitalization for heart failure is incomplete resolution of volume overload despite use of parenteral diuretics. Therefore, ultrafiltration (UF) has been investigated as an alternative strategy of treating fluid retention in patients with acute decompensated heart failure (ADHF).[3] Venovenous UF can remove up to 500 mL/h via peripheral intravenous access.[3] An unblinded trial that randomized 200 patients with ADHF to either loop diuretic therapy or UF showed that rehospitalization for heart failure was less frequent after treatment with UF than after diuretic therapy (hazard ratio 0.56; $P = .04$).[4]

Acute cardiorenal syndrome type I, defined as worsening renal function in patients with ADHF, occurs in 25% to 33% of patients hospitalized with ADHF.[5] Intravenous diuretic therapy may precipitate acute cardiorenal syndrome in patients with ADHF. The National Heart, Lung, and Blood Institute–sponsored Heart Failure Network conducted the Cardiorenal Rescue Study in Acute Decompensated Heart Failure (CARRESS-HF) to compare UF with diuretic-based stepped pharmacologic therapy in patients with heart failure and worsening renal function. The CARRESS-HF trial randomized 188 patients with ADHF, worsened renal function, and persistent congestion to either ultrafiltration (n = 94) or a strategy of stepped pharmacologic therapy (n = 94). Enrollment was terminated before the planned 200 patients were enrolled because UF was associated with an excess of adverse events and no evidence of benefit. UF was inferior to pharmacologic therapy because of a statistically significant increase in the serum creatinine 96 hours after enrollment. Nevertheless, the mean increase in the serum creatinine 96 hours after enrollment was only 0.23 ± 0.70 mg/dL in the UF group. Also, there was no significant difference in the changes from baseline serum creatinine between the UF group and the pharmacologic therapy group at 7 days or 30 days after enrollment. There was no difference in weight loss at 96 hours. Also, death or rehospitalization for heart failure during the 60-day follow-up period was not significantly different.

Refractory congestion not responsive to medical therapy is a Class IIa indication for UF according to the American College of Cardiology/American Heart Association Guidelines for the Management of Heart Failure in Adults,[6] but the results of the CARRESS-HF do not serve as evidence for a major role for ultrafiltration in the management of ADHF with cardiorenal syndrome.

S. W. Werns, MD

References

1. Vaduganathan M, Bonow RO, Gheorghiade M. Thirty-day readmissions: the clock is ticking. *JAMA.* 2013;309:345-346.
2. Dharmarajan K, Hsieh AF, Lin Z, et al. Diagnoses and timing of 30-day readmissions after hospitalization for heart failure, acute myocardial infarction, or pneumonia. *JAMA.* 2013;309:355-363.
3. Felker GM, Mentz RJ. Diuretics and ultrafiltration in acute decompensated heart failure. *J Am Coll Cardiol.* 2012;59:2145-2153.
4. Costanzo MR, Guglin ME, Saltzberg MT, et al. Ultrafiltration versus intravenous diuretics for patients hospitalized for acute decompensated heart failure. *J Am Coll Cardiol.* 2007;49:675-683.
5. Ronco C, Cicoira M, McCullough PA. Cardiorenal syndrome type 1: pathophysiological crosstalk leading to combined heart and kidney dysfunction in the setting of acutely decompensated heart failure. *J Am Coll Cardiol.* 2012;60:1031-1042.
6. Hunt SA, Abraham WT, Chin MH, et al. 2009 focused update incorporated into the ACC/AHA 2005 guidelines for the diagnosis and management of heart failure in adults: a report of the American College of Cardiology Foundation/American Heart Association Task Force on Practice Guidelines Developed in Collaboration with the International Society for Heart and Lung Transplantation. *J Am Coll Cardiol.* 2009;53:e1-e90.

Long-Term Prognosis Following Resuscitation From Out of Hospital Cardiac Arrest: Role of Percutaneous Coronary Intervention and Therapeutic Hypothermia

Dumas F, White L, Stubbs BA, et al (Emergency Med Services Division of Public Health for Seattle and King County, Seattle, WA; et al)

J Am Coll Cardiol 60:21-27, 2012

Objectives.—The aim of the study was to assess the influence of percutaneous coronary intervention (PCI) and therapeutic hypothermia (TH) on long-term prognosis.

Background.—Although hospital care consisting of TH and/or PCI in particular patients resuscitated following out-of-hospital cardiac arrest (OHCA) can improve survival to hospital discharge, there is little evidence regarding how these therapies may impact long-term prognosis.

Methods.—We performed a cohort investigation of all persons >18 years of age who suffered nontraumatic OHCA and were resuscitated and discharged alive from the hospital between January 1, 2001, and December 31, 2009, in a metropolitan emergency medical service (EMS) system. We reviewed EMS and hospital records, state death certificates, and the national death index to determine clinical characteristics and vital status. Survival analyses were conducted using Kaplan-Meier estimates and multivariable Cox regression. Analyses of TH were restricted to those patients who were comatose at hospital admission.

Results.—Of the 5,958 persons who received EMS-attempted resuscitation, 1,001 (16.8%) were discharged alive from the hospital. PCI was performed in 384 of 1,001 (38.4%), whereas TH was performed in 241 of 941 (25.6%) persons comatose at hospital admission. Five-year survival was 78.7% among those treated with PCI compared with 54.4% among those not receiving PCI and 77.5% among those treated with TH compared with 60.4% among those not receiving TH (both $p < 0.001$). After adjustment for confounders, PCI was associated with a lower risk of death (hazard ratio [HR]: 0.46 [95% confidence interval [CI]: 0.34 to 0.61]; $p < 0.001$). Likewise, TH was associated with a lower risk of death (HR: 0.70 [95% CI: 0.50 to 0.97]; $p < 0.04$).

Conclusions.—The findings suggested that effects of acute hospital interventions for post-resuscitation treatment extend beyond hospital survival and can positively influence prognosis following the arrest hospitalization.

▶ More than 10 years have elapsed since the publication of 2 small, randomized trials that showed that therapeutic hypothermia improved neurologic recovery and 6-month mortality after cardiac arrest caused by ventricular fibrillation or pulseless ventricular tachycardia.[1,2] A French study that was published in 1997 showed that a coronary artery occlusion was present in 40 of 84 patients who underwent immediate coronary angiography after surviving an out-of-hospital cardiac arrest.[3] Successful angioplasty was an independent predictor of in-hospital survival.[3] Clinical and electrocardiographic findings were not reliable predictors of a recent coronary artery occlusion, which was present in 9 of the 35 patients who had neither chest pain nor ST-segment elevation.[3] Another French registry study that enrolled 435 patients who underwent immediate coronary angiography after out-of-hospital cardiac arrest found that successful immediate coronary angioplasty was an independent predictor of improved hospital survival in patients with or without ST-segment elevation on the postresuscitation electrocardiogram.[4] Therapeutic hypothermia was used in 92% of survivors and 82% of nonsurvivors ($P = .006$).[4]

Dumas et al performed an analysis of the 5-year survival of 1001 patients who were discharged alive after hospitalization for nontraumatic out-of-hospital cardiac arrest. Both percutaneous coronary intervention (PCI) and therapeutic hypothermia were independently associated with improved 5-year survival. PCI was associated with improved survival in patients with and without ST-segment elevation after resuscitation from cardiac arrest. Patients who were treated with both PCI and therapeutic hypothermia had the highest 1-year and 5-year survival estimates, whereas those who received neither treatment had the lowest survival estimates.

The 2013 ACCF/American Heart Association Guideline for the Management of ST-Elevation Myocardial Infarction includes the following class I recommendation: "Therapeutic hypothermia should be started as soon as possible in comatose patients with STEMI and out-of-hospital cardiac arrest caused by ventricular fibrillation or pulseless ventricular tachycardia, including patients who undergo primary PCI."[5] Nevertheless, it is evident that therapeutic hypothermia is underutilized. In the study by Dumas et al only 245 of 941 patients (26%) who were eligible for treatment with therapeutic hypothermia received it. Both PCI and therapeutic hypothermia were administered to only 86 of the 941 patients who were eligible for therapeutic hypothermia. A strategy designed to increase access to therapeutic hypothermia was reported by Mooney et al.[6] A regional network of hospitals that was implemented for treatment of patients with ST-segment elevation myocardial infarction (STEMI) found that it is feasible to provide concurrent therapeutic hypothermia and emergency coronary angiography to patients who have been resuscitated after out-of-hospital cardiac arrest.[6] During the initial 4 years of the program, the median time between return of spontaneous circulation and attainment of the target core temperature was reduced from 345 minutes to 258 minutes. Each 1-hour delay in the initiation of cooling was associated with a 20% reduction in the survival of resuscitated victims of out-of-hospital cardiac arrest.

The potential cardiac effects of therapeutic hypothermia were reviewed in a recent publication.[7] Experimental studies have indicated that therapeutic hypothermia may exert beneficial cardiac effects in addition to the salutary effect on neurologic outcomes.[7] Hypothermia has been found to limit myocardial infarct size in experimental animals subjected to coronary occlusion followed by reperfusion if hypothermia is achieved before reperfusion.[7] The results of small clinical trials have been mixed. Two studies failed to demonstrate an overall reduction of infarct size in patients with anterior or large inferior STEMIs who were randomly assigned to endovascular cooling.[7] A pilot study that enrolled 20 patients with STEMI showed that achievement of a core temperature less than 35°C before reperfusion was associated with a 38% reduction of infarct size measured by magnetic resonance imaging.[8]

One cause for concern is a suggestion that therapeutic hypothermia may be associated with an increased risk of stent thrombosis after PCI.[9,10] Ibrahim[9] reported a 14.8% rate of stent thrombosis among 27 patients who underwent therapeutic hypothermia and PCI after sudden death. Penela et al[10] reported the outcomes of 11 patients who underwent both therapeutic hypothermia and PCI after an out-of-hospital cardiac arrest. Five of the patients had a subsequent myocardial infarction caused by stent thrombosis that was documented by angiography in 4 patients and autopsy in 1 patient. In both reports, dual antiplatelet after PCI consisted of aspirin and clopidogrel. Ibrahim[9] measured platelet inhibition 24 hours after the loading dose of clopidogrel and found that 81% of the patients treated with hypothermia satisfied the criterion for clopidogrel nonresponsiveness. The author speculated that hepatic conversion of clopidogrel, an inactive prodrug, to an active metabolite may be impaired in patients who are treated with hypothermia. Future pharmacokinetic and pharmacodynamic studies are needed to assess clopidogrel metabolism and platelet inhibition in patients treated with therapeutic hypothermia. Meanwhile, it might be prudent to use alternative inhibitors of the platelet P2Y12 receptor that are not prodrugs, such as prasugrel or ticagrelor, in patients who undergo concurrent PCI and therapeutic hypothermia.

S. W. Werns, MD

References

1. Hypothermia after Cardiac Arrest Study Group. Mild therapeutic hypothermia to improve the neurologic outcome after cardiac arrest. *N Engl J Med.* 2002;346: 549-556.
2. Bernard SA, Gray TW, Buist MD, et al. Treatment of comatose survivors of out-of-hospital cardiac arrest with induced hypothermia. *N Engl J Med.* 2002;346: 557-563.
3. Spaulding M, Joly L-M, Rosenberg A, et al. Immediate coronary angiography in survivors of out-of-hospital cardiac arrest. *N Engl J Med.* 1997;336:1629-1633.
4. Dumas F, Cariou A, Manzo-Silberman S, et al. Immediate percutaneous coronary intervention is associated with better survival after out-of-hospital cardiac arrest: insights from the PROCAT (Parisian Region Out of hospital Cardiac ArresT) registry. *Circ Cardiovasc Interv.* 2010;3:200-207.
5. O'Gara PT, Kushner FG, Ascheim DD, et al. 2013 ACCF/AHA guideline for the management of ST-elevation myocardial infarction: a report of the America College of Cardiology Foundation/American Heart Association Task Force on Practice Guidelines. *Circulation.* In press.
6. Mooney MR, Unger BT, Boland LL, et al. Therapeutic hypothermia after out-of-hospital cardiac arrest: evaluation of a regional system to increase access to cooling. *Circulation.* 2011;124:206-214.
7. Schwartz BG, Kloner RA, Thomas JL, et al. Therapeutic hypothermia for acute myocardial infarction and cardiac arrest. *Am J Cardiol.* 2012;110:461-466.
8. Götberg M, Olivecrona GK, Koul S, et al. A pilot study of rapid cooling by cold saline and endovascular cooling before reperfusion in patients with ST-elevation myocardial infarction. *Circ Cardiovasc Interv.* 2010;3:400-407.
9. Ibrahim K. Increased rate of stent thrombosis due to clopidogrel resistance in therapeutic hypothermia after sudden cardiac death. *Eur Heart J.* 2011;32:252.
10. Penela D, Magaldi M, Fontanals J, et al. Hypothermia in acute coronary syndrome: brain salvage versus stent thrombosis? *J Am Coll Cardiol.* In press.

Prevalence of acute myocardial infarction in patients with presumably new left bundle-branch block
Mehta N, Huang HD, Bandeali S, et al (Univ of Texas Med Branch, Galveston, TX; Baylor College of Medicine, Houston, TX)
J Electrocardiol 45:361-367, 2012

Objectives.—We assessed the prevalence of true acute myocardial infarction and the need for emergent revascularization among patients with new or presumably new left bundle branch block (nLBBB) for whom the primary percutaneous coronary intervention protocol was activated.

Methods and Results.—Among 802 patients, 69 (8.6%) had nLBBB. The chief presenting symptom was chest pain or cardiac arrest in 36 patients (52.2%) and shortness of breath in 15 (21.7%). Less than 30% of the patients had elevated cardiac troponin-I, and less than 10% had elevated creatine kinase—MB. Only 11.6% of the patients underwent emergent revascularization; the rate was higher for patients who presented with chest pain or cardiac arrest or shortness of breath than for patients who presented with other symptoms.

Conclusions.—Acute myocardial infarction and the need for emergent revascularization are relatively uncommon among patients who present with nLBBB, especially when symptoms are atypical. Current guidelines for primary percutaneous coronary intervention protocol activation for nLBBB should be reconsidered.

▶ A bundle branch block was present on the admission electrocardiogram (ECG) in 4% of the patients with a suspected acute myocardial infarction (MI) who were included in a meta-analysis of 9 trials that randomly assigned 58 600 patients to either fibrinolytic therapy or a control group.[1] The mortality rate at 35 days for patients who were assigned to the control groups was substantially higher among patients who presented with a bundle branch block (23.6%) compared with patients who had ST-segment elevation in the anterior leads (16.9%) or inferior leads (8.4%) or ST-segment depression (13.8%).[1] Fibrinolytic therapy was associated with a 25% reduction in mortality rate among patients who presented with a bundle branch block on ECG, which translates to 49 lives saved per thousand patients treated compared with 37 and 8 lives saved per thousand treated for patients who presented with ST-segment elevation in the anterior or inferior leads, respectively.[1] The publication did not specify, however, whether the meta-analysis was limited to patients with a left bundle branch block (LBBB) or also included patients with a right bundle branch block.[1] Also, no information regarding the age of the bundle branch block was provided.

A new or presumably new LBBB in patients with symptom onset within the prior 12 hours was designated as a class I indication for either fibrinolytic therapy or primary percutaneous coronary intervention (PCI) in the guidelines for the management of acute MI that were issued by the American College of Cardiology/American Heart Association Task Force on Practice Guidelines in 2004.[2] According to an expert consensus document entitled "Third Universal Definition of Myocardial Infarction" that was published in 2012, acute MI can be diagnosed when there is a new LBBB and an increase and/or decrease of cardiac biomarker values (preferably cardiac troponin) with at least one value above the 99th percentile upper reference limit.[3] Unfortunately, the electrocardiographic diagnosis of acute MI in the presence of LBBB is problematic, and according to the most recent revision of the practice guidelines for ST-elevation MI, a new or presumably new LBBB "should not be considered diagnostic of acute MI in isolation."[4]

Angiographic studies have documented the low prevalence of acute MI among patients with a new LBBB.[5-7] Among 36 patients with a suspected ST-segment elevation MI and a new or presumably new LBBB, coronary angiography did not show a culprit coronary artery in 16 patients (44%), and 10 patients (27%) had no significant coronary artery disease.[5] An analysis of the Mayo Clinic's regional primary PCI network database found that only 12 of 36 patients with a new LBBB and clinical symptoms suspicious for an MI met troponin criteria for an MI, resulting in emergency activation of the cardiac catheterization laboratory for a false-positive diagnosis of acute MI in 2 of 3 patients with a new LBBB.[6] Mehta et al reported that the primary PCI team was activated for 69 patients with a new or presumably new LBBB between January 1, 2007 and June 30, 2010. Only 19 patients (28%) had an elevated cardiac troponin-I, and an occluded culprit coronary artery was found in only 8 of the 37 patients (22%) who underwent coronary angiography.

Sgarbossa et al[8] devised an algorithm for the diagnosis of acute MI in patients with LBBB that used 3 electrocardiographic criteria: ≥1 mm ST segment elevation concordant with the QRS complex; ≥1 mm ST-segment depression in leads V1, V2, or V3; and ≥5 mm ST-segment elevation discordant with the QRS complex. Several subsequent studies investigated the utility of the so-called Sgarbossa criteria. A study that enrolled 83 patients with LBBB and symptoms suggestive of acute MI found that the ECG algorithm based on the Sgarbossa criteria had a sensitivity of only 10%.[9] The criteria were applied to a cohort of 253 patients with suspected MI who had both an LBBB on the baseline ECG and peak creatine kinase (CK) and MB fraction (CK-MB) data available for analysis and were enrolled in the Assessment of the Safety and Efficacy of a New Thrombolytic (ASSENT) 2 and 3 trials.[10] Either ≥1 mm ST-segment elevation concordant with the QRS complex or ≥1 mm ST-segment depression in leads V1, V2, or V3 was present in 48.7% of patients with an LBBB and a peak CK/CK-MB > 2x the upper limit of normal, compared with 12.6% of patients without a CK/CK-MB increase (P < .001). A large clinical trial that included 98 patients with suspected ST-segment elevation MI and LBBB who underwent coronary angiography found that both an occluded infarct-related artery and positive cardiac biomarkers were seen in 60.2% of patients, 71.4% of patients with ST-segment elevation ≥1 mm concordant with the QRS complex, compared with 44.1% of patients without concordant ST-segment elevation ≥1 mm (P = .027).[7]

Based on the published literature, one can draw several conclusions regarding MI and LBBB. First, patients with an acute MI who present with LBBB that is new or of indeterminate age have a worse prognosis than patients without LBBB.[11] Multivariate logistic regression analysis of 3053 patients who were enrolled in the Primary Angioplasty in Myocardial Infarction trials found that an LBBB was an independent predictor of in-hospital death (odds ratio, 5.53; 95% confidence interval, 1.89–16.1; P = .002).[11] Second, it is common for patients with LBBB and acute MI to have no chest pain at the time of presentation. Among 29 585 patients with LBBB and acute MI who were enrolled in the National Registry of Myocardial 2 registry, 13 872 (47%) did not report chest pain.[12] Patients who presented without chest pain were 4 times less likely to receive reperfusion therapy (odds ratio, 0.25) and were also less likely to receive aspirin or a β-blocker.[12] Consequently, patients with acute MI and LBBB who presented without chest pain had a 47% greater in-hospital mortality rate than patients who presented with chest pain (27% vs 18%; P < .001).[12] Third, the electrocardiographic criteria for the diagnosis of acute MI in patients with LBBB are quite specific, but their sensitivity is fairly low. Fourth, the risks of fibrinolytic therapy may be increased in patients with LBBB because of older age and a higher prevalence of hypertension. Therefore, immediate coronary angiography may be the most prudent approach for patients with LBBB and suspected acute MI, both to diagnose an acute coronary artery occlusion that warrants intervention and to avoid the risk of fibrinolytic therapy in patients who cannot benefit from it; that is, patients with a non—ST-segment elevation MI or a noncardiac condition. A more detailed discussion of the management of patients with LBBB and suspected MI can be found in an excellent review article that was published in 2012.[13]

S. W. Werns, MD

References

1. Indications for fibrinolytic therapy in suspected acute myocardial infarction: collaborative overview of early mortality and major morbidity results from all randomised trials of more than 1000 patients. Fibrinolytic Therapy Trialists' (FTT) Collaborative Group. *Lancet.* 1994;343:311-322.
2. Antman EM, Anbe DT, Armstrong PW, et al. ACC/AHA guidelines for the management of patients with ST-elevation myocardial infarction: a report of the American College of Cardiology/American Heart Association Task Force on Practice Guidelines (Committee to Revise the 1999 Guidelines for the Management of Patients with Acute Myocardial Infarction). *Circulation.* 2004; 110:e82-e292.
3. Thygesen K, Alpert JS, Jaffe JS, et al. Third universal definition of myocardial infarction. *J Am Coll Cardiol.* 2012;60:1581-1598.
4. O'Gara PT, Kushner FG, Ascheim DD, et al. 2013 ACCF/AHA guideline for the management of ST-elevation myocardial infarction: a report of the America College of Cardiology Foundation/American Heart Association Task Force on Practice Guidelines. *Circulation.* In press.
5. Larson DM, Menssen KM, Sharkey SW, et al. "False-positive" cardiac catheterization laboratory activation among patients with suspected ST-segment elevation myocardial infarction. *JAMA.* 2007;298:2754-2760.
6. Jain S, Ting HT, Bell M, et al. Utility of left bundle branch block as a diagnostic criterion for acute myocardial infarction. *Am J Cardiol.* 2011;107:1111-1116.
7. Lopes RD, Siha H, Fu Y, et al. Diagnosing acute myocardial infarction in patients with left bundle branch block. *Am J Cardiol.* 2011;108:782-788.
8. Sgarbossa EB, Pinski SL, Barbagelata A, et al. Electrocardiographic diagnosis of evolving acute myocardial infarction in the presence of left bundle-branch block. GUSTO-1 (Global Utilization of Streptokinase and Tissue Plasminogen Activator for Occluded Coronary Arteries) Investigators. *N Engl J Med.* 1996;334: 481-487.
9. Shlipak MG, Lyons WL, Go AS, Chou TM, Evans GT, Browner WS. Should the electrocardiogram be used to guide therapy for patients with left bundle-branch block and suspected myocardial infarction? *JAMA.* 1999;281:714-719.
10. Al-Faleh H, Fu Y, Wagner G, et al. Unraveling the spectrum of left bundle branch block in acute myocardial infarction: insights from the Assessment of the Safety and Efficacy of a New Thrombolytic (ASSENT 2 and 3) trials. *Am Heart J.* 2006; 151:10-15.
11. Guerrero M, Harjai K, Stone GW, et al. Comparison of the prognostic effect of left versus right versus no bundle branch block on presenting electrocardiogram in acute myocardial infarction patients treated with primary angioplasty in the primary angioplasty in myocardial infarction trials. *Am J Cardiol.* 2005;96: 482-488.
12. Shlipak MG, Go AS, Frederick PD, Malmgren J, Barron HV, Canto JG. Treatment and outcomes of left bundle-branch block patients with myocardial infarction who present without chest pain. National Registry of Myocardial Infarction 2 Investigators. *J Am Coll Cardiol.* 2000;36:706-712.
13. Neeland KJ, Kontos MC, de Lemos JA. Evolving considerations in the management of patients with left bundle branch block and suspected myocardial infarction. *J Am Coll Cardiol.* 2012;60:96-105.

Bedside Monitoring to Adjust Antiplatelet Therapy for Coronary Stenting

Collet J-P, for the ARCTIC Investigators (Institut de Cardiologie Hôpital Pitié—Salpêtrière and Université Pierre et Marie Curie, Paris, France; et al)

N Engl J Med 367:2100-2109, 2012

Background.—Patients' responses to oral antiplatelet therapy are subject to variation. Bedside monitoring offers the opportunity to improve outcomes after coronary stenting by individualizing therapy.

Methods.—We randomly assigned 2440 patients scheduled for coronary stenting at 38 centers to a strategy of platelet-function monitoring, with drug adjustment in patients who had a poor response to antiplatelet therapy, or to a conventional strategy without monitoring and drug adjustment. The primary end point was the composite of death, myocardial infarction, stent thrombosis, stroke, or urgent revascularization 1 year after stent implantation. For patients in the monitoring group, the Verify-Now P2Y12 and aspirin point-of-care assays were used in the catheterization laboratory before stent implantation and in the outpatient clinic 2 to 4 weeks later.

Results.—In the monitoring group, high platelet reactivity in patients taking clopidogrel (34.5% of patients) or aspirin (7.6%) led to the administration of an additional bolus of clopidogrel, prasugrel, or aspirin along with glycoprotein IIb/IIIa inhibitors during the procedure. The primary end point occurred in 34.6% of the patients in the monitoring group, as compared with 31.1% of those in the conventional-treatment group (hazard ratio, 1.13; 95% confidence interval [CI], 0.98 to 1.29; $P = 0.10$). The main secondary end point, stent thrombosis or any urgent revascularization, occurred in 4.9% of the patients in the monitoring group and 4.6% of those in the conventional-treatment group (hazard ratio, 1.06; 95% CI, 0.74 to 1.52; $P = 0.77$). The rate of major bleeding events did not differ significantly between groups.

Conclusions.—This study showed no significant improvements in clinical outcomes with platelet-function monitoring and treatment adjustment for coronary stenting, as compared with standard antiplatelet therapy without monitoring. (Funded by Allies in Cardiovascular Trials Initiatives and Organized Networks and others; ARCTIC ClinicalTrials.gov number, NCT00827411.)

▶ Clinical trials have demonstrated that compared with aspirin alone, the combination of aspirin and clopidogrel, a thienopyridine antagonist of the P2Y12 receptor, reduces the risk of ischemic events and stent thrombosis in acute coronary syndrome (ACS) patients, with or without ST-segment elevation, whether they are treated medically or with percutaneous coronary intervention (PCI).[1-4] Therefore, dual antiplatelet therapy with aspirin and an antagonist of the platelet P2Y12 receptor is the standard of care for patients with ACS with or without ST-segment elevation[5,6] and for patients who undergo PCI.[7]

The response to clopidogrel, a prodrug that must be converted to an active metabolite, is affected by a variety of factors, including genetic polymorphisms, drug interactions, and cigarette smoking.[8-11] The enzymatic activities that convert clopidogrel from an inactive pro-drug to an active metabolite are reduced in patients with loss-of-function cytochrome P450 alleles, resulting in increased risk of cardiovascular events, including stent thrombosis and death.[8-10] On March 12, 2010, the US Food and Drug Administration approved a revised label for clopidogrel that includes a boxed warning about the reduced efficacy of clopidogrel in patients with impaired ability to convert clopidogrel to its active metabolite.[12] Subsequently the American College of Cardiology Foundation and American Heart Association published a Clinical Expert Consensus document that reviewed potential solutions to the decreased efficacy of clopidogrel in patients who are hypo-responders.[13]

High residual platelet reactivity during treatment with clopidogrel is associated with an increased risk of both short-term and long-term ischemic events after PCI.[14] Therefore, several studies have evaluated alternative treatment strategies in patients with high residual platelet activity during clopidogrel treatment after PCI.[15-17] Increased loading and maintenance doses of clopidogrel produce greater platelet inhibition in patients who are heterozygous for the CYP2C19*2 loss of function allele.[18,19] The Gauging Responsiveness with a VerifyNow Assay-Impact on Thrombosis and Safety (GRAVITAS) trial was a double-blind study that randomized 2214 patients with high on-treatment platelet reactivity 12 to 24 hours after PCI to either standard-dose clopidogrel (75 mg daily maintenance dose) or high-dose clopidogrel (600 mg loading dose and 150 mg daily maintenance dose).[15] Platelet function was assessed with the VerifyNow P2Y12 test (Accumetrics, San Diego, CA) 12 to 24 hours after PCI, and 30 days and 6 months after PCI. The test measures adenosine diphosphate—induced platelet agglutination as an increase in light transmittance. The GRAVITAS trial demonstrated that high-dose clopidogrel did not reduce the incidence of the primary end point, cardiovascular death, nonfatal myocardial infarction (MI), or stent thrombosis, among patients with high on-treatment platelet reactivity after PCI with drug-eluting stents.[15] Although high-dose clopidogrel induced a 22% absolute reduction in the rate of high on-treatment platelet reactivity at 30 days after PCI (62% vs 40%; $P < .001$), at 6 months the primary end point occurred in 25 of 1109 patients (2.3%) treated with high-dose clopidogrel compared with 25 of 1105 patients (2.3%) treated with standard-dose clopidogrel (hazard ratio 1.01; 95% CI 0.58-1.76; $P = .97$).[15]

Prasugrel was shown to exert greater inhibition of platelets than high-dose clopidogrel in patients with high platelet reactivity during treatment with standard dose clopidogrel.[20] A randomized trial that compared clopidogrel with prasugrel in patients with high platelet reactivity on clopidogrel after PCI was terminated prematurely after enrollment of only 423 patients because the incidence of the primary end point was lower than expected.[16] Collet et al[17] designed a study to test the hypothesis that platelet-function monitoring with adjustment of therapy in patients with high on-treatment platelet reactivity would be superior to a conventional strategy without monitoring or drug adjustment in patients who undergo coronary artery stenting. The VerifyNow aspirin and P2Y12 assays were used to assess platelet function in the patients who were randomized to the monitoring group. Aspirin hypo-responders received intravenous aspirin before PCI, and clopidogrel hypo-responders received both an intravenous glycoprotein IIb/IIIa inhibitor and either high-dose clopidogrel (a loading dose ≥600 mg and daily maintenance dose of 150 mg) or a 60-mg loading dose of prasugrel before PCI and a 10-mg daily maintenance dose after PCI. Platelet function testing was not performed in the conventional treatment group, and the use of clopidogrel, prasugrel, and glycoprotein IIb/IIIa inhibitors was left to the physician's discretion. The primary end point, a composite of death, MI, stent thrombosis, stroke, or urgent revascularization 1 year after PCI was similar for the 2 groups (hazard ratio 1.13; 95% CI 0.98-1.29; $P = .10$). Also, there was no significant difference in the main secondary end point, stent thrombosis, or urgent revascularization.

The doses of antihypertensive and lipid-lowering medications are adjusted to achieve reductions in blood pressure or serum cholesterol that are believed to optimally reduce the risk of clinical events such as MI and stroke. It seems logical to suppose that platelet function monitoring and adjustment of antiplatelet therapy in patients with high platelet reactivity during treatment with standard-dose clopidogrel would reduce the risk of thrombotic events, such as acute MI or stent thrombosis, in patients with ACS or coronary stents. Unfortunately, recent studies have been unable to demonstrate the utility of such a strategy in patients undergoing PCI. A large study that used the VerifyNow device to measure platelet function confirmed that prasugrel was associated with lower platelet reactivity than clopidogrel, but there was not an independent association between platelet reactivity and the incidence of ischemic outcomes among 2564 patients with ACS who were randomly assigned to treatment with either clopidogrel or prasugrel.[21]

Cytochrome P450 genetic polymorphisms do not affect drug metabolite concentrations, inhibition of platelet aggregation, or clinical event rates in patients treated with prasugrel[22,23] or ticagrelor.[24] Also, compared with the combination of aspirin and clopidogrel, the combination of aspirin and ticagrelor reduced the risk of death in patients with ACS.[25] The class I recommendations of the most recent update of the practice guidelines for PCI include both prasugrel and ticagrelor as alternatives to clopidogrel to inhibit the platelet P2Y12 receptor.[7] Unfortunately, the recent clinical studies discussed here have not established a definitive role for platelet function monitoring to guide the selection of a P2Y12 inhibitor in patients who have undergone PCI.

S. W. Werns, MD

References

1. The Clopidogrel in Unstable Angina to Prevent Recurrent Events Trial Investigators. Effects of clopidogrel in addition to aspirin in patients with acute coronary syndromes without ST-Segment Elevation. *N Engl J Med*. 2001;345:494-502.
2. Mehta SR, Yusuf S, Peters RJG, et al. Effects of pretreatment with clopidogrel and aspirin followed by long-term therapy in patients undergoing percutaneous coronary intervention: the PCI-CURE study. *Lancet*. 2001;358:527-533.
3. Sabatine MS, Cannon CP, Gibson CM, et al. Addition of clopidogrel to aspirin and fibrinolytic therapy for myocardial infarction with ST-segment elevation. *N Engl J Med*. 2005;352:1179-1189.
4. Desai NR, Bhatt DL. The state of the periprocedural antiplatelet therapy after recent trials. *JACC Cardiovasc Interv*. 2010;3:571-583.

5. O'Gara PT, Kushner FG, Ascheim DD, et al. 2013 ACCF/AHA guideline for the management of ST-elevation myocardial infarction: a report of the American College of Cardiology Foundation/American Heart Association Task Force on Practice Guidelines. *Circulation.* 2013;127:e362-e425.
6. Jneid H, Anderson JL, Wright RS, et al. 2012 ACCF/AHA focused update of the guideline for the management of patients with UA/non-ST-elevation myocardial infarction (updating the 2007 guideline and replacing the 2011 focused update): a report of the American College of Cardiology Foundation/American Heart Association Task Force on Practice Guidelines. *J Am Coll Cardiol.* 2012;60: 645-681.
7. Levine GN, Bates ER, Blankenship JC, et al. 2011 ACCF/AHA/SCAI guideline for percutaneous coronary intervention: a report of the American College of Cardiology Foundation/American Heart Association Task Force on Practice Guidelines and the Society for Cardiovascular Angiography and Interventions. *J Am Coll Cardiol.* 2011;58:e44-e122.
8. Shuldiner AR, O'Connell JR, Bliden KP, et al. Association of cytochrome P450 2C19 genotype with the antiplatelet effect and clinical efficacy of clopidogrel therapy. *JAMA.* 2009;302:849-858.
9. Mega JL, Close SL, Wiviott SD, et al. Genetic variants in ABCB1 and CYP2C19 and cardiovascular outcomes after treatment with clopidogrel and prasugrel in the TRITON-TIMI 38 trial: a pharmacogenetic analysis. *Lancet.* 2010;376: 1312-1319.
10. Mega JL, Simon T, Colleg J-P, et al. Reduced-function CYP2C19 genotype and risk of adverse clinical outcomes among patients treated with clopidogrel predominantly for PCI. A meta-analysis. *JAMA.* 2010;304:1821-1830.
11. Gurbel PA, Nolin TD, Tantry US. Clopidogrel efficacy and cigarette smoking status. *JAMA.* 2012;307:2495-2496.
12. FDA Drug Safety Communication: reduced effectiveness of Plavix (clopidogrel) in patients who are poor metabolizers of the drug: http://www.fda.gov/Drugs/DrugSafety/PostmarketDrugSafetyInformationforPatientsandProviders/ucm203888.htm. Accessed January 30, 2013.
13. Holmes DR Jr, Dehmer GJ, Kaul S, et al. ACCF/AHA clopidogrel clinical alert: approaches to the FDA "Boxed Warning": a report of the American College of Cardiology Foundation Task Force on Clinical Expert Consensus Documents and the American Heart Association. *J Am Coll Cardiol.* 2010;56:321-341.
14. Parodi G, Marcucci R, Valenti R, et al. High residual platelet reactivity after clopidogrel loading and long-term cardiovascular events among patients with acute coronary syndromes undergoing PCI. *JAMA.* 2011;306:1215-1223.
15. Price MJ, Berger PB, Teirstein PS, et al. Standard- vs high-dose clopidogrel based on platelet function testing after percutaneous coronary intervention. The GRAVITAS randomized trial. *JAMA.* 2011;305:1097-1105.
16. Trenk D, Stone GW, Gawaz M, et al. A randomized trial of prasugrel versus clopidogrel in patients with high platelet reactivity on clopidogrel after elective percutaneous coronary intervention with implantation of drug-eluting stents. *J Am Coll Cardiol.* 2012;59:2159-2164.
17. Collet J-P, Cuisset T, Range G, et al. Bedside monitoring to adjust antiplatelet therapy for coronary stenting. *N Engl J Med.* 2012;367:2100-2109.
18. Bonello L, Armero S, Mokhtar OA, et al. Clopidogrel loading dose adjustment according to platelet reactivity monitoring in patients carrying the 2C19 2* loss of function polymorphism. *J Am Coll Cardiol.* 2010;56:1630-1636.
19. Mega JL, Hochholzer W, Frelinger A, et al. Dosing clopidogrel based on CYP2C19 genotype and the effect on platelet reactivity in patients with stable cardiovascular disease. *JAMA.* 2011;306:2221-2228.
20. Alexopoulos D, Xanthopoulou I, Davlouros P, et al. Prasugrel overcomes high on-clopidogrel platelet reactivity in chronic coronary artery disease patients more effectively than high dose (150 mg) clopidogrel. *Am Heart J.* 2011;162: 733-739.

21. Gurbel PA, Erlinge D, Ohman EM, et al. Platelet function during extended prasugrel and clopidogrel therapy for patients with ACS treated without revascularization. *JAMA.* 2012;308:1785-1794.
22. Varenhorst C, James S, Erlinge D, et al. Genetic variation of CYP2C19 affects both pharmacokinetic and pharmacodynamic responses to clopidogrel but not prasugrel in aspirin-treated patients with coronary artery disease. *Eur Heart J.* 2009;30:1744-1752.
23. Mega JL, Close SL, Wiviott SD, et al. Cytochrome P450 genetic polymorphisms and the response to prasugrel. *Circulation.* 2009;119:2553-2556.
24. Wallentin L, James S, Storey RF, et al. Effect of CYP2C19 and ABCB1 single nucleotide polymorphisms on outcomes of treatment with ticagrelor versus clopidogrel for acute coronary syndromes: a genetic substudy of the PLATO trial. *Lancet.* 2010;376:1320-1328.
25. Wallentin L, Becker RC, Budaz A, et al. Ticagrelor versus clopidogrel in patients with acute coronary syndromes. *N Engl J Med.* 2009;361:1045-1057.

Rivaroxaban in Patients with a Recent Acute Coronary Syndrome

Mega JL, for the ATLAS ACS 2—TIMI 51 Investigators (Brigham and Women's Hosp and Harvard Med School, Boston, MA; et al)

N Engl J Med 366:9-19, 2012

Background.—Acute coronary syndromes arise from coronary atherosclerosis with superimposed thrombosis. Since factor Xa plays a central role in thrombosis, the inhibition of factor Xa with low-dose rivaroxaban might improve cardiovascular outcomes in patients with a recent acute coronary syndrome.

Methods.—In this double-blind, placebo-controlled trial, we randomly assigned 15,526 patients with a recent acute coronary syndrome to receive twice-daily doses of either 2.5 mg or 5 mg of rivaroxaban or placebo for a mean of 13 months and up to 31 months. The primary efficacy end point was a composite of death from cardiovascular causes, myocardial infarction, or stroke.

Results.—Rivaroxaban significantly reduced the primary efficacy end point, as compared with placebo, with respective rates of 8.9% and 10.7% (hazard ratio in the rivaroxaban group, 0.84; 95% confidence interval [CI], 0.74 to 0.96; $P = 0.008$), with significant improvement for both the twice-daily 2.5-mg dose (9.1% vs. 10.7%, $P = 0.02$) and the twice-daily 5-mg dose (8.8% vs. 10.7%, $P = 0.03$). The twice-daily 2.5-mg dose of rivaroxaban reduced the rates of death from cardiovascular causes (2.7% vs. 4.1%, $P = 0.002$) and from any cause (2.9% vs. 4.5%, $P = 0.002$), a survival benefit that was not seen with the twice-daily 5-mg dose. As compared with placebo, rivaroxaban increased the rates of major bleeding not related to coronary-artery bypass grafting (2.1% vs. 0.6%, $P < 0.001$) and intracranial hemorrhage (0.6% vs. 0.2%, $P = 0.009$), without a significant increase in fatal bleeding (0.3% vs. 0.2%, $P = 0.66$) or other adverse events. The twice-daily 2.5-mg dose resulted in fewer fatal bleeding events than the twice-daily 5-mg dose (0.1% vs. 0.4%, $P = 0.04$).

Conclusions.—In patients with a recent acute coronary syndrome, rivaroxaban reduced the risk of the composite end point of death from cardiovascular causes, myocardial infarction, or stroke. Rivaroxaban increased the risk of major bleeding and intracranial hemorrhage but not the risk of fatal bleeding. (Funded by Johnson & Johnson and Bayer Healthcare; ATLAS ACS 2—TIMI 51 ClinicalTrials.gov number, NCT00809965.)

▶ The spectrum of acute coronary syndrome (ACS) encompasses unstable angina (UA), non—ST-segment elevation myocardial infarction (NSTEMI), and ST-segment elevation myocardial infarction (STEMI). The current practice guidelines for patients with ACS include several class I recommendations for dual antiplatelet therapy with aspirin and an inhibitor of the platelet P2Y12 receptor.[1,2] For patients with UA or NSTEMI who are treated medically without stent placement, aspirin should be prescribed indefinitely and clopidogrel or ticagrelor should be prescribed for up to 12 months.[1] For patients with UA or NSTEMI who are treated with a coronary stent, aspirin should be prescribed indefinitely and clopidogrel, prasugrel, or ticagrelor should be prescribed for at least 12 months after a drug-eluting stent and up to 12 months after a bare metal stent.[1] For patients with STEMI who undergo percutaneous coronary intervention (PCI), aspirin should be continued indefinitely, and clopidogrel, prasugrel, or ticagrelor should be given for 1 year.[2] For patients with STEMI who receive fibrinolytic therapy, aspirin should be continued indefinitely, and clopidogrel should be continued for at least 14 days and up to 1 year.[2]

The role of oral anticoagulants in patients with ACS is less certain and remains an area of active investigation. A meta-analysis that included 5938 patients with ACS who did not undergo PCI with stents and who were enrolled in 10 clinical trials, concluded that, compared with aspirin alone, aspirin plus warfarin was associated with a decreased risk of myocardial infarction (MI) or revascularization, an increased risk of major bleeding, and no significant effect on mortality.[3] Several trials have found, however, that aspirin plus warfarin is less effective than dual antiplatelet therapy after coronary stent placement.[4-6] The Stent Anticoagulation Restenosis Study randomly assigned 1653 patients to aspirin alone, aspirin and warfarin, or aspirin and ticlopidine after coronary stent placement.[6] The primary endpoint, death, revascularization of the target lesion, stent thrombosis, or MI within 30 days, was observed in 20 patients (3.6%) assigned to aspirin alone, 15 patients (2.7%) assigned to receive aspirin plus warfarin, and only 3 patients (0.5%) assigned to receive aspirin and ticlopidine ($P = .001$).[6]

Recent clinical trials have tested the efficacy and safety of several new oral anticoagulants in patients with a variety of disorders, including atrial fibrillation and ACS.[7-10] Ximelagatran, an oral direct thrombin inhibitor, reduced the incidence of major cardiovascular events during 6 months of therapy after a recent STEMI or NSTEMI, but the drug was not marketed because of hepatotoxicity.[7] Large clinical trials have been conducted to investigate 2 oral factor Xa inhibitors, apixaban and rivaroxaban, in patients with ACS.[8] A trial that randomized patients with a recent ACS to either apixaban or placebo was terminated prematurely after the recruitment of 7392 patients because apixaban was associated with an increase in the number of major bleeding events but no significant reduction in recurrent ischemic events.[8] Mega et al conducted a trial that randomly assigned 15 526 patients with a recent ACS to rivaroxaban 2.5 mg twice daily, rivaroxaban 5 mg twice daily, or placebo. Approximately 99% of patients received aspirin, and approximately 93% also received a thienopyridine. The primary efficacy endpoint, a composite of stroke, MI, or cardiovascular death, was reduced by both the low dose (9.1% vs 10.7%, $P = .02$) and high dose (8.8% vs 10.7%, $P = .03$) of rivaroxaban. The 2.5-mg twice-daily dose, but not the 5-mg twice-daily dose, also reduced the rates of death from cardiovascular causes (2.7% vs 4.1%, $P = .002$) and from any cause (2.9% vs 4.5%, $P = .002$). The patients who received the lower dose of rivaroxaban also exhibited a lower risk of stent thrombosis, an important observation. Patients who were randomly assigned to rivaroxaban also experienced higher rates of major bleeding and intracranial hemorrhage but not fatal bleeding. It is important to note that the doses of rivaroxaban that were used in the latter study were either 2.5 mg or 5 mg twice daily, less than the dose of 15 or 20 mg daily that was noninferior to warfarin in patients with nonvalvular atrial fibrillation.[9] A meta-analysis was performed to pool the results of 7 randomized, placebo-controlled clinical trials that evaluated the effects of direct thrombin inhibitors or anti-Xa inhibitors in 31 286 patients who received antiplatelet therapy after an ACS.[10] The new oral anticoagulants significantly reduced the risk of MI and the risk of definite or probable stent thrombosis, but the risk of major bleeding events was 2 to 3 times greater. Consequently, there was no difference in overall mortality or the net clinical benefit.

The increased bleeding risk of combining an oral anticoagulant with dual antiplatelet therapy has been investigated extensively.[10-13] Analysis of a nationwide Danish registry that included 40 812 patients who were hospitalized for a first MI found that therapy with a combination of aspirin, clopidogrel, and a vitamin K antagonist after hospital discharge was associated with a 12% annual incidence of readmission for bleeding, compared with only 2.6% among patients who received aspirin alone and 3.7% for aspirin plus clopidogrel.[11] A similar analysis used the Danish registry to study the outcomes of 82 854 patients who were discharged after a first-time hospitalization for atrial fibrillation.[12] During a mean follow-up period of 3.3 years, the incidence of fatal bleeding or hospitalization for nonfatal bleeding was 3.9% per patient-year for warfarin monotherapy, 3.7% per patient-year for aspirin monotherapy, and 5.6% per patient-year for clopidogrel monotherapy. The combinations of warfarin and anti-platelet therapy were associated with an increased incidence of fatal or nonfatal bleeding: 6.9% per patient-year for warfarin and aspirin, 13.9% per patient-year for warfarin and clopidogrel, and 15.7% per patient-year for aspirin, clopidogrel, and warfarin.[12] Using warfarin monotherapy as a reference, the hazard ratios for nonfatal and fatal bleeding were 1.83 for warfarin and aspirin; 3.08 for warfarin and clopidogrel; and 3.70 for warfarin, aspirin, and clopidogrel.[12] The outcomes of several clinical trials showed that patients with ACS who have bleeding complications are at increased risk of both short-term and long-term adverse events, including an increased risk of 30-day and 6-month mortality.[14-17]

Warfarin is not popular with either patients or physicians because of the high rate of bleeding complications, the numerous interactions with food and medications, and the need for frequent monitoring of the international normalized ratio. Although drugs like rivaroxaban may obviate many of those considerations, the safety and efficacy of triple antithrombotic therapy, such as the combination of rivaroxaban with aspirin and a P2Y12 inhibitor, requires further study. Triple antithrombotic therapy with aspirin, a P2Y12 inhibitor, and an oral anticoagulant such as rivaroxaban, may be indicated in patients with coronary stents and a high risk of stroke due to atrial fibrillation despite the increased risk of bleeding.[18] Patients with ACS who are at low risk of bleeding and increased risk of recurrent ischemic events may derive benefit from triple antithrombotic therapy. Populations of ACS patients who are at increased risk of bleeding complications during triple antithrombotic therapy, such as the elderly and patients with a history of cerebrovascular disease, might be harmed by triple antithrombotic therapy. The challenge will be to discover the characteristics that can reliably distinguish both groups of patients to target appropriate ACS patients for triple antithrombotic therapy.

S. W. Werns, MD

References

1. Jneid H, Anderson JL, Wright RS, et al. 2012 ACCF/AHA focused update of the guideline for the management of patients with unstable angina/non-ST-elevation myocardial infarction (updating the 2007 guideline and replacing the 2011 focused update): a report of the American College of Cardiology Foundation/American Heart Association Task Force on Practice Guidelines. *J Am Coll Cardiol.* 2012;60:645-681.
2. O'Gara PT, Kushner FG, Ascheim DD, et al. 2013 ACCF/AHA guideline for the management of ST-elevation myocardial infarction: a report of the American College of Cardiology Foundation/American Heart Association Task Force on Practice Guidelines. *Circulation.* In press.
3. Rothberg MB, Celestin C, Fiore LD, Lawler E, Cook JR. Warfarin plus aspirin after myocardial infarction or the acute coronary syndrome: meta-analysis with estimates of risk and benefit. *Ann Intern Med.* 2005;143:241-250.
4. Schömig A, Neumann F-J, Kastrati A, et al. A randomized comparison of antiplatelet and anticoagulant therapy after the placement of coronary-artery stents. *N Engl J Med.* 1996;334:1084-1089.
5. Bertrand ME, Legrand V, Boland J, et al. Randomized multicenter comparison of conventional anticoagulation versus antiplatelet therapy in unplanned and elective coronary stenting. The full anticoagulation versus aspirin and ticlopidine (fantastic) study. *Circulation.* 1998;98:1597-1603.
6. Leon MB, Baim DS, Popma JJ, et al. A clinical trial comparing three antithrombotic-drug regimens after coronary-artery stenting. Stent Anticoagulation Restenosis Study Investigators. *N Engl J Med.* 1998;339:1665-1671.
7. Wallentin L, Wilcox RG, Weaver WD, et al. Oral ximelagatran for secondary prophylaxis after myocardial infarction: the ESTEEM randomised controlled trial. *Lancet.* 2003;362:789-797.
8. Alexander JH, Lopes RD, James S, et al. Apixaban with antiplatelet therapy after acute coronary syndrome. *N Engl J Med.* 2011;365:699-708.
9. Patel MR, Mahaffey KW, Garg J, et al. Rivaroxaban versus warfarin in nonvalvular atrial fibrillation. *N Engl J Med.* 2011;365:883-891.
10. Komócsi A, Vorobcsuk A, Kehl D, Aradi D. Use of new-generation oral anticoagulant agents in patients receiving antiplatelet therapy after an acute coronary syndrome. *Arch Intern Med.* 2012;172:1537-1545.
11. Sørensen R, Hansen ML, Abildstrom SZ, et al. Risk of bleeding in patients with acute myocardial infarction treated with different combinations of aspirin, clopidogrel, and vitamin K antagonists in Denmark: a retrospective analysis of nationwide registry data. *Lancet.* 2009;374:1967-1974.

12. Hansen ML, Sørensen R, Clausen MT, et al. Risk of bleeding with single, dual, or triple therapy with warfarin, aspirin, and clopidogrel in patients with atrial fibrillation. *Arch Intern Med.* 2010;170:1433-1441.
13. Ruiz-Nodar JM, Marín F, Roldán V, et al. Should we recommend oral anticoagulation therapy in patients with atrial fibrillation undergoing coronary artery stenting with a high HAS-BLED bleeding risk score? *Circ Cardiovasc Interv.* 2012;5:459-466.
14. Rao SV, O'Grady K, Pieper KS, et al. Impact of bleeding severity on clinical outcomes among patients with acute coronary syndromes. *Am J Cardiol.* 2005; 96:1200-1206.
15. Eikelboom JW, Mehta SR, Anand SS, Xie C, Fox KA, Yusuf S. Adverse impact of bleeding on prognosis in patients with acute coronary syndromes. *Circulation.* 2006;114:774-782.
16. Manoukian SV, Feit F, Mehran R, et al. Impact of major bleeding on 30-day mortality and clinical outcomes in patients with acute coronary syndromes: an analysis from the ACUITY Trial. *J Am Coll Cardiol.* 2007;49:1362-1368.
17. Budaj A, Eikelboom JW, Mehta SR, et al. Improving clinical outcomes by reducing bleeding in patients with non-ST-elevation acute coronary syndromes. *Eur Heart J.* 2009;30:655-661.
18. Coppens M, Eikelboom JW. Antithrombotic therapy after coronary artery stenting in patients with atrial fibrillation. *Circ Cardiovasc Interv.* 2012;5:454-455.

Intraaortic Balloon Support for Myocardial Infarction with Cardiogenic Shock

Thiele H, for the IABP-SHOCK II Trial Investigators (Univ of Leipzig—Heart Ctr, Germany; et al)

N Engl J Med 367:1287-1296, 2012

Background.—In current international guidelines, intraaortic balloon counterpulsation is considered to be a class I treatment for cardiogenic shock complicating acute myocardial infarction. However, evidence is based mainly on registry data, and there is a paucity of randomized clinical trials.

Methods.—In this randomized, prospective, open-label, multicenter trial, we randomly assigned 600 patients with cardiogenic shock complicating acute myocardial infarction to intraaortic balloon counterpulsation (IABP group, 301 patients) or no intraaortic balloon counterpulsation (control group, 299 patients). All patients were expected to undergo early revascularization (by means of percutaneous coronary intervention or bypass surgery) and to receive the best available medical therapy. The primary efficacy end point was 30-day all-cause mortality. Safety assessments included major bleeding, peripheral ischemic complications, sepsis, and stroke.

Results.—A total of 300 patients in the IABP group and 298 in the control group were included in the analysis of the primary end point. At 30 days, 119 patients in the IABP group (39.7%) and 123 patients in the control group (41.3%) had died (relative risk with IABP, 0.96; 95% confidence interval, 0.79 to 1.17; $P = 0.69$). There were no significant differences in secondary end points or in process-of-care measures, including the time to hemodynamic stabilization, the length of stay in the intensive care unit, serum lactate levels, the dose and duration of catecholamine therapy, and renal function. The IABP group and the control group did not differ significantly with respect to the rates of major bleeding (3.3% and 4.4%, respectively; $P = 0.51$), peripheral ischemic complications (4.3% and 3.4%, $P = 0.53$), sepsis (15.7% and 20.5%, $P = 0.15$), and stroke (0.7% and 1.7%, $P = 0.28$).

Conclusions.—The use of intraaortic balloon counterpulsation did not significantly reduce 30-day mortality in patients with cardiogenic shock complicating acute myocardial infarction for whom an early revascularization strategy was planned. (Funded by the German Research Foundation and others; IABP-SHOCK II ClinicalTrials.gov number, NCT00491036.)

▶ Cardiogenic shock (CS) is a relatively infrequent complication of acute coronary syndromes (ACS). CS occurred in only 2992 of 65 119 patients (4.6%) who were hospitalized with ACS and were enrolled in the Global Registry of Acute Coronary Events (GRACE) between 1999 and 2007.[1] Nevertheless, CS is an important complication of ACS because the mortality remains high. In the GRACE registry, the in-hospital mortality rate was 59.4% among patients with CS compared with 2.3% among patients who did not have CS ($P < .001$).

The SHOCK (Should We Emergently Revascularize Occluded Coronaries for Cardiogenic Shock) trial was a landmark randomized study to evaluate early revascularization in patients with CS.[2-4] Patients with an acute myocardial infarction (MI) complicated by CS due to left ventricular failure were randomly assigned to either emergency revascularization (n = 152 patients) or initial medical stabilization (n = 150 patients). The SHOCK trial found that myocardial revascularization, via percutaneous coronary intervention (PCI) or coronary artery bypass surgery (CABG), improved 6-month, 1-year, and 6-year survival among patients with acute MI complicated by CS.[2-4] Therefore, according to the 2013 American College of Cardiology Foundation/American Heart Association Guideline for the Management of ST-Elevation Myocardial Infarction, MI complicated by CS due to pump failure is a class I indication for emergency revascularization with either PCI or CABG.[5]

In the SHOCK trial, which enrolled patients from 1993 to 1998, an intra-aortic balloon pump (IABP) was used in 86% of the patients in both treatment groups, reflecting the prevalent consensus regarding treatment of CS.[2] CS not quickly reversed with pharmacologic therapy was designated a class I indication for an IABP in the guidelines for the management of MI that were issued jointly by the American College of Cardiology and American Heart Association in 1996 and 2004.[6,7] The evidence base for that recommendation, however, was never strong and has grown weaker since the SHOCK trial was conducted and the 2004 guideline was formulated. In 2009 Sjauw et al[8] performed a meta-analysis of 9 cohort studies of IABP use in MI patients with CS. An adjunctive IABP was associated with an absolute decrease in 30-day mortality rate of 18% (95% confidence interval [CI], 16%–20%; $P < .0001$) among the patients who were enrolled in 7 studies that used fibrinolytic therapy as the mode of reperfusion, perhaps a result of less frequent reocclusion of the infarct-related artery in patients who received an IABP.[9] In the 2 studies that utilized primary PCI as the mode of reperfusion, however, treatment with an IABP was associated with an absolute increase in 30-day mortality rate of 6% (95% CI, 3%–10%; $P = .0008$). The larger PCI cohort study, MRMI-2 (National Registry of Myocardial Infarction 2), found that IABP therapy was an independent predictor of higher 30-day mortality after multivariate adjustment for multiple factors.[10] Nevertheless, it is impossible to exclude bias caused by preferential use of an IABP in the sicker patients.

Unfortunately, studies that were published in 2011 and 2012 did not provide evidence that the IABP improves outcomes in patients with ACS, with or without CS.[11,12] The Counterpulsation to Reduce Infarct Size Pre-PCI Acute Myocardial Infarction (CRISP AMI) trial was a prospective, multicenter, randomized trial to determine if routine insertion of an IABP before primary PCI reduces infarct size in patients with an acute anterior ST-segment elevation MI without CS.[11] Insertion of an IABP was not associated with a reduction of infarct size as measured by cardiac magnetic resonance imaging 3 to 5 days after PCI. The CRISP AMI trial was included in a meta-analysis of 6 trials that randomly assigned 1054 patients with acute MI without CS to either an IABP or no IABP.[12] Insertion of an IABP did not reduce the incidence of reinfarction, congestive heart failure, or all-cause death, whereas the risk of bleeding (21.4% vs 16.1%, odds ratio 1.46, $P = .02$) and stroke (2% vs 0.3%, odds ratio 4.39, $P = .03$) were both increased.[12]

The IABP-SHOCK II Trial was a randomized, multicenter trial that randomly assigned 600 patients with acute MI complicated by CS. Primary PCI was performed in 287 of 301 patients who were randomly assigned to the IABP group (95.3%) and 288 of 299 patients in the control group (96.3%; $P = .55$). The primary efficacy endpoint, 30-day all-cause mortality, was 39.7% for the IABP group and 41.3% for the control group ($P = .69$). The recommendation for the use of an IABP in patients with CS after MI has been downgraded to class IIa according to the updated MI guidelines issued in 2013.[5]

The revised guidelines also include a class IIb recommendation for alternative left ventricular assist devices for circulatory support in patients with refractory CS.[5] Recent reviews of percutaneous circulatory support devices for patients with CS have provided detailed descriptions of the alternatives to the IABP.[13,14] The TandemHeart (CardiacAssist, Inc, Pittsburgh, PA) is a percutaneous, left atrial-femoral bypass centrifugal pump that can provide up to 4.5 L/min of cardiac output.[13] Among 18 patients with CS after MI, use of the TandemHeart was associated with an increase in cardiac index from 1.7 ± 0.3 L to 2.4 ± 0.6 L/min/m^2 ($P < .001$), an increase in mean blood pressure from 63 ± 8 to 80 ± 9 mm Hg ($P < .001$), and a decrease in pulmonary capillary wedge pressure from 21 ± 4 to 14 ± 4 mm Hg ($P < .001$).[15] Thiele and colleagues[16] conducted a trial that randomly assigned 41 patients with CS after an acute MI to an IABP or Tandem-Heart. Although there was greater improvement of hemodynamic and metabolic parameters among the patients who received the TandemHeart compared with an IABP, there was no difference in 30-day mortality rate, and more patients treated with the TandemHeart had severe bleeding and limb ischemia.[16] The TandemHeart also has been used as a right ventricular assist device to treat CS caused by right ventricular infarction.[17] A right atrial inflow cannula and a pulmonary artery outflow catheter were inserted percutaneously via the femoral veins.

The Impella 2.5 (Abiomed Inc, Danvers, MA) can be inserted percutaneously and is capable of augmenting cardiac output by 2.5 L/min.[13] A randomized trial compared the Impella 2.5 with the IABP in 26 patients with acute MI complicated by CS.[18] The cardiac index after 30 minutes of support was increased by 0.49 ± 0.46 L/min/m^2 among the patients with an Impella (n = 12), compared with an increase of only 0.11 ± 0.31 L/min/m^2 among patients with an IABP (n = 13; P = .02). Six patients within each group died within 30 days. The Impella 5.0 (Abiomed, Inc, Danvers, MA), which can be inserted via a cutdown on the axillary or femoral artery, can augment cardiac output by 5.0 L/min and has been used in patients with MI complicated by CS.[19]

It is difficult to formulate strong recommendations regarding hemodynamic support devices for patients with acute MI complicated by CS because the limited number of clinical trials constitute an inadequate evidence base. A meta-analysis of 3 trials that randomly assigned patients with CS to an IABP or a left ventricular assist device, the Impella 2.5 in 1 trial[18] and the TandemHeart in 2 trials,[16,20] found that 30-day mortality was not significantly different, but the total number of patients was only 100, and one study included 16 patients with chronic decompensated heart failure.[21] Clearly, further clinical trials are desirable to define the impact of the Impella and TandemHeart on mortality, but the required sample sizes represent a formidable obstacle. Thiele et al[22] calculated the sample sizes that would be needed to detect various reductions in mortality. Assuming a 45% mortality rate in the control group, a sample size of 396 patients per group would be needed to show a 10% absolute mortality reduction with an alpha of 5% and power of 80%.[22] It took 3 years for 37 centers in Germany to randomly assign patients with acute MI complicated by CS to an IABP or no IABP. Therefore, it is possible that there may never be a study that has adequate power to assess the impact of the Impella or TandemHeart on mortality in patients with CS.

S. W. Werns, MD

References

1. Awad HH, Anderson FA, Gore JM, Goodman SG, Goldberg RJ. Cardiogenic shock complicating acute coronary syndromes: insights from the Global Registry of Acute Coronary Events. *Am Heart J.* 2012;163:963-967.
2. Hochman JS, Sleeper LA, Webb JG, et al; Early revascularization in acute myocardial infarction complicated by cardiogenic shock. SHOCK Investigators. Should We Emergently Revascularize Occluded Coronaries for Cardiogenic Shock. *N Engl J Med.* 1999;341:625-634.
3. Hochman JS, Sleeper LA, White HD, et al. One-year survival following early revascularization for cardiogenic shock. *JAMA.* 2001;285:190-192.
4. Hochman JS, Sleeper LA, Webb JG, et al. Early revascularization and long-term survival in cardiogenic shock complicating acute myocardial infarction. *JAMA.* 2006;295:2511-2515.
5. O'Gara PT, Kushner FG, Ascheim DD, et al. 2013 ACCF/AHA guideline for the management of ST-elevation myocardial infarction: a report of the America College of Cardiology Foundation/American Heart Association Task Force on Practice Guidelines. *Circulation.* In press.
6. Ryan TJ, Anderson JL, Antman EM, et al. ACC/AHA guidelines for the management of patients with acute myocardial infarction. A report of the American College of Cardiology/American Heart Association Task Force on Practice Guidelines (Committee on Management of Acute Myocardial Infarction). *J Am Coll Cardiol.* 1996;28:1328-1428.

7. Antman EM, Anbe DT, Armstrong PW, et al. ACC/AHA guidelines for the management of patients with ST-elevation myocardial infarction: a report of the American College of Cardiology/American Heart Association Task Force on Practice Guidelines (Committee to Revise the 1999 Guidelines for the Management of Patients with Acute Myocardial Infarction). *Circulation*. 2004; 110:e82-e292.

8. Sjauw KD, Engström AE, Vis MM, et al. A systematic review and meta-analysis of intra-aortic balloon pump therapy in ST-elevation myocardial infarction: should we change the guidelines? *Eur Heart J*. 2009;30:459-468.

9. Ohman EM, George BS, White CJ, et al. Use of aortic counterpulsation to improve sustained coronary artery patency during acute myocardial infarction. Results of a randomized trial. The Randomized IABP Study Group. *Circulation*. 1994;90:792-799.

10. Barron HV, Every NR, Parsons LS, et al. The use of intra-aortic balloon counterpulsation in patients with cardiogenic shock complicating acute myocardial infarction: data from the National Registry of Myocardial Infarction 2. *Am Heart J*. 2001;141:933-939.

11. Patel MR, Smalling RW, Thiele H, et al. Intra-aortic balloon counterpulsation and infarct size in patients with acute anterior myocardial infarction without shock: the CRISP AMI randomized trial. *JAMA*. 2011;306:1329-1337.

12. Cassese S, de Waha A, Ndrepepa G, et al. Intra-aortic balloon counterpulsation in patients with acute myocardial infarction without cardiogenic shock. A meta-analysis of randomized trials. *Am Heart J*. 2012;164:58-65.e1.

13. Kar B, Basra S, Shah N, Loyalka P. Percutaneous circulatory support in cardiogenic shock: interventional bridge to recovery. *Circulation*. 2012;125:1809-1817.

14. Ouweneel DM, Henriques JPS. Percutaneous cardiac support devices for cardiogenic shock: current indications and recommendations. *Heart*. 2012;98: 1246-1254.

15. Thiele H, Lauer B, Hambrecht R, Boudriot E, Cohen HA, Schuler G. Reversal of cardiogenic shock by percutaneous left atrial-to-femoral arterial bypass assistance. *Circulation*. 2001;104:2917-2922.

16. Thiele H, Sick P, Boudriot E, et al. Randomized comparison of intra-aortic balloon support with a percutaneous left ventricular assist device in patients with revascularized acute myocardial infarction complicated by cardiogenic shock. *Eur Heart J*. 2005;26:1276-1283.

17. Giesler GM, Gomez JS, Letsou G, Vooletich M, Smalling RW. Initial report of percutaneous right ventricular assist for right ventricular shock secondary to right ventricular infarction. *Catheter Cardiovasc Interv*. 2006;68:263-266.

18. Seyfarth M, Sibbing D, Bauer I, et al. A randomized clinical trial to evaluate the safety and efficacy of a percutaneous left ventricular assist device versus intra-aortic balloon pumping for treatment of cardiogenic shock caused by myocardial infarction. *J Am Coll Cardiol*. 2008;52:1584-1588.

19. Engström AE, Cocchieri R, Driessen AH, et al. The Impella 2.5 and 5.0 devices for ST-elevation myocardial infarction patients presenting with severe and profound cardiogenic shock: the Academic Medical Center intensive care unit experience. *Crit Care Med*. 2011;39:2072-2079.

20. Burkhoff D, Cohen H, Brunckhorst C, O'Neill WW. A randomized multicenter clinical study to evaluate the safety and efficacy of the TandemHeart percutaneous ventricular assist device versus conventional therapy with intraaortic balloon pumping for treatment of cardiogenic shock. *Am Heart J*. 2006;152: 469.e1-469.e8.

21. Cheng JM, den Uil CA, Hoeks SE, et al. Percutaneous left ventricular assist devices vs. intra-aortic balloon pump counterpulsation for treatment of cardiogenic shock: a meta-analysis of controlled trials. *Eur Heart J*. 2009;30: 2102-2108.

22. Thiele H, Allam B, Chatellier G, Schuler G, Lafont A. Shock in acute myocardial infarction: the Cape Horn for trials? *Eur Heart J*. 2010;31:1828-1835.

Fast-track practice in cardiac surgery: results and predictors of outcome
Haanschoten MC, van Straten AHM, ter Woorst JF, et al (Catharina Hosp, Eindhoven, Netherlands; et al)
Interact Cardiovasc Thorac Surg 15:989-994, 2012

Objectives.—Various studies have shown different parameters as independent risk factors in predicting the success of fast-track postoperative management in cardiac surgery. In the present study, we evaluated our 7-year experience with the fast-track protocol and investigated the preoperative predictors of successful outcome.

Methods.—Between 2004 and 2010, 5367 consecutive patients undergoing cardiac surgery were preoperatively selected for postoperative admission in the postanaesthesia care unit (PACU) and were included in this study. These patients were then transferred to the ordinary ward on the same day of the operation. The primary end-point of the study was the success of the PACU protocol, defined as discharge to the ward on the same day, no further admission to the intensive care unit and no operative mortality. Logistic regression analysis was performed to detect the independent risk factors for failure of the PACU pathway.

Results.—Of 11 895 patients undergoing cardiac surgery, 5367 (45.2%) were postoperatively admitted to the PACU. The protocol was successful in 4510 patients (84.0%). Using the multivariate logistic regression analysis, older age and left ventricular dysfunction were found to be independent risk factors for failure of the PACU protocol [odds ratio of 0.98/year (0.97–0.98) and 0.31 (0.14–0.70), respectively].

Conclusions.—Our fast-track management, called the PACU protocol, is efficient and safe for the postoperative management of selected patients undergoing cardiac surgery. Age and left ventricular dysfunction are significant preoperative predictors of failure of this protocol (Fig 1, Table 5).

▶ Given the current and expanding efforts for reducing health care costs, this article by Haanschoten and colleagues is very timely. It highlights the success of a fast-track protocol in cardiac surgery that used the postanesthesia care unit (PACU) for the initial phase of care for a subset of cardiac surgical patients. The authors report their experience between 2004 and 2007, having had the fast-track protocol in place since 2001. The goal of the protocol was to have the patient discharged to the regular ward on the same day after their PACU stay. They describe success of the protocol using a composite outcome that includes: same-day discharge to the ward, no readmission to the intensive care unit (ICU), and survival. There is later mention that reoperation was also included in the composite. They report that using their baseline inclusion and exclusion criteria that 84% of the PACU admissions are successful; this group constitutes approximately 45% of their entire cardiac surgery population. Using multivariate logistic regression, they identified older age and left ventricular ejection fraction < 35% as independent predictors of the failure of the protocol (Table 5, Fig 1).

Fast-track programs are not new—they have been around for a couple of decades. There certainly are data supporting that there is a select group of

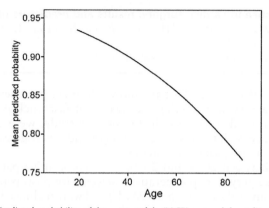

FIGURE 1.—Predicted probability of the success of the PACU protocol depending on age. (Reprinted from Haanschoten MC, van Straten AHM, ter Woorst JF, et al. Fast-track practice in cardiac surgery: results and predictors of outcome. *Interact Cardiovasc Thorac Surg.* 2012;15:989-994, © 2012 European Association for Cardio-Thoracic Surgery.)

TABLE 5.—Results of Logistic Regression Analyses for Outcome of the PACU Protocol

Variables	Univariate Analyses OR (95% CI)	P	Multivariate Analysis OR (95% CI)	P
Male	1.18 (0.99–1.40)	0.052		
Age[a]	0.97 (0.97–0.98)[c]	<0.0001	0.98 (0.97–0.98)[c]	<0.0001
Diabetes	0.93 (0.77–1.11)	0.460		
COPD	0.86 (0.67–1.10)	0.239		
Peripheral vascular disease	0.91 (0.73–1.14)	0.443		
Hypertension	0.83 (0.72–0.96)	0.016	0.86 (0.74–1.00)	0.058
Renal dysfunction	0.60 (0.38–0.94)	0.028	0.69 (0.44–1.08)	0.111
BMI > 35 kg m^{-2}	0.89 (0.59–1.32)	0.568		
EF < 35%	0.32 (0.14–0.70)	0.004	0.31 (0.14–0.70)	0.005
AVR	1.08 (0.84–1.37)	0.532		
AVR + CABG[b]	0.30 (0.16–0.54)	<0.0001		
Other procedures[b]	0.73 (0.35–1.52)	0.407		
Logistic EuroSCORE[a]	0.94 (0.92–0.97)	<0.0001		
Additive EuroSCORE[a]	0.89 (0.86–0.92)	<0.0001		

AVR: aortic valve replacement; BMI: body mass index; CABG: coronary artery bypass grafting; CI: confidence interval; COPD: chronic obstructive pulmonary disease; EF: ejection fraction; PACU: postanaesthesia care unit; PCI: percutaneous coronary intervention.
[a]Entered as a continuous variable.
[b]Compared with CABG.
[c]OR is per year.

patients for whom fast-track anesthesia is appropriate, and we have learned a significant amount on how to manage such patients from these fast-track programs. However, it is important to consider that this methodology of using the PACU, although potentially freeing up ICU beds, may have unintended consequences and may not save costs or personnel depending on how a local cost center is determined. This may just reflect a shifting of costs and resources. For example, some centers elect to admit all patients to the ICU and then transfer those "fast-track" patients to the ward from the ICU. However, depending on what time of day/night the patient is discharged and/or when a hospital cost/ location is calculated for charges, costs savings may not be realized. Furthermore, there are fixed costs, charged by a day or in personnel for a day (such as a respiratory therapist), that can't always be impacted, depending on the system. Furthermore, in the PACU, there is an assumption that these patients require one-on-one nursing coverage, which may equal the cost of a nurse in the ICU. The potential upside is that with the opening of beds in the PACU for a fast-track program, the center has essentially opened more short-term cardiac beds.

Although this report revisits the fast-track programs in cardiac anesthesia and demonstrates the relative safety of such a program, the findings are limited. The data are only from a single center with unknown resources in the PACU, and they only report on the cohort that was admitted to the PACU and do not compare these to the overall patient population outcomes. However, having said that, the outcomes are good mortality 0/4% (24 patients of the 5367 patients). One important limitation is that they do not report a measure of cost savings. As we continue to face value-based care payment programs, we need to continue to develop optimal management programs for cardiac surgical programs and the use of a fast-track program appears to be a viable option. When developing new programs or pathways, it is imperative to define and understand what success looks like and identify and monitor for unintended consequences. Finally, it is important to accurately understand and develop accurate methods to assess net cost savings.

E. A. Martinez, MD, MHS

The Cardiopulmonary Effects of Vasopressin Compared With Norepinephrine in Septic Shock

Gordon AC, Wang N, Walley KR, et al (Imperial College London, England, UK; St Paul's Hosp and Univ of British Columbia, Vancouver, Canada)
Chest 142:593-605, 2012

Background.—Vasopressin is known to be an effective vasopressor in the treatment of septic shock, but uncertainty remains about its effect on other hemodynamic parameters.

Methods.—We examined the cardiopulmonary effects of vasopressin compared with norepinephrine in 779 adult patients with septic shock recruited to the Vasopressin and Septic Shock Trial. More detailed cardiac output data were analyzed for a subset of 241 patients managed with a pulmonary artery catheter, and data were collected for the first 96 h after randomization. We compared the effects of vasopressin vs norepinephrine in all patients and according to severity of shock (<15 or ≥15 µg/min of norepinephrine) and cardiac output at baseline.

Results.—Equal BPs were maintained in both treatment groups, with a significant reduction in norepinephrine requirements in the patients treated with vasopressin. The major hemodynamic difference between the two groups was a significant reduction in heart rate in the patients treated with vasopressin ($P < .0001$), and this was most pronounced in the less severe shock stratum (treatment × shock stratum interaction, $P = .03$). There were no other major cardiopulmonary differences between treatment groups, including no difference in cardiac index or stroke volume index between patients treated with vasopressin and those treated with norepinephrine. There was significantly greater use of inotropic drugs in the vasopressin group than in the norepinephrine group.

Conclusions.—Vasopressin treatment in septic shock is associated with a significant reduction in heart rate but no change in cardiac output or other measures of perfusion.

Trial Registry.—ISRCTN Register; No.: ISRCTN94845869; URL: www.isrctn.org.

▶ These authors use the extensive data from the Vasopressin And Septic Shock Trial (VASST) in which low-dose vasopressin is compared with norepinephrine in addition to standard vasopressors in the treatment of adult septic shock.[1,2] The VASST trial found no overall treatment difference between the vasopressin and norepinephrine study groups. It is interesting to note, however, that patients with less severe shock had significantly lower 28-day mortality with vasopressin compared with norepinephrine. There was no difference in outcome for patients with more severe shock as assessed by the amount of norepinephrine required at baseline.

This trial examines the impact of vasopressin and norepinephrine on cardiac output with these drugs administered according to target blood pressure. A subset of approximately 200 patients was used. These individuals had pulmonary artery catheters in place.

There was no evidence of metabolic difference between vasopressin and norepinephrine as reflected in mixed venous oxygen saturation or lactate levels. It is interesting to note that the rate-pressure product as an indicator of myocardial workload and oxygen consumption was lower in the vasopressin group. However, inotrope use was increased with vasopressin.

The clinician is provided additional cardiopulmonary data to determine the role of vasopressin as opposed to norepinephrine in septic shock patients. Relative vasopressin deficiency in septic shock has been found and a role for vasopressin clearly can be supported in this setting.[2] We should also note that a second agent (dobutamine in this study) will frequently be necessary.

D. J. Dries, MSE, MD

References

1. Russell JA, Walley KR, Singer J, et al; VASST Investigators. Vasopressin versus norepinephrine infusion in patients with septic shock. *N Engl J Med.* 2008;358: 877-887.
2. Holmes CL, Patel BM, Russell JA, Walley KR. Physiology of vasopressin relevant to management of septic shock. *Chest.* 2001;120:989-1002.

Percutaneous Coronary Intervention at Centers With and Without On-Site Surgery: A Meta-Analysis

Singh M, Holmes DR Jr, Dehmer GJ, et al (Mayo Clinic, Rochester, MN; Scott & White Healthcare, Temple, TX; et al)

JAMA 306:2487-2494, 2011

Context.—Percutaneous coronary interventions are performed at centers without onsite surgery, despite current guidelines discouraging this.

Objective.—To assess literature comparing rates of in-hospital mortality and emergency coronary artery bypass grafting surgery at centers with and without on-site surgery.

Data Sources.—A systematic search of studies published between January 1990 and May 2010 was conducted using MEDLINE, EMBASE, and Cochrane Review databases.

Study Selection.—English-language studies of percutaneous coronary intervention performed at centers with and without on-site surgery providing data on in-hospital mortality and emergency bypass were identified. Two study authors independently reviewed the 1029 articles originally identified and selected 40 for analysis.

Data Extraction.—Study title, time period, indication for angioplasty, and outcomes were extracted manually from all selected studies, and quality of each study was assessed using the strengthening the reporting of observational studies in epidemiology (STROBE) checklist.

Data Synthesis.—High-quality studies of percutaneous coronary interventions performed at centers with and without on-site surgery were included. Pooled-effect estimates were calculated with random-effects models. Analyses of primary percutaneous coronary intervention for ST-segment elevation myocardial infarction of 124 074 patients demonstrated no increase in in-hospital mortality (no on-site surgery vs on-site surgery: observed risk, 4.6% vs 7.2%; odds ratio [OR], 0.96; 95% CI, 0.88-1.05; $I^2 = 0\%$) or emergency bypass (observed risk, 0.22% vs 1.03%; OR, 0.53; 95% CI, 0.35-0.79; $I^2 = 20\%$) at centers without on-site surgery. For non-primary percutaneous coronary interventions (elective and urgent, n = 914 288), the rates of in-hospital mortality (observed risk, 1.4% vs 2.1%; OR, 1.15; 95% CI, 0.93-1.41; $I^2 = 46\%$) and emergency bypass (observed risk, 0.17% vs 0.29%; OR, 1.21; 95% CI, 0.52-2.85; $I^2 = 5\%$) were not significantly different at centers without or with on-site surgery.

Conclusion.—Percutaneous coronary interventions performed at centers without onsite surgery, compared with centers with on-site surgery, were not associated with a higher incidence of in-hospital mortality or emergency bypass surgery.

▶ This important article indicates that the absence of cardiac surgery onsite is not a contraindication to having a center perform percutaneous coronary interventions. Because many of these catheterizations are outpatient procedures and well tolerated, the need for urgent surgery is small. Patients can easily be transferred to centers having surgical capability if this resource is justified. For patients with complex coronary artery disease, it appears that bypass grafting is still favored, particularly from the standpoint of improved cardiovascular outcomes. Quality of life also favors surgery in patients with complex disease.[1-3]

An obvious strength of this article is the large dataset. There are several weaknesses, however. The definition of emergency bypass surgery and complications of these procedures vary with studies performed. In addition, because of inconsistent terminology in the manuscripts reviewed, key questions such as the quality of percutaneous coronary intervention outcomes at low-volume centers without on-site surgery remain unclear. Clinical stratification of cases by ventricular function or severity of coronary artery disease is also unavailable. Thus, we may not be considering a comparison of equivalent percutaneous coronary intervention programs.

D. J. Dries, MSE, MD

References

1. Serruys PW, Morice MC, Kappetein AP, et al. Percutaneous coronary intervention versus coronary-artery bypass grafting for severe coronary artery disease. *N Engl J Med*. 2009;360:961-972.
2. Cohen DJ, Van Hout B, Serruys PW, et al. Quality of life after PCI with drug-eluting stents or coronary-artery bypass surgery. *N Engl J Med*. 2011;364: 1016-1026.
3. Park SJ, Kim YH, Park DW, et al. Randomized trial of stents versus bypass surgery for left main coronary artery disease. *N Engl J Med*. 2011;364:1718-1727.

Pulmonary Embolism/Pulmonary Artery

Pulmonary Embolism: The Weekend Effect

Nanchal R, from the Milwaukee Initiative in Critical Care Outcomes Research (MICCOR) Group of Investigators (Med College of Wisconsin, Milwaukee; et al)

Chest 142:690-696, 2012

Background.—Pulmonary embolism is a common, often fatal condition that requires timely recognition and rapid institution of therapy. Previous studies have documented worse outcomes for weekend admissions for a variety of time-sensitive medical conditions. This phenomenon has not been clearly demonstrated for pulmonary embolism.

Methods.—We used the Healthcare Cost and Utilization Project Nationwide Inpatient Sample for the years 2000 to 2008 to identify people with a principal discharge diagnosis of pulmonary embolism. We classified admissions as weekend if they occurred between midnight Friday and midnight Sunday. We compared all-cause in-hospital mortality between weekend and weekday admissions and investigated the timing of inferior vena cava (IVC) filter placement and thrombolytic infusion as potential explanations for differences in mortality.

Results.—Unadjusted mortality was higher for weekend admissions than weekday admissions (OR, 1.19; 95% CI, 1.13-1.24). This increase in

TABLE 4.—Complications in Pulmonary Embolism-Related Admissions

Complication	Weekday	Weekend	OR (95% CI)[a]
Upper-GI bleed[b]	13,705 (1.5)	4,093 (1.7)	1.1 (1.03-1.17)
Blood[b]	42,208 (4.7)	12,438 (5.0)	1.06 (1.02-1.11)
Cardiac arrest[b]	7,705 (0.9)	2,697 (1.1)	1.26 (1.14-1.39)
Cardiogenic shock[b]	2182 (0.24)	797 (0.32)	1.31 (1.10-1.58)
Mechanical ventilation[b]	23,371 (2.6)	8,012 (3.2)	1.24 (1.17-1.31)
Mechanical ventilation >96 h[b]	7,887 (0.9)	2,674 (1.1)	1.22 (1.10-1.34)

Data are presented as No. (%), unless otherwise indicated.
[a]Using univariate logistic regression.
[b]Significant difference at $P < .05$ using χ^2 test.

mortality remained statistically significant after controlling for potential confounding variables (OR, 1.17; 95% CI, 1.11-1.22). Among patients who received an IVC filter, a larger proportion of those admitted on a weekday than on the weekend received it on their first hospital day (38% vs 29%, $P < .001$). The timing of thrombolytic therapy did not differ between weekday and weekend admissions.

Conclusions.—Weekend admissions for pulmonary embolism were associated with higher mortality than weekday admissions. Our finding that IVC filter placement occurred later in the hospital course for patients admitted on weekends with pulmonary embolism suggests differences in the timeliness of diagnosis and treatment between weekday and weekend admissions. Regardless of cause, physicians should be aware that weekend admissions for pulmonary embolism have a 20% increased risk of death and warrant closer attention than provided during the week (Table 4).

▶ A variety of studies suggest that in the setting of critical illness, the day of the week for admission may have an effect on resource utilization and outcome.[1] This article uses a national database developed by the Agency for Healthcare Research and Quality to examine the impact of day of admission on outcomes and relevant resource utilization in patients with pulmonary embolism. It is important to emphasize that this is administrative data and details of care are absent.[2] The attached table (Table 4) suggests that more than management of pulmonary embolism could be different in patients admitted on the weekend. Nonetheless, the authors examine the Charlson-Deyo comorbidity index and noted that this parameter was higher in patients admitted on weekdays.

I can infer reduced availability of advanced imaging and interventional procedures on weekends when I see a comparable use of thrombolytic therapy but delays in placement of vena cava filters in patients admitted on the weekend.

Despite a reduction in mortality associated with pulmonary embolism during the period examined in this study, the weekend effect persisted. The authors calculate that there were 1200 excess deaths associated with weekend admission for pulmonary emboli across the United States during 2008, the final year of data analyzed (Fig 1 in the original article).

D. J. Dries, MSE, MD

References

1. Bendavid E, Kaganova Y, Needleman J, Gruenberg L, Weissman JS. Complication rates on weekends and weekdays in US hospitals. *Am J Med.* 2007;120:422-428.
2. Wynn A, Wise M, Wright MJ, et al. Accuracy of administrative and trauma registry databases. *J Trauma.* 2001;51:464-468.

Usefulness of Preemptive Anticoagulation in Patients With Suspected Pulmonary Embolism: A Decision Analysis

Blondon M, Righini M, Aujesky D, et al (Univ Hosps of Geneva, Switzerland; Bern Univ Hosp, Switzerland; et al)
Chest 142:697-703, 2012

Background.—The diagnostic workup of pulmonary embolism (PE) may take several hours. The usefulness of anticoagulant treatment while awaiting the results of diagnostic tests has not been assessed. The objective of this study was to compare the risks and benefits of bid low-molecular-weight heparin vs no treatment in patients with suspected PE.

Methods.—We developed a decision tree with the following outcomes: mortality related to untreated and treated PE, mortality due to major hemorrhage, and intracranial bleeding. The timeframe extended from the suspicion of PE to its confirmation or exclusion. Most probabilities were derived from data from the Computerized Registry of Patients with VTE (RIETE). We estimated the incidence of bleeding by categories of clinical prediction rules of PE from a recent diagnostic management study of PE. Uncertainty was assessed through one-way and probabilistic sensitivity analyses.

Results.—The model favored preemptive anticoagulation if the diagnostic delay was > 6.3 h, > 2.3 h, and > 0.3 h (Revised Geneva low, intermediate, and high probability) and > 8.1 h and > 1.7 h (Wells unlikely and likely). With a diagnostic delay of 6 h, the absolute mortality reduction with anticoagulation was 0%, 0.02%, and 0.1% for low, intermediate, and high clinical probability, respectively. In one-way sensitivity analyses, the mortality of untreated PE was the most critical variable. Probabilistic

TABLE 2.—Preferred Strategy According to Diagnostic Delay

Category of PE Probability	No Treatment Superior	Time to Definite Diagnosis Preemptive Anticoagulation Superior
Low RGS	<6.3 h	>6.3 h
Intermediate RGS	<2.3 h	>2.3 h
High RGS	<20 min	>20 min
Unlikely Wells Score	<8.1 h	>8.1 h
Likely Wells Score	<1.7 h	>1.7 h

See Table 1 legend for expansion of abbreviations.

analyses reinforced the superiority of anticoagulation in intermediate- and high-probability patients and suggested that low-probability patients might not benefit from treatment after diagnostic delays of < 6 to 8 h.

Conclusions.—Our model suggests that patients with intermediate and high/likely probabilities of PE benefit from preemptive anticoagulation. With a low probability, the decision to treat may rely on the expected diagnostic delay (Table 2).

▶ Years ago during training, we were all taught the importance of early administration of anticoagulation in patients where pulmonary embolism was suspected.[1] Using extensive venous thromboembolism datasets, these authors provide additional data strongly supporting early administration of anticoagulation in patients with moderate to high risk of pulmonary emboli based on clinical evaluation.

These results are in agreement with the recent statements of American College of Chest Physicians, which also recommends anticoagulation for patients at high risk for pulmonary emboli.[2]

Bleeding risk should also be considered. Patients with greater age, history of bleeding, female gender, malignancy, anemia, thrombocytopenia, and preexisting coagulopathy may benefit from delayed administration of anticoagulation or administration of anticoagulants after a diagnosis is made. However, these data lend support to the view that anticoagulation is appropriate if diagnostic testing needed to confirm pulmonary embolism will be delayed in high- or moderate-risk patients.[3]

The table and figure from the original article demonstrate the time intervals for appropriate administration of preemptive anticoagulation in patients with moderate to high risk for pulmonary embolism based on clinical parameters (Table 2, Fig 3 in the original article). The figure demonstrates the results of the simulation model using the extensive datasets available to these authors.[1,3,4]

D. J. Dries, MSE, MD

References

1. Ceriani E, Combescure C, Le Gal G, et al. Clinical prediction rules for pulmonary embolism: a systematic review and meta-analysis. *J Thromb Haemost.* 2010;8: 957-970.
2. Kearon C, Kahn SR, Agnelli G, et al. Antithrombotic therapy for venous thromboembolic disease: American College of Chest Physicians Evidence-Based Clinical Practice Guidelines (8th Edition). *Chest.* 2008;133:454S-545S.
3. Nieto JA, Solano R, Ruiz-Ribó MD, et al; Riete Investigators. Fatal bleeding in patients receiving anticoagulant therapy for venous thromboembolism: findings from the RIETE registry. *J Thromb Haemost.* 2010;8:1216-1222.
4. Laporte S, Mismetti P, Décousus H, et al. Clinical predictors for fatal pulmonary embolism in 15,520 patients with venous thromboembolism: findings from the Registro Informatizado de la Enfermedad TromboEmbolica venosa (RIETE) Registry. *Circulation.* 2008;117:1711-1716.

Creation and Validation of a Simple Venous Thromboembolism Risk Scoring Tool for Thermally Injured Patients: Analysis of the National Burn Repository

Pannucci CJ, Osborne NH, Wahl WL (Univ of Michigan, Ann Arbor)
J Burn Care Res 33:20-25, 2012

Venous thromboembolism (VTE) has been identified as a major patient safety issue. The authors report their use of the National Burn Repository (NBR) to create and validate a weighted risk scoring system for VTE. Adult patients with thermal injury from the NBR admitted between 1995 and 2009 were included. Independent variables were either known or could be derived at the time of admission, including TBSA burned, inhalation injury, gender, and age. The dependent variable was VTE, a composite variable of patients with deep venous thrombosis, and pulmonary embolus. The dataset was split into working and validation sets using a random number generator. Multivariable logistic regression identified independent predictors. β-coefficients for independent predictors were used to generate a weighted risk score. The NBR contained 22,618 patients who met inclusion criteria. The working and validation sets were not statistically different for demographics or risk factors. In the working set, the presence of inhalation injury and increased TBSA were independent predictors of VTE. Adjusted β-coefficients were used to generate a weighted risk score, which showed excellent discrimination for VTE in both the working (c-statistic 0.774) and the validation (c-statistic 0.750) sets. As risk score increased, a linear increase in observed VTE rate was demonstrated in both working and validation sets. The authors have created and validated a simple risk score model to predict VTE risk in thermally injured patients using the NBR. The model is based on risk factors that are easily identified during initial patient contact.

▶ This work by Pannucci et al is an important step forward in the quest to answer this question: what is the risk of a deep vein thrombosis (DVT) in this particular burn patient? As the authors point out, much of the previous work that has been published regarding the occurrence of DVT, prevention, and risk factors has focused on surgical patients not at all similar in disease or treatment processes to burn patients. Although even the most critically ill surgical patient is anticipated to have 1 or at the most 2 surgical interventions, a patient with a large body surface area burn will undergo multiple, frequent, lengthy operative procedures during the initial hospitalization. The next issue requiring clarification is that of burn size. From a teleological perspective, it makes sense that the larger the burn, the higher the risk of developing a DVT. But what is the jumping off point at which a burn patient is at higher risk for developing a DVT? And finally, how does body mass index (BMI) relate to risk of DVT development? We know that patients with a BMI $\geq$ 35 have a significantly higher chance of dying from a burn injury than those with a BMI < 35 (eg, they are above the "tilt point").[1] How does this all fit into the equation?

Another unknown, as partially discussed in this article, is how and when to administer chemoprophylaxis. Again, it makes intuitive sense that the patient is at highest risk for developing a DVT when he or she is on the operating room table, immobile for long hours. Should we administer DVT prophylaxis on the day of surgery and have more potential surgical site bleeding? The authors point out that a significant risk score that can be calculated at the time of admission is required, and I agree. The main weakness of using the American Burn Association's National Burn Repository as the tool to define risk for DVT is that unless one is examining every patient, every extremity, at predetermined times throughout the hospital stay using Doppler (noninvasive and painless but expensive and usually difficult to obtain during off hours), then the real DVT risk remains unknown. The recommended next study is a logical next step in our understanding of this multifactorial adverse event. Antifactor Xa levels will provide a more rational dosing scheme for burn patients in the future. Until then, based on a favorable risk:benefit ratio, I will continue to provide DVT chemoprophylaxis to my burn patients, including the morning of surgery, using enoxaparin 0.5 mg/kg twice daily, increasing the dose for patients who have burns ≥ 40% total body surface area.

B. A. Latenser, MD, FACS

Reference

1. Ghanem AM, Sen S, Philp B, Dziewulski P, Shelley OP. Body Mass Index (BMI) and mortality in patients with severe burns: is there a "tilt point" at which obesity influences outcome? *Burns.* 2011;37:208-214.

3 Hemodynamics and Monitoring

Comparison of hemodynamic measurements from invasive and noninvasive monitoring during early resuscitation

Tchorz KM, Chandra MS, Markert RJ, et al (Miami Valley Hosp, Dayton, OH; Miami Valley Cardiologists, Inc, Dayton, OH; Miami Valley Hosp-Boonshoft School of Medicine, Dayton, OH)

J Trauma Acute Care Surg 72:852-860, 2012

Background.—Measurements obtained from the insertion of a pulmonary artery catheter (PAC) in critically ill and/or injured patients have traditionally assisted with resuscitation efforts. However, with the recent utilization of ultrasound in the intensive care unit setting, transthoracic echocardiography (TTE) has gained popularity. The purpose of this study is to compare serial PAC and TTE measurements and document levels of serum biomarkers during resuscitation.

Methods.—Over a 25-month period, critically ill and/or injured patients admitted to a Level I adult trauma center were enrolled in this 48-hour intensive care unit study. Serial PAC and TTE measurements were obtained every 12 hours (total = 5 points/patient). Serial levels of lactate, Δ base, troponin-1, and B-type natriuretic peptide were obtained. Pearson correlation coefficient and intraclass correlation (ICC) assessed relationship and agreement, respectively, between PAC and TTE measures of cardiac output (CO) and stroke volume (SV). Analysis of variance with post hoc pairwise determined differences over time.

Results.—Of the 29 patients, 69% were male, with a mean age of 47.4 years ± 19.5 years and 79.3% survival. Of these, 25 of 29 were trauma with a mean Injury Severity Score of 23.5 ± 10.7. CO from PAC and TTE was significantly related (Pearson correlations, 0.57–0.64) and agreed with moderate strength (ICC, 0.66–0.70). SV from PAC and TTE was significantly related (Pearson correlations, 0.40–0.58) and agreed at a weaker level (ICC, 0.41–0.62). Tricuspid regurgitation was noted in 80% and mitral regurgitation in 50% to 60% of patients.

Conclusion.—Measurements of CO and SV were moderately strong in correlation and agreement which may suggest PAC measurements overestimate actual values. The significance of tricuspid regurgitation and mitral regurgitation during early resuscitation is unknown.

▶ Goal-directed resuscitation in the intensive care unit is aided by hemodynamic monitoring and at times by assessment of cardiac function parameters. Pulmonary artery catheters (PAC) allow for direct measurement of many variables that can be targeted for intervention during resuscitation. However, PACs are invasive and therefore prone to complications. This small, single-center observational study compared PAC measurements to transthoracic echocardiography (TTE) measurements in 44 critically ill patients. The greatest correlation between the 2 modalities involved cardiac output, with weaker correlations noted when measuring stroke volume. This was a novel study in that TTE measurements were performed and compared with PAC measurements at 5 time points during the initial 48 hours of resuscitation. Other findings of note were a large number of patients with mitral regurgitation and tricuspid regurgitation, which is known to affect PAC measurements. The study had a number of weaknesses, including its observational nature and small number of patients. All TTE measurements were performed by a certified echocardiographer, but several patients had problems with either the PAC (3 patients) or with inadequate TTE images (8 patients). Bedside TTE is a challenging examination, and ideally any study looking at this would involve clinicians performing the ultrasound themselves. This study paves the way for a larger, perhaps randomized, multicenter study. Until then, we are left with the very imperfect status quo.

R. T. Bourdon, MD

Comparison of hemodynamic measurements from invasive and noninvasive monitoring during early resuscitation

Tchorz KM, Chandra MS, Markert RJ, et al (Wright State Univ-Boonshoft School of Medicine, Dayton, OH; Wright State Univ, Dayton, OH; et al)
J Trauma 72:852-860, 2012

Background.—Measurements obtained from the insertion of a pulmonary artery catheter (PAC) in critically ill and/or injured patients have traditionally assisted with resuscitation efforts. However, with the recent utilization of ultrasound in the intensive care unit setting, transthoracic echocardiography (TTE) has gained popularity. The purpose of this study is to compare serial PAC and TTE measurements and document levels of serum biomarkers during resuscitation.

Methods.—Over a 25-month period, critically ill and/or injured patients admitted to a Level I adult trauma center were enrolled in this 48-hour intensive care unit study. Serial PAC and TTE measurements were obtained every 12 hours (total = 5 points/patient). Serial levels of lactate, Δ base, troponin-1, and B-type natriuretic peptide were obtained. Pearson correlation coefficient and intraclass correlation (ICC) assessed relationship and agreement, respectively, between PAC and TTE measures of cardiac output

(CO) and stroke volume (SV). Analysis of variance with post hoc pairwise determined differences over time.

Results.—Of the 29 patients, 69% were male, with a mean age of 47.4 years ± 19.5 years and 79.3% survival. Of these, 25 of 29 were trauma with a mean Injury Severity Score of 23.5 ± 10.7. CO from PAC and TTE was significantly related (Pearson correlations, 0.57—0.64) and agreed with moderate strength (ICC, 0.66—0.70). SV from PAC and TTE was significantly related (Pearson correlations, 0.40—0.58) and agreed at a weaker level (ICC, 0.41—0.62). Tricuspid regurgitation was noted in 80% and mitral regurgitation in 50% to 60% of patients.

Conclusion.—Measurements of CO and SV were moderately strong in correlation and agreement which may suggest PAC measurements overestimate actual values. The significance of tricuspid regurgitation and mitral regurgitation during early resuscitation is unknown.

▶ Transthoracic echocardiography and thermodilution measurements with a late generation pulmonary artery catheter are compared in seriously injured patients. Biochemical parameters, including lactate and hemoglobin, decreased, consistent with resuscitation. Correlation was identified between parameters obtained with thermodilution and ultrasound. The clinical significance of a high incidence of mitral and tricuspid regurgitation is unknown at this time.

A number of summary observations can be made. First, technical problems with the pulmonary artery catheter affected 4 patients in this small study group. Details of these problems were not provided. Eight of the 44 patients originally enrolled had very poor echocardiographic images and were excluded from the trial. This is disappointing as an experienced echocardiographic technician and senior cardiology reader were consulted. Thus, echocardiography results in these patients are probably the best results available. Use of either monitoring technology in critically ill patients is not straightforward.

Recent studies have demonstrated the difficulties associated with consistent use of the pulmonary artery catheter.[1] These include complications related to insertion and interpretation of data. Although this report also demonstrates that echocardiography has clear limitations, I prefer to combine episodic echocardiogram data with biochemical results, urine output, and vital signs to assess resuscitation in my patients.[2] Although historical data associate pulmonary artery catheter use with reduced mortality in injured patients, a mechanism for this benefit has not been demonstrated.[3]

D. J. Dries, MSE, MD

References

1. Pinsky MR, Vincent JL. Let us use the pulmonary artery catheter correctly and only when we need it. *Crit Care Med.* 2005;33:1119-1122.
2. Husain FA, Martin MJ, Mullenix PS, Steele SR, Elliott DC. Serum lactate and base deficit as predictors of mortality and morbidity. *Am J Surg.* 2003;185:485-491.
3. Friese RS, Shafi S, Gentilello LM. Pulmonary artery catheter use is associated with reduced mortality in severely injured patients: a National Trauma Data Bank analysis of 53,312 patients. *Crit Care Med.* 2006;34:1597-1601.

The Deleterious Effect of Admission Hyperglycemia on Survival and Functional Outcome in Patients With Intracerebral Hemorrhage

Béjot Y, Aboa-Eboulé C, Hervieu M, et al (Univ of Burgundy, France)
Stroke 43:243-245, 2012

Background and Purpose.—We aimed to evaluate the association between blood glucose (BG) levels at admission and both functional outcome at discharge and 1-month mortality after intracerebral hemorrhage (ICH).

Methods.—All cases of first-ever ICH were identified from the population-based Stroke Registry of Dijon, France from 1985 to 2009. Clinical and radiological information was recorded. BG was measured at admission. Multivariate analyses were performed using logistic and Cox regression models. Multiple imputation was used as a sensitivity analysis.

Results.—We recorded 465 first-ever ICH. BG at admission was obtained in 416 patients (89.5%) with a median value of 6.92 mmol/L. In multivariate analyses, BG in the highest tertile ($\geq$ 8.6 mmol/L) was an independent predictor of functional handicap (odds ratio, 2.51; 95% CI, 1.43—4.40; $P = 0.01$) and 1-month mortality (hazard ratio, 2.51; 95% CI, 1.23—2.43; $P = 0.002$). The Results were consistent with those obtained from multiple imputation analyses.

Conclusions.—Admission hyperglycemia is associated with poor functional recovery at discharge and 1-month mortality after ICH. These results suggest a need for trials that evaluate strategies to lower BG in acute ICH.

▶ This article sought to investigate the relationship between admission hyperglycemia and poor outcome in patients with spontaneous intracerebral hemorrhage (ICH). The authors looked to improve on previous reports, which were limited by either (1) small population size, (2) a hospital-based setting, or (3) a lack of control for potentially confounding factors. Some limitations to the current study include the delay between ICH onset and blood glucose measurement, and the variability in this delay between patients. Additionally, 10.5% of patients had missing blood glucose data, for which the authors performed multiple imputation sensitivity analyses. These imputation sensitivity analyses were found to be consistent with their complete-case analyses. Other methods for accounting for missing data exist, but given the correlation between their imputed and non-imputed results, it is unlikely that this statistical analysis merits intense scrutiny. Other limitations demonstrated by the authors include the hematoma volume and the National Institutes of Health stroke scale, neither of which were used in their determination of functional outcome. Of concern is that hematoma value is the most powerful determinant of outcome after ICH. Hence, the relationship between hyperglycemia and hematoma growth could not be studied.

D. Yaron, MD

Multimodality Monitoring for Cerebral Perfusion Pressure Optimization in Comatose Patients With Intracerebral Hemorrhage

Ko S-B, Choi HA, Parikh G, et al (Columbia Univ College of Physicians and Surgeons, NY; et al)
Stroke 42:3087-3092, 2011

Background and Purpose.—Limited data exist to recommend specific cerebral perfusion pressure (CPP) targets in patients with intracerebral hemorrhage. We sought to determine the feasibility of brain multimodality monitoring for optimizing CPP and potentially reducing secondary brain injury after intracerebral hemorrhage.

Methods.—We retrospectively analyzed brain multimodality monitoring data targeted at perihematomal brain tissue in 18 comatose intracerebral hemorrhage patients (median monitoring, 164 hours). Physiological measures were averaged over 1-hour intervals corresponding to each microdialysis sample. Metabolic crisis was defined as a lactate/pyruvate ratio > 40 with a brain glucose concentration < 0.7 mmol/L. Brain tissue hypoxia (BTH) was defined as $P_{bt}O_2 < 15$ mm Hg. Pressure reactivity index and oxygen reactivity index were calculated.

Results.—Median age was 59 years, median Glasgow Coma Scale score was 6, and median intracerebral hemorrhage volume was 37.5 mL. The risk of BTH, and to a lesser extent metabolic crisis, increased with lower CPP values. Multivariable analyses showed that CPP < 80 mm Hg was associated with a greater risk of BTH (odds ratio, 1.5; 95% confidence interval, 1.1−2.1; $P = 0.01$) compared to CPP > 100 mm Hg as a reference range. Six patients died (33%). Survivors had significantly higher CPP and $P_{bt}O_2$ and lower ICP values starting on postbleed day 4, whereas lactate/pyruvate ratio and pressure reactivity index values were persistently lower, indicating preservation of aerobic metabolism and pressure autoregulation.

Conclusions.—$P_{bt}O_2$ monitoring can be used to identify CPP targets for optimal brain tissue oxygenation. In patients who do not undergo multimodality monitoring, maintaining CPP > 80 mm Hg may reduce the risk of BTH.

▶ In the setting of intraparenchymal hemorrhage and intraventricular hemorrhage, blood pressure control and cerebral perfusion pressure (CPP) management are of paramount importance in preventing expansion of the hemorrhage and in optimizing blood flow in perihemorrhagic areas. If CPP is too low, infarcted areas may expand; if CPP is too high, the hemorrhage could expand. There have not been enough data published to establish firm guidelines on what optimal perfusion pressures may be. This retrospective study seeks to determine whether multimodality monitoring (MMM) of intracerebral hemorrhage (ICP), $P_{bt}O_2$, and microdialysis monitoring (of metabolic status) could be helpful in establishing optimal CPP goals. The retrospective study included 18 patients, of whom 6 died. ICP, CPP, and PO_2 goals were less than 20 mmHg, greater than 60 mmHg, and greater than 94%, respectively. The results of the study showed that patients were less likely to suffer brain tissue hypoxia with higher CPP levels. Interestingly, there was no independent predictor of metabolic crisis as measured by lactate or pyruvate levels. According to the study, survivors had markedly higher CPP and $P_{bt}O_2$ values on postbleed day 4 and lower ICP measurements on postbleed day 5 than nonsurvivors. The study is somewhat limited in the low enrollment (N = 18); however, the results do intimate that such monitoring could be quite helpful in heralding a poor outcome and consequently in trying to avoid such an outcome. Using MMM to achieve such specific goals may be difficult given the myriad equipment currently required. In the coming years, the data gathered by all this equipment will hopefully become much more streamlined. Currently, MMM may prove useful in determining when care may be appropriately withdrawn.

T. Clark, MD

Accuracy of an expanded early warning score for patients in general and trauma surgery wards
Smith T, Den Hartog D, Moerman T, et al (Univ Med Centre Rotterdam, The Netherlands)
Br J Surg 99:192-197, 2012

Background.—Early warning scores (EWS) may aid the prediction of major adverse events in hospitalized patients. Recently, an expanded EWS was introduced in the Netherlands. The aim of this study was to assess the relationship between this EWS and the occurrence of major adverse clinical events during hospitalization of patients admitted to a general and trauma surgery ward.

Methods.—This was a prospective cohort study of consecutive patients admitted to the general and trauma surgery ward of a university medical centre (March–September 2009). Follow-up was limited to the time the patient was hospitalized. Logistic regression analysis was used to assess the relationship between the EWS and the occurrence of the composite endpoint consisting of death, reanimation, unexpected intensive care unit admission, emergency surgery and severe complications. Performance of the EWS was analysed using sensitivity, specificity, predictive values and receiver operating characteristic (ROC) curves.

Results.—A total of 572 patients were included. During a median follow-up of 4 days, 46 patients (8.0 per cent) reached the composite endpoint (two deaths, two reanimations, 17 intensive care unit admissions, 44 severe complications, one emergency operation). An EWS of at least 3, adjusted for baseline American Society of Anesthesiology classification, was associated with a significantly higher risk of reaching the composite endpoint (odds ratio 11·3, 95 per cent confidence interval (c.i.) 5·5 to 22·9). The area under the ROC curve was 0·87 (95 per cent c.i. 0·81 to 0·93). When considering an EWS of at least 3 to be a positive test result, sensitivity was 74 per cent and specificity was 82 per cent.

Early warning signs for vitally threatened patients							
Score	3	2	1	0	1	2	3
Heart rate (bpm)		< 40	40-50	51-100	101-110	111-130	> 130
Systolic blood pressure (mmHg)	< 70	70-80	81-100	101-200		> 200	
Breath rate (breaths/min)		< 9		9-14	15-20	21-30	> 30
Temperature (°C)		< 35.1	35.1-36.5	36.6-37.5	> 37.5		
Consciousness				A	V	P	U

A=Alert   V=Reaction when verbally addressed   P=Response to pain   U=No reaction

If you are uneasy with the patient's condition: add 1 point

Urinary production < 75 mL during at least 4 hours: add 1 point

Saturation < 90 despite therapy: → 3 points

Erasmus MC
University Medical Center Rotterdam

Patient scores 3 points or higher

→ Call the attending physician

FIGURE 1.—The expanded early warning score flow chart. (Reprinted from Smith T, Den Hartog D, Moerman T, et al. Accuracy of an expanded early warning score for patients in general and trauma surgery wards. *Br J Surg.* 2012;99:192-197. British Journal of Surgery Society Ltd. Reproduced with permission. Permission is granted by John Wiley & Sons Ltd on behalf of the BJSS Ltd.)

Conclusion.—An EWS of 3 or more is an independent predictor of major adverse events in patients admitted to a general and trauma surgery ward (Fig 1).

▶ This article is a follow-up to an early-warning score initially reported from the Netherlands in 2009. The score is composed of heart rate, systolic blood pressure, respiratory rate, temperature, level of consciousness, urine production, and nursing staff evaluation of the patient. These authors show effective detection of patients with mortality or major morbidity if a score of 3 is obtained (Fig 1).[1]

This work parallels major studies from the National Trauma Data Bank in the United States, which demonstrate that among trauma centers, high mortality hospitals have similar rates of major complications but higher likelihood of failure to rescue compared with low mortality hospitals.[2] As a result, treatment strategies focusing on the prevention of complications must be supplemented by efforts to reduce mortality in patients who experience complications. Thus, this Dutch work is only half of the answer. Once we identify patients at risk for major complications, we must intervene appropriately. Failure to rescue in this setting is defined as death after a major complication. Failure to rescue may be a more sensitive measure of hospital quality as opposed to complication rates that do not strongly correlate with mortality. The likelihood that a patient is rescued after developing a major complication tests the ability of physicians and nursing staff to minimize the impact of potentially life-threatening events.[3-5]

Limitations of this work must be reported. Physicians involved in the study were not blinded to the use of the early warning system. Second, nurses making decisions about outcome were not blinded to the early warning system. Therefore, a significant possibility of bias is present. Additional blinded research using this methodology could be compared with work done in the American trauma system.

D. J. Dries, MSE, MD

References

1. Subbe CP, Kruger M, Rutherford P, Gemmel L. Validation of a modified early warning score in medical admissions. *QJM*. 2001;94:521-526.
2. Glance LG, Dick AW, Meredith JW, Mukamel DB. Variation in hospital complication rates and failure-to-rescue for trauma patients. *Ann Surg*. 2011;253:811-816.
3. Silber JH, Williams SV, Krakauer H, Schwartz JS. Hospital and patient characteristics associated with death after surgery. A study of adverse occurrence and failure to rescue. *Med Care*. 1992;30:615-629.
4. Ghaferi AA, Birkmeyer JD, Dimick JB. Variation in hospital mortality associated with inpatient surgery. *N Engl J Med*. 2009;361:1368-1375.
5. Silber JH, Romano PS, Rosen AK, Wang Y, Even-Shoshan O, Volpp KG. Failure-to-rescue: comparing definitions to measure quality of care. *Med Care*. 2007;45:918-925.

4 Infectious Disease

Nosocomial/Ventilator-Acquired Pneumonia

Linezolid in Methicillin-Resistant *Staphylococcus aureus* Nosocomial Pneumonia: A Randomized, Controlled Study

Wunderink RG, Niederman MS, Kollef MH, et al (Northwestern Univ Feinberg School of Medicine, Chicago, IL; Winthrop-Univ Hosp, Mineola, NY; Washington Univ School of Medicine, St Louis, MO; et al)
Clin Infect Dis 54:621-629, 2012

Background.—Post hoc analyses of clinical trial data suggested that linezolid may be more effective than vancomycin for treatment of methicillin-resistant *Staphylococcus aureus* (MRSA) nosocomial pneumonia. This study prospectively assessed efficacy and safety of linezolid, compared with a dose-optimized vancomycin regimen, for treatment of MRSA nosocomial pneumonia.

Methods.—This was a prospective, double-blind, controlled, multicenter trial involving hospitalized adult patients with hospital-acquired or healthcare—associated MRSA pneumonia. Patients were randomized to receive intravenous linezolid (600 mg every 12 hours) or vancomycin (15 mg/kg every 12 hours) for 7—14 days. Vancomycin dose was adjusted on the basis of trough levels. The primary end point was clinical outcome at end of study (EOS) in evaluable per-protocol (PP) patients. Prespecified secondary end points included response in the modified intent-to-treat (mITT) population at end of treatment (EOT) and EOS and microbiologic response in the PP and mITT populations at EOT and EOS. Survival and safety were also evaluated.

Results.—Of 1184 patients treated, 448 (linezolid, n = 224; vancomycin, n = 224) were included in the mITT and 348 (linezolid, n = 172; vancomycin, n = 176) in the PP population. In the PP population, 95 (57.6%) of 165 linezolid-treated patients and 81 (46.6%) of 174 vancomycin-treated patients achieved clinical success at EOS (95% confidence interval for difference, 0.5%—21.6%; $P = .042$). All-cause 60-day mortality was similar (linezolid, 15.7%; vancomycin, 17.0%), as was incidence of adverse events. Nephrotoxicity occurred more frequently with vancomycin (18.2%; linezolid, 8.4%).

Conclusions.—For the treatment of MRSA nosocomial pneumonia, clinical response at EOS in the PP population was significantly higher with linezolid than with vancomycin, although 60-day mortality was similar.

▶ In recent years, retrospective studies of clinical trial data have suggested that linezolid may be superior to vancomycin in the treatment of nosocomial methicillin-resistant *Staphylococcus aureus* (MRSA) pneumonia.[1] However, these analyses have not been entirely convincing given their retrospective nature, suboptimal dosing of vancomycin, and that mortality was often similar between the groups even if clinical cure was superior with linezolid. This is one of the first large double-blind randomized studies to directly compare linezolid and vancomycin for nosocomial MRSA pneumonia. Although linezolid showed superiority with respect to clinical response, 60-day mortality was similar. A recent meta-analysis similarly failed to show superiority of linezolid for ventilator-associated pneumonia resulting from MRSA.[2] Given these results, it is not possible to definitively recommend linezolid as the preferred treatment option. Economic analyses may be needed to define the optimal regimen. If linezolid generates shorter intensive care unit times and overall costs despite similar mortality rates, it may still be the best available antibiotic option.

A. Kumar, MD

References

1. Wunderink RG, Rello J, Cammarata SK, Croos-Dabrera RV, Kollef MH. Linezolid vs vancomycin: analysis of two double-blind studies of patients with methicillin-resistant *Staphylococcus aureus* nosocomial pneumonia. *Chest.* 2003;124: 1789-1797.
2. Walkey AJ, O'Donnell MR, Wiener RS. Linezolid vs glycopeptide antibiotics for the treatment of suspected methicillin-resistant *Staphylococcus aureus* nosocomial pneumonia: a meta-analysis of randomized controlled trials. *Chest.* 2011;139: 1148-1155.

Other

Hospital Admission Decision for Patients With Community-Acquired Pneumonia: Variability Among Physicians in an Emergency Department
Dean NC, Jones JP, Aronsky D, et al (Univ of Utah, Salt Lake City; Kaiser Permanente Los Angeles, CA; Vanderbilt Hosp Dept of Biomedical Informatics and Emergency Medicine, Nashville, TN; et al)
Ann Emerg Med 59:35-41, 2012

Study Objective.—We examine variability among emergency physicians in rate of hospitalization for patients with pneumonia and the effect of variability on clinical outcomes.

Methods.—We studied 2,069 LDS Hospital emergency department (ED) patients with community-acquired pneumonia who were aged 18 years or older during 1996 to 2006, identified by *International Classification of Diseases, Ninth Revision* coding and compatible chest radiographs. We extracted vital signs, laboratory and radiographic results, hospitalization, and outcomes from the electronic medical record. We defined "low severity" as PaO_2/FiO_2 ratio greater than or equal to 280 mm Hg, predicted mortality less than 5% by an electronic version of CURB-65 that uses continuous and weighted elements (eCURB), and less than 3 Infectious Disease Society of America-American Thoracic Society 2007 severe pneumonia minor criteria. We adjusted hospitalization decisions and outcomes for illness severity and patient demographics.

Results.—Initial hospitalization rate was 58%; 10.7% of patients initially treated as outpatients were secondarily hospitalized within 7 days. Median age of admitted patients was 63 years; median eCURB predicted mortality was 2.65% (mean 6.8%) versus 46 years and 0.93% for outpatients. The 18 emergency physicians (average age 44.9 [standard deviation 7.6] years; years in practice 8.4 [standard deviation 6.9]) objectively calculated and documented illness severity in 2.7% of patients. Observed 30-day mortality for inpatients was 6.8% (outpatient mortality 0.34%) and decreased over time. Individual physician admission rates ranged from 38% to 79%, with variability not explained by illness severity, time of day, day of week, resident care in conjunction with an attending physician, or patient or physician demographics. Higher hospitalization rates were not associated with reduced mortality or fewer secondary hospital admissions.

Conclusion.—We observed a 2-fold difference in pneumonia hospitalization rates among emergency physicians, unexplained by objective data.

▶ Over the past few years, the issue of quality has come to the forefront of the national discussion of health care in the United States. One indicator of high quality is low variability. Conversely, high variability in clinical practice generally implies that some patients are receiving good care while others are receiving suboptimal care. This article focuses on the issue by examining variability in physician practice when deciding whether to admit a given patient with community-acquired pneumonia (CAP) to the hospital. The authors calculated the admission rates of 18 attending physicians who had cared for at least 10 patients diagnosed with radiograph-confirmed pneumonia. The admission rate varied from 38% to 79%. Additionally, they applied an evidence-based rule called CURB-65, which had been previously validated to predict mortality in patients with CAP. As expected, there were many patients classified by the decision rule as low mortality risk who were admitted to the hospital. On the other hand, there were also a number of patients classified as high mortality risk who were actually discharged. The variability did not correlate with illness severity, time of day, day of week, resident working with an attending, or patient or physician demographics. Higher hospitalization rates did not decrease mortality or reduce secondary hospital admissions. By pointing out the variability and lack of utilization of validated evidence-based tools, this study takes the first step in improving quality of care in a given disease. It appropriately shows that there are physicians on both sides of the ideal—those who admit patients with a very low likelihood of death and those who send patients home with a high mortality risk. This is the type of research that will lead to the end of the good old days of managing patients based on what a physician's gut tells him or her, which is just what patients and the ailing health care system need.

M. D. Zwank, MD

Cerium nitrate treatment prevents progressive tissue necrosis in the zone of stasis following burn
Eski M, Ozer F, Firat C, et al (Gulhane Military Med Academy and Med School, Etlik, Ankara, Turkey)
Burns 38:283-289, 2012

Cerium nitrate (CN) was used as a topical antiseptic agent for the treatment of burn wounds and found to reduce the number of anticipated death in burn. This decreased burn related mortality cannot be explained by the control of wound infection alone. In the studies performed to elucidate the unexplained effects of CN treatment, it was shown that CN treatment reduced the alarm cytokine levels, decreased leukocyte activation, reduced macromolecular leakage and finally burn edema formation. We hypothesized that CN treatment prevents the conversion of the zone of stasis to progressive tissue necrosis by decreasing leukocyte activation and reducing macromolecular leakage and burn edema.

This was investigated on a well-described burn comb model in the rats. Fifty-four rats were randomly divided into control and CN treatment groups. Each rat in CN treatment group received 0.04 M CN bathing 30 min after burn whereas rats in control group received 0.09% saline bathing. Viability of zone of stasis is assessed with ^{99m}Tc-sestamibi scintigraphy. Nine rats in each group were scintigraphically evaluated at the 3rd and 7th day after burn and remaining 9 rats had macroscopic and histological examination at the 21st day after burn to confirm the scintigraphic results.

In CN treatment groups, the scintigraphic uptake ratios were higher both at post burn day 3rd and 7th when compared to that of control groups. This was statistically significant ($p \le 0.05$). In the CN treatment group, the results of the average percentage of the re-epithelialization in the zone of stasis were higher than that of control groups. The difference between the groups was also statistically significant ($p \le 0.05$).

These results were accepted that CN treatment prevents progressive tissue necrosis in the zone of stasis. This study further elucidates the unexplained effects of CN treatment on burn.

▶ Cerium nitrate (CN) has been available outside of the United States to burn care providers for several decades. The most well-known preparation is Flammacerium, in which CN is simply mixed with silver sulfadiazine. There are other products available, depending on your country/continent. Although previous work has been published showing some of the effects of CN at the molecular level, it is nice to finally see something so relevant to the burn care provider as well as the patient: there is no progressive tissue loss in the zone of stasis in a burn wound. Application of CN to an indeterminate or deep partial thickness burn will result in the most tissue saved without skin grafting. Having used the product outside of the United States but not having been involved in any of this research until now, I could provide only anecdotal support. Although a recent Cochran review did not support the use of silver sulfadiazine in acute burn wound management, the many new agents currently available for topical wound care are beyond the financial means for many of those in low- and middle-income countries, as well as those who are uninsured or underinsured in the United States. Perhaps companies manufacturing topical burn care treatments will again approach the US Food and Drug Administration and investigate the opportunity to make CN-containing compounds more readily available.

B. A. Latenser, MD, FACS

The prevalence of genes encoding leukocidins in *Staphylococcus aureus* strains resistant and sensitive to methicillin isolated from burn patients in Taleghani hospital, Ahvaz, Iran
Khosravi AD, Hoveizavi H, Farshadzadeh Z (Ahvaz Jundishapur Univ of Med Sciences, Iran; Islamic Azad Univ, Jahrom, Iran)
Burns 38:247-251, 2012

Background.—*Staphylococcus aureus* has been recognized as an important human pathogen and is the major cause of nosocomial infections. Various strains of *S. aureus* produce bicomponent toxins such as *LukE/D*, and PVL. The toxins subunits bind to leukocyte cell membrane inducing trans-membrane pore formation and subsequent cell lysis. PVL is an example of these toxins and causes leukocyte destruction and tissue necrosis. It seems that S. aureus strains comprising *LukE/D* and PVL genes are more important in the disease process and associated with severe skin diseases, fatal pneumonia and osteomyelitis with high morbidity and mortality.

Objective.—The aim of this study was to determine the prevalence of genes encoding leukocidins in *S. aureus* strains resistant and sensitive to methicillin isolated from burn patients in Taleghani hospital, Ahvaz, Iran.

Methods.—In an 11-month study, 203 staphylococci isolates were collected from burn patients. The isolates were examined by traditional culture method for detecting *S. aureus* strains and further confirmation with standard biochemical tests including catalase, coagulase and DNase. DNA was extracted from bacterial colony by simple boiling method. Using template DNA, the polymerase chain reaction technique (PCR) was used to detect *mecA* gene for detecting methicillin resistant *S. aureus* strains (MRSA), PVL and *LukE/D* genes.

Results.—Ninety-five (46.8%) out of total tested isolates were identified as *S. aureus*. Based on the results from PCR, 83 strains (87.36%), were *mecA* positive, so they were resistant to methicillin and the rest were sensitive to methicillin (MSSA). The prevalence of PVL and *LukE/D* genes in MRSA strains were (7.23%) and (66.26%) respectively. While this prevalence were (33.3%) for both genes in MSSA strains.

Conclusion.—There were PVL and *LukE/D* positive MRSA isolates with high prevalence in evaluated hospital. Since resulting diseases from these bacteria are severe and may even lead to death, the prevention of disease progress is desired by early diagnosis and proper treatment.

▶ *Staphylococcus aureus* has been recognized for decades as a major pathogen in burn units. Endemic in many hospital settings, it is transmitted by the hands of health care workers. There are various strains of *S. aureus*, largely grouped together into those who are sensitive to methicillin and those who are methicillin-resistant (MRSA). MRSA infections, along with the other commonly acquired pathogens in patients with major burns, cause around 75% to 80% of burn deaths in burn units today. Knowledge of pathogen patterns in each burn unit aids the clinician in the earliest treatment against the most likely pathogen. Pseudomonas infections, previously the scourge of burn centers, have by and large been relegated to burn wounds that stay open for extended periods of time. In this study, wounds were cultured either at the time of admission or when clinical signs of infection occurred. Of all the isolates cultured in this study, 95 of 203 (nearly 47%) were *S. aureus*. Wounds cultured on admission may reveal those patients serving as MRSA reservoirs, but I doubt there are meaningful data provided here, and sadly, we are not provided with information on which patients were *S. aureus* positive on admission and which patients developed wound cultures positive for *S. aureus*. In this burn center, the vast majority of *S. aureus* cultures were MRSA, much higher than in other published studies. Having said that, the polymerase chain reaction (PCR) method of evaluating cultures for staph, either MRSA positive or negative, is easily performed, available within hours, and can prevent wound colonization from becoming wound infections. With the ease and affordability of the PCR method of evaluating cultures for *S. aureus*, I recommend testing patients for being a repository for *S. aureus* (nasal swab) and any open burn areas on admission and then weekly.

B. A. Latenser, MD, FACS

Prevalence and Outcomes of Antimicrobial Treatment for *Staphylococcus aureus* Bacteremia in Outpatients with ESRD
Chan KE, Warren HS, Thadhani RI, et al (Fresenius Med Care North America, Waltham, MA; Massachusetts General Hosp, Boston)
J Am Soc Nephrol 23:1551-1559, 2012

Staphylococcus bacteremia is a common and life-threatening medical emergency, but it is treatable with appropriate antibiotic therapy. To identify opportunities that may reduce morbidity and mortality associated with *S. aureus*, we analyzed data from 293,094 chronic hemodialysis outpatients to characterize practices of antibiotic selection. In the study population, the overall rate of bacteremia was 15.4 per 100 outpatient-years; the incidence rate for methicillin-sensitive (MSSA) was 2.1 per 100 outpatient-years, and the incidence rate for methicillin-resistant (MRSA) *S. aureus* was 1.9 per

100 outpatient-years. One week after the collection of the index blood culture, 56.1% of outpatients with MSSA bacteremia were receiving vancomycin, and 16.7% of outpatients with MSSA were receiving cefazolin. Among MSSA-bacteremic patients who did not die or get hospitalized 1 week after blood culture collection, use of cefazolin was associated with a 38% lower risk for hospitalization or death compared with vancomycin (adjusted HR = 0.62, 95% CI = 0.46−0.84). In conclusion, vancomycin is commonly used to treat MSSA bacteremia in outpatients receiving chronic dialysis, but there may be more risk of treatment failure than observed among those individuals who receive a β-lactam antibiotic such as cefazolin.

▶ Dialysis-dependent end-stage renal failure patients with severe sepsis or septic shock due to infections caused by *Staphylococcus aureus* are common in the intensive care unit (ICU). In fact, uncontrolled infection with sepsis is one of the leading causes of mortality in such patients. In addition, many infected patients with acute renal failure requiring dialysis are treated in the ICU. The clinical course of a significant fraction of these patients will be complicated by *S. aureus* infection.

The uncritical use of intravenous vancomycin for all potential *S. aureus* infections in patients with renal failure due to its convenient dosing schedule (single dose followed by intermittent blood levels until repeat dose required) has become disturbingly common. While vancomycin may be appropriate for renal failure patients with methicillin-resistant *S. aureus* (MRSA) infection, it is clearly an inferior agent for methicillin-sensitive *S. aureus* infections (MSSA) compared with β-lactam antibiotics such as semisynthetic penicillins (eg, oxacillin, cloxacillin) and early-generation cephalosporins.

This study, like others to examine this issue,[1] shows that indiscriminant vancomycin use for MSSA infections in patients with dialysis-dependent renal failure is associated with lower clinical cure and survival. Intensivists must be aware of the inferiority of vancomycin for serious MSSA infections. A convenient dosing scheme is no reason to utilize vancomycin as the sole agent when *S. aureus* infection is suspected. In these situations, the authors suggest using a combination of a *S. aureus*–active β-lactam with vancomycin until sensitivity results are available. This allows the most potent possible therapy in case of MSSA while ensuring early appropriate therapy in case of MRSA. Once sensitivities are available, therapy can be narrowed to the single appropriate agent.

A. Kumar, MD

Reference

1. Stryjewski ME, Szczech LA, Benjamin DK Jr, et al. Use of vancomycin or first-generation cephalosporins for the treatment of hemodialysis-dependent patients with methicillin-susceptible staphylococcus aureus bacteremia. *Clin Infect Dis.* 2007;44:190-196.

Prospective Observational Study Comparing Three Different Treatment Regimes in Patients with *Clostridium difficile* Infection

Wenisch JM, Schmid D, Kuo H-W, et al (Med Univ of Vienna, Austria; Austrian Agency for Health and Food Safety, Vienna, Austria; et al)
Antimicrob Agents Chemother 56:1974-1978, 2012

In a hospital-based, prospective cohort study, the effects of the three standard treatment regimens for mild *Clostridium difficile* infection (CDI), oral (p.o.) metronidazole at 500 mg three times/day, intravenous (i.v.) metronidazole at 500 mg three times/day, and oral (p.o.) vancomycin at 250 mg four times/day, were compared with respect to the risk of occurrence of complications, sequelae, and all-cause death within 30 days after the date of starting treatment. Differences in the incidence of these outcomes were tested by χ^2 or Fisher's exact tests. A Poisson regression model was performed to control for possible confounding effects of sex, age, and severity of comorbidity categorized according to the Charlson comorbidity index. The highest mortality was observed in the metronidazole i.v. group, with a mortality rate 38.1% (16/42) compared to mortality rates of 7.4% (9/121) in the metronidazole p.o. group and 9.5% (4/42) in the vancomycin p.o. group ($P < 0.001$). After adjustment for possible effects of sex, age (> 65 years), and severity of comorbidity, the relative risk of a 30-day fatal outcome for patients receiving metronidazole i.v. was 4.3 (95% confidence interval [CI] = 1.92 to 10; $P < 0.0001$) compared to patients treated with metronidazole p.o. and 4.0 (95% CI = 1.31 to 5.0; $P < 0.015$) compared to patients treated with vancomycin p.o. There were no significant differences in the risk of complications between the three treatment groups. This study generates the hypothesis that treatment with i.v. metronidazole is inferior to the oral alternatives metronidazole and vancomycin.

▶ *Clostridium difficile* colitis is an emerging problem in intensive care units (ICUs) of the developed world. A novel clone with enhanced exotoxin production and elevated virulence has rapidly disseminated around the globe.[1,2] As a consequence, outbreaks of severe disease requiring ICU admission are being seen with greater frequency. The standard therapy for *C. difficile* colitis is discontinuation of any systemic antibiotics that may be driving or aggravating the process and initiation of one of several antibiotics effective for *C. difficile* infection (preferably orally). On occasion, surgical source control with an emergency colectomy may be required with severe disease.

Although fidaxomicin has recently been introduced to practice as a specific anti–*C. difficile* colitis treatment,[3,4] the standard therapy has consisted of either oral vancomycin or oral metronidazole. Intravenous metronidazole has also been utilized frequently, particularly if there is an impediment to oral administration. Although oral administration of anti–*C. difficile* therapy has been preferred for reasons of reduced expense (and based on the localized intraluminal origin of the infection/injury), there has been limited direct evidence of inferiority of intravenous metronidazole relative to oral metronidazole or vancomycin.

This retrospective cohort study provides evidence that intravenous metronidazole may be inferior to oral therapy with either metronidazole or vancomycin. This retrospective study is flawed by the fact that patients receiving intravenous metronidazole may be selected for gastrointestinal dysfunction. Although the authors do attempt to adjust for severity of illness in their regression model, such matching may not entirely capture differences in the subject populations. Nonetheless, the study does reinforce the need to try to deliver oral therapy wherever possible for *C. difficile* colitis and points to the potential need for a randomized trial to properly address this issue.

A. Kumar, MD

References

1. Warny M, Pepin J, Fang A, et al. Toxin production by an emerging strain of *Clostridium difficile* associated with outbreaks of severe disease in North America and Europe. *Lancet.* 2005;366:1079-1084.
2. Pépin J, Valiquette L, Cossette B. Mortality attributable to nosocomial *Clostridium difficile*-associated disease during an epidemic caused by a hypervirulent strain in Quebec. *CMAJ.* 2005;173:1037-1042.
3. Crook DW, Walker AS, Kean Y, et al. Fidaxomicin versus vancomycin for *Clostridium difficile* infection: meta-analysis of pivotal randomized controlled trials. *Clin Infect Dis.* 2012;55:S93-S103.
4. Cornely OA, Crook DW, Esposito R, et al. Fidaxomicin versus vancomycin for infection with *Clostridium difficile* in Europe, Canada, and the USA: a double-blind, non-inferiority, randomised controlled trial. *Lancet Infect Dis.* 2012;12: 281-289.

Performance of *Candida* Real-time Polymerase Chain Reaction, β-D-Glucan Assay, and Blood Cultures in the Diagnosis of Invasive Candidiasis
Nguyen MH, Wissel MC, Shields RK, et al (Univ of Pittsburgh, PA; Viracor-IBT Laboratories, Lee's Summit, MO)
Clin Infect Dis 54:1240-1248, 2012

Background.—The sensitivity of blood cultures for diagnosing invasive candidiasis (IC) is poor.

Methods.—We performed a validated *Candida* real-time polymerase chain reaction (PCR) and the Fungitell 1,3-β-D-glucan (BDG) assay on blood samples collected from prospectively identified patients with IC (n = 55) and hospitalized controls (n = 73). Patients with IC had candidemia (n = 17), deep-seated candidiasis (n = 33), or both (n = 5). Controls had mucosal candidiasis (n = 5), *Candida* colonization (n = 48), or no known *Candida* colonization (n = 20).

Results.—PCR using plasma or sera was more sensitive than whole blood for diagnosing IC (*P* = .008). Plasma or sera PCR was more sensitive than BDG in diagnosing IC (80% vs 56%; *P* = .03), with comparable specificity (70% vs 73%; *P* = .31). The tests were similar in diagnosing candidemia (59% vs 68%; *P* = .77), but PCR was more sensitive for deep-seated candidiasis (89% vs 53%; *P* = .004). PCR and BDG were more sensitive than blood cultures among patients with deep-seated candidiasis (88% and 62% vs 17%; $P = .0005$ and .003, respectively). PCR and culture identified the same *Candida* species in 82% of patients. The sensitivity of blood cultures combined with PCR or BDG among patients with IC was 98% and 79%, respectively.

Conclusions.—*Candida* PCR and, to a lesser extent, BDG testing significantly enhanced the ability of blood cultures to diagnose IC.

▶ Real-time polymerase chain reaction (RT-PCR) has evolved into an increasingly user-friendly, cost-effective, rapid, and accurate diagnostic tool available to many mainstream clinical laboratories. Timely and accurate diagnosis of invasive candidal infections is critical in order to treat patients with early, appropriate antifungal therapy as well as to direct clinicians toward identifying and controlling sources of infection. Given the inherent limitations of the currently available tests, scoring systems were developed as adjunctive measures to predict patients at greatest risk for invasive candidiasis.[1] Although clinical scoring systems are appealing, a laboratory-based test would be ideal. The most broadly available test is the 1,3 β-D-glucan assay. As the authors of this article point out, the sensitivity of the *Candida* RT-PCR used in this study appears to have greatly improved sensitivity over the 1,3 β-D-glucan assay to identify invasive disease (not isolated blood stream infection) without compromising specificity. The authors are correct to point out that although the RT-PCR is an important and useful test, it is perhaps best used in conjunction with blood cultures. Clinicians should anticipate PCR-based pathogen assays to become broadly available in the next few years.

S. Kethireddy, MD

Reference

1. Posteraro B, De Pascale G, Tumbarello M, et al. Early diagnosis of candidemia in intensive care unit patients with sepsis: a prospective comparison of $(1 \rightarrow 3)$ β-D-glucan assay, *Candida* score, and colonization index. *Crit Care.* 2011;15:R249.

The Frequency of Autoimmune *N*-Methyl-D-Aspartate Receptor Encephalitis Surpasses That of Individual Viral Etiologies in Young Individuals Enrolled in the California Encephalitis Project
Gable MS, Sheriff H, Dalmau J, et al (California Dept of Public Health, Richmond; Univ of Barcelona, Spain; et al)
Clin Infect Dis 54:899-904, 2012

Background.—In 2007, the California Encephalitis Project (CEP), which was established to study the epidemiology of encephalitis, began identifying cases of anti-N-methyl-D-aspartate receptor (anti-NMDAR) encephalitis. Increasing numbers of anti-NMDAR encephalitis cases have been identified at the CEP, and this form rivals commonly known viral etiologies as a causal agent. We report here the relative frequency and differences among encephalitides caused by anti-NMDAR and viral etiologies within the CEP experience.

Methods.—Demographic, frequency, and clinical data from patients with anti-NMDAR encephalitis are compared with those with viral encephalitic agents: enterovirus, herpes simplex virus type 1 (HSV-1), varicella-zoster virus (VZV), and West Nile virus (WNV). All examined cases presented to the CEP between September 2007 and February 2011 and are limited to individuals aged ≤ 30 years because of the predominance of anti-NMDAR encephalitis in this group. The diagnostic costs incurred in a single case are also included.

Results.—Anti-NMDAR encephalitis was identified > 4 times as frequently as HSV-1, WNV, or VZV and was the leading entity identified in our cohort. We found that 65% of anti-NMDAR encephalitis occurred in patients aged ≤ 18 years. This disorder demonstrated a predilection, which was not observed with viral etiologies, for females ($P < 01$). Seizures, language dysfunction, psychosis, and electroencephalographic abnormalities were significantly more frequent in patients with anti-NMDAR encephalitis ($P < 05$), and autonomic instability occurred exclusively in this group.

Discussion.—Anti-NMDAR encephalitis rivals viral etiologies as a cause of encephalitis within the CEP cohort. This entity deserves a prominent place on the encephalitic differential diagnosis to avoid unnecessary diagnostic and treatment costs, and to permit a more timely treatment.

▶ Acute encephalitis syndromes result in a significant burden of disease. Analysis of the National Hospital Discharge Survey data identified acute encephalitis as accounting for nearly 19 000 hospitalizations, 230 000 hospital days, 1400 deaths, and $650 million in hospitalization costs annually.[1] A substantial number of these cases, however, lack an etiologic diagnosis. Many of these cases have been assumed to represent unidentified viral syndromes. The California Encephalitis Project provided us with valuable epidemiologic data and raised awareness of a noninfectious disease entity not previously recognized. Autoimmune N-methyl-D-aspartate receptor encephalitis, an immune-mediated and occasionally tumor-associated encephalitis, characteristically affects children and young adults and is more likely to occur among females. The constellation of seizures, language dysfunction, and psychosis along with autonomic instability should raise a clinician's suspicion to this disease entity. Its consideration is critical in potential cases as antiviral therapy will not alter the progression of this illness. Earlier diagnosis of this entity could lead to timely immunologic therapy, associated tumor identification and removal, and also help avoid unnecessary and expensive testing.

S. Kethireddy, MD

Reference

1. Khetsuriani N, Holman RC, Anderson LJ. Burden of encephalitis-associated hospitalizations in the United States, 1988-1997. *Clin Infect Dis.* 2002;35: 175-182.

Chlorhexidine Bathing to Reduce Central Venous Catheter-associated Bloodstream Infection: Impact and Sustainability

Montecalvo MA, McKenna D, Yarrish R, et al (Westchester Med Ctr, Valhalla, NY; Sound Shore Med Ctr, New Rochelle, NY; et al)
Am J Med 125:505-511, 2012

Background.—Chlorhexidine bathing has been associated with reductions in healthcare-associated bloodstream infection. To determine the impact and sustainability of the effect of chlorhexidine bathing on central venous catheter-associated bloodstream infection, we performed a prospective, 3-phase, multiple-hospital study.

Methods.—In the medical intensive care unit and the respiratory care unit of a tertiary care hospital and the medical-surgical intensive care units of 4 community hospitals, rates of central venous catheter-associated bloodstream infection were collected prospectively for each period. Pre-intervention (phase 1) patients were bathed with soap and water or nonmedicated bathing cloths; active intervention (phase 2) patients were bathed with 2% chlorhexidine gluconate cloths with the number of baths administered and skin tolerability assessed; post-intervention (phase 3) chlorhexidine bathing was continued but without oversight by research personnel. Central venous catheter-associated bloodstream infection rates were compared over study periods using Poisson regression.

Results.—Compared with pre-intervention, during active intervention there were significantly fewer central venous catheter-associated bloodstream infections (6.4/1000 central venous catheter days vs 2.6/1000 central venous catheter days, relative risk, 0.42; 95% confidence interval, 0.25-0.68; $P < .001$), and this reduction was sustained during post-intervention (2.9/1000 central venous catheter days; relative risk, 0.46; 95% confidence interval, 0.30-0.70; $P < .001$). During the active intervention period, compliance with chlorhexidine bathing was 82%. Few adverse events were observed.

Conclusion.—In this multiple-hospital study, chlorhexidine bathing was associated with significant reductions in central venous catheter-associated bloodstream infection, and these reductions were sustained post-intervention when chlorhexidine bathing was unmonitored. Chlorhexidine bathing was well tolerated and is a useful adjunct to reduce central venous catheter-associated bloodstream infection.

▶ Catheter-associated bloodstream infection has been a persistent problem in hospitals and in intensive care units (ICUs) in particular since their introduction to practice. Catheter-associated infection has a substantial adverse effect on morbidity and, arguably, mortality in the ICU. Infection of central catheters is thought to typically occur from sequential migration of pathogenic organisms from the skin, onto the catheter, and along the tunnel site. From there, pathogens may disseminate into the bloodstream.

Many efforts to eliminate catheter-associated bloodstream infections have focused on the use of novel (and relatively expensive) antimicrobial or antibiotic-bonded catheters. However, a simpler and more broadly applicable approach may be the use of antimicrobial baths. In this study, Montecalvo and colleagues demonstrate that the routine topical application of a chlorhexidine (2%) bath halved the risk of catheter-associated bloodstream infection in a mixed group of ICUs. Critically, this reduction was sustained after the active intervention period when chlorhexidine bathing was no longer followed.

These data suggest that chlorhexidine bathing is an effective adjunct to other measures to reduce catheter-associated bloodstream infection. In fact, it may be worthwhile to assess whether other ICU-acquired nosocomial infections associated with skin colonization (wound/skin and soft-tissue infections) may also be reduced.

A. Kumar, MD

Fidaxomicin Versus Vancomycin for *Clostridium difficile* Infection: Meta-Analysis of Pivotal Randomized Controlled Trials
Crook DW, for the Study 003/004 Teams (Oxford Univ, UK; et al)
Clin Infect Dis 55:S93-S103, 2012

Two recently completed phase 3 trials (003 and 004) showed fidaxomicin to be noninferior to vancomycin for curing *Clostridium difficile* infection (CDI) and superior for reducing CDI recurrences. In both studies, adults with active CDI were randomized to receive blinded fidaxomicin 200 mg twice daily or vancomycin 125 mg 4 times a day for 10 days. Post hoc exploratory intent-to-treat (ITT) time-to-event analyses were undertaken on the combined study 003 and 004 data, using fixed-effects meta-analysis and Cox regression models. ITT analysis of the combined 003/004 data for 1164 patients showed that fidaxomicin reduced persistent diarrhea, recurrence, or death by 40% (95% confidence interval [CI], 26%−51%; $P < .0001$) compared with vancomycin through day 40. A 37% (95% CI, 2%−60%; $P = .037$) reduction in persistent diarrhea or death was evident through day 12 (heterogeneity $P = .50$ vs 13−40 days), driven by 7 (1.2%) fidaxomicin versus 17 (2.9%) vancomycin deaths at < 12 days. Low albumin level, low eosinophil count, and CDI treatment preenrollment were risk factors for persistent diarrhea or death at 12 days, and CDI in the previous 3 months was a risk factor for recurrence (all $P < .01$). Fidaxomicin has the potential to substantially improve outcomes from CDI.

▶ *Clostridium difficile* is a growing nosocomial problem. A new variant with enhanced toxin production and virulence has undergone rapid global spread and is greatly increasing morbidity and mortality.[1] Metronidazole has been the first-line agent but often fails with severe illness. Oral vancomycin may be more clinically effective, but widespread use may be problematic in terms of driving the emergence of vancomycin-resistant enterococci and, most recently, a few isolates of *Staphylococcus aureus*. With both drugs, there is a relatively high rate of recurrence.

Fidaxomicin is the first of a new macrocyclic class antibiotic with very high fecal concentrations and minimal systemic absorption. In addition, although it is highly active for *C. difficile*, it possesses little activity against other bowel flora. This meta-analysis integrates patients from 2 blinded randomized trials comparing vancomycin with fidaxomicin. Fidaxomicin was associated with a substantial reduction in persistence or recurrence of *C. difficile* symptoms or death compared with vancomycin therapy.

Given that the most severe cases of *C. difficile* enterocolitis can develop organ failure and shock, intensive care unit admission is common, especially the new virulent variant. Early data suggest that fidaxomicin may become the treatment of choice for such severe disease.

A. Kumar, MD

Reference

1. Warny M, Pepin J, Fang A, et al. Toxin production by an emerging strain of Clostridium difficile associated with outbreaks of severe disease in North America and Europe. *Lancet*. 2005;366:1079-1084.

Variability of antibiotic concentrations in critically ill patients receiving continuous renal replacement therapy: A multicentre pharmacokinetic study
Roberts DM, on behalf of the RENAL Replacement Therapy Study Investigators (The Univ of Queensland, Brisbane, Australia; et al)
Crit Care Med 40:1523-1528, 2012

Objectives.—In critically ill patients receiving continuous renal replacement therapy, we aimed to assess the variability of antibiotic trough concentrations, the influence of effluent flow rates on such concentrations, and the incidence of suboptimal antibiotic dosage.

Design.—Prospective, observational, multicenter, pharmacokinetic study.

Setting.—Four tertiary intensive care units within the multicenter RENAL randomized controlled trial of continuous renal replacement therapy intensity.

Patients.—Twenty-four critically ill adult patients with acute kidney injury receiving ciprofloxacin, meropenem, piperacillin/tazobactam, or vancomycin during continuous renal replacement therapy.

Interventions.—We obtained trough blood samples and measured antibiotic concentrations.

Measurements and Main Results.—We obtained data from 40 dosing intervals and observed wide variability in trough concentrations (6.7-fold for meropenem, 3.8-fold for piperacillin, 10.5-fold for tazobactam, 1.9-fold for vancomycin, and 3.9-fold for ciprofloxacin). The median (interquartile range) trough concentrations (mg/L) for meropenem was 12.1 (7.8–18.4), 105.0 (74.4–204.0)/3.8 (3.4–21.8) for piperacillin/tazobactam, 12.0 (9.8–16.0) for vancomycin, and 3.7 (3.0–5.6) for ciprofloxacin. Overall,

15% of dosing intervals did not meet predetermined minimum therapeutic target concentrations, 40% did not achieve the higher target concentration, and, during 10% of dosing intervals, antibiotic concentrations were excessive. No difference, however, was found between patients on the basis of the intensity of continuous renal replacement therapy; this effect may have been obscured by differences in dosing regimens, time off the filter, or altered pharmacokinetics.

Conclusions.—There is significant variability in antibiotic trough concentrations in critically ill patients receiving continuous renal replacement therapy, which did not only appear to be influenced by effluent flow rate. Here, empirical dosing of antibiotics failed to achieve the target trough antibiotic concentration during 25% of the dosing intervals.

▶ Deficiencies of antimicrobial dosing resulting in suboptimal plasma antimicrobial levels are becoming a well-known phenomenon in the critically ill. Critically ill patients have rapidly developing and substantial alternations in volume of distribution and elimination kinetics so that antimicrobial drug levels may exhibit an exceptional degree of variability. In this article, the authors extend such observations to critically ill patients on continuous renal replacement therapy using a variety of antimicrobials. The study demonstrates that > 50% of critically ill patients on continuous renal replacement therapy exhibited suboptimal drug levels for at least some portion of the dosing interval. In most cases, drug levels were lower than required for optimal clinical response. This study makes a strong argument in favor of therapeutic drug monitoring of antimicrobials in the critically ill.

A. Kumar, MD

Estimated global mortality associated with the first 12 months of 2009 pandemic influenza A H1N1 virus circulation: a modelling study
Dawood FS, Iuliano AD, Reed C, et al (Ctrs for Disease Control and Prevention, Atlanta, GA; et al)
Lancet Infect Dis 12:687-695, 2012

Background.—18 500 laboratory-confirmed deaths caused by the 2009 pandemic influenza A H1N1 were reported worldwide for the period April, 2009, to August, 2010. This number is likely to be only a fraction of the true number of the deaths associated with 2009 pandemic influenza A H1N1. We aimed to estimate the global number of deaths during the first 12 months of virus circulation in each country.

Methods.—We calculated crude respiratory mortality rates associated with the 2009 pandemic influenza A H1N1 strain by age (0—17 years, 18—64 years, and > 64 years) using the cumulative (12 months) virus-associated symptomatic attack rates from 12 countries and symptomatic case fatality ratios (sCFR) from five high-income countries. To adjust crude mortality rates for differences between countries in risk of death from influenza, we developed a respiratory mortality multiplier equal to the ratio of the median lower respiratory tract infection mortality rate in each WHO region mortality stratum to the median in countries with very low mortality. We calculated cardiovascular disease mortality rates associated with 2009 pandemic influenza A H1N1 infection with the ratio of excess deaths from cardiovascular and respiratory diseases during the pandemic in five countries and multiplied these values by the crude respiratory disease mortality rate associated with the virus. Respiratory and cardiovascular mortality rates associated with 2009 pandemic influenza A H1N1 were multiplied by age to calculate the number of associated deaths.

Findings.—We estimate that globally there were 201 200 respiratory deaths (range 105 700–395 600) with an additional 83 300 cardiovascular deaths (46 000–179 900) associated with 2009 pandemic influenza A H1N1. 80% of the respiratory and cardiovascular deaths were in people younger than 65 years and 51% occurred in southeast Asia and Africa.

Interpretation.—Our estimate of respiratory and cardiovascular mortality associated with the 2009 pandemic influenza A H1N1 was 15 times higher than reported laboratory-confirmed deaths. Although no estimates of sCFRs were available from Africa and southeast Asia, a disproportionate number of estimated pandemic deaths might have occurred in these regions. Therefore, efforts to prevent influenza need to effectively target these regions in future pandemics.

▶ The 2009 influenza A/H1N1 pandemic was the first such pandemic in more than 40 years. Although a severe event, pandemic morbidity and mortality was held down by aggressive public educational efforts and health measures, an aggressive program of vaccination, and modern antiviral and general medical therapy. Compared with previous epidemics, reports of confirmed deaths were remarkably low. However, early reports are invariably based on laboratory-confirmed cases. This is one of the first reports to attempt to quantify worldwide mortality using an epidemiologic modeling approach. Their result suggesting that there were between 150 000 and 600 000 deaths globally from influenza A/H1N1—associated cardiorespiratory failure (a value 25× greater than laboratory H1N1-confirmed deaths) points to the peril of using laboratory-confirmed deaths as a measure of how seriously future influenza control and management efforts should be taken. Although the 2009 influenza pandemic yielded a significantly lower mortality rate than previous pandemics, much of the credit for that should go to the efficacy of control and treatment measures that were available and used during this event. Further epidemiologic studies using data from underdeveloped countries may well continue to push up estimated mortality rates during this pandemic.

A. Kumar, MD

Impact of Treatment Strategy on Outcomes in Patients with Candidemia and Other Forms of Invasive Candidiasis: A Patient-Level Quantitative Review of Randomized Trials

Andes DR, for the Mycoses Study Group (Univ of Wisconsin, Madison; et al)
Clin Infect Dis 54:1110-1122, 2012

Background.—Invasive candidiasis (IC) is an important healthcare-related infection, with increasing incidence and a crude mortality exceeding 50%. Numerous treatment options are available yet comparative studies have not identified optimal therapy.

Methods.—We conducted an individual patient-level quantitative review of randomized trials for treatment of IC and to assess the impact of host-, organism-, and treatment-related factors on mortality and clinical cure. Studies were identified by searching computerized databases and queries of experts in the field for randomized trials comparing the effect of ≥ 2 antifungals for treatment of IC. Univariate and multivariable analyses were performed to determine factors associated with patient outcomes.

Results.—Data from 1915 patients were obtained from 7 trials. Overall mortality among patients in the entire data set was 31.4%, and the rate of treatment success was 67.4%. Logistic regression analysis for the aggregate data set identified increasing age (odds ratio [OR], 1.01; 95% confidence interval [CI], 1.00−1.02; $P = .02$), the Acute Physiology and Chronic Health Evaluation II score (OR, 1.11; 95% CI, 1.08−1.14; $P = .0001$), use of immunosuppressive therapy (OR, 1.69; 95% CI, 1.18−2.44; $P = .001$), and infection with *Candida tropicalis* (OR, 1.64; 95% CI, 1.11−2.39; $P = .01$) as predictors of mortality. Conversely, removal of a central venous catheter (CVC) (OR, 0.50; 95% CI, .35−.72; $P = .0001$) and treatment with an echinocandin antifungal (OR, 0.65; 95% CI, .45−.94; $P = .02$) were associated with decreased mortality. Similar findings were observed for the clinical success end point.

Conclusions.—Two treatment-related factors were associated with improved survival and greater clinical success: use of an echinocandin and removal of the CVC.

▶ Invasive *Candida* is a serious problem among patients who are immunocompromised. Although we usually think of the group at risk as those with classic immunosuppression (neutropenia, leukemia, bone marrow transplant, acquired immunodeficiency syndrome [AIDS]), immunocompromised patients include those with vascular or urinary catheters that breach anatomical barriers, chronic organ failure that impairs cellular immunity, and a variety of other conditions often found in intensive care unit (ICU) patients. Not surprisingly, apart from the hematology/oncology wards, the ICUs (particularly surgical ICUs) are the sites where most serious *Candida* infections are found.

The optimal antimicrobial therapy for invasive candidiasis and candidemia is uncertain. Amphotericin and its various formulations are highly active (fungicidal) and have a very broad spectrum of activity. However, even the lipid and colloidal formulations retain a significant amount of nephrotoxicity that can be highly problematic in critically ill patients who are already at risk for or exhibit renal injury. Azoles have a somewhat more restricted spectrum of activity and less potency (fungistatic) but minimal toxicity. Finally, the newest antifungal class, the echinocandins, have both minimal toxicity and a high degree of cidality.

This quantitative review, similar to a meta-analysis of randomized trials, combines available data comparing the efficacy of all 3 agent classes in logistic regression. Among the key predictors of survival were the use of an echinocandin and the removal of central venous catheters. This study demonstrates a superiority of echinocandins in the treatment of invasive *Candida* in critically ill patients and strongly supports a primary role for this class of drugs.

A. Kumar, MD

Concurrent Use of Warfarin and Antibiotics and the Risk of Bleeding in Older Adults

Baillargeon J, Holmes HM, Lin Y-L, et al (Univ of Texas Med Branch, Galveston; Univ of Texas, MD Anderson Cancer Ctr, Houston)
Am J Med 125:183-189, 2012

Background.—Antibiotic medications are associated with an increased risk of bleeding among patients receiving warfarin. The recent availability of data from the Medicare Part D prescription drug program provides an opportunity to assess the association of antibiotic medications and the risk of bleeding in a national population of older adults receiving warfarin.

Methods.—We conducted a case-control study nested within a cohort of 38,762 patients aged 65 years and older who were continuous warfarin users, using enrollment and claims data for a 5% national sample of Medicare beneficiaries with Part D benefits. Cases were defined as patients hospitalized for a primary diagnosis of bleeding and were matched with 3 control subjects on age, race, sex, and indication for warfarin. Logistic regression analysis was used to calculate adjusted odds ratios (aORs) and 95% confidence intervals (CIs) for the risk of bleeding associated with prior exposure to antibiotic medications.

Results.—Exposure to any antibiotic agent within the 15 days of the event/index date was associated with an increased risk of bleeding (aOR 2.01; 95% CI, 1.62-2.50). All 6 specific antibiotic drug classes examined (azole antifungals [aOR, 4.57; 95% CI, 1.90-11.03], macrolides [aOR, 1.86; 95% CI, 1.08-3.21], quinolones [aOR, 1.69; 95% CI, 1.09-2.62], cotrimoxazole [aOR, 2.70; 95% CI, 1.46-5.05], penicillins [aOR, 1.92; 95% CI, 1.21-2.07], and cephalosporins [aOR, 2.45; 95% CI, 1.52-3.95]) were associated with an increased risk of bleeding.

Conclusion.—Among older continuous warfarin users, exposure to antibiotic agents—particularly azole antifungals—was associated with an increased risk of bleeding.

▶ With the increasing number of older patients being admitted for intensive care unit (ICU) support, more patients will experience the kind of drug interaction issues that are typical of a geriatric practice. Unfortunately, most intensivists may not be as attuned to this issue to the extent that geriatric practitioners are. This article represents an excellent example of this issue.

Since the acceptance of long-term anticoagulation therapy to prevent thrombotic strokes in chronic atrial fibrillation, many more elderly patients are admitted on warfarin therapy compared with the past. Because most patients in the ICU receive at least one course of antimicrobials, the possibility of significant drug interactions with warfarin resulting in adverse outcomes is more than a passing risk.

In this excellent case-control study, Baillargeon and colleagues show that among older (age > 65 y) hospitalized patients on warfarin, the use of any antimicrobial within 2 weeks of admission was associated with twice the risk of serious bleeding. The effect was particularly strong for use of azoles (4.5x risk), but it was present for every antimicrobial group assessed.

Intensivists should be aware of this phenomenon given the frequency with which critically ill elderly patients on warfarin are managed with antimicrobials in the ICU setting.

A. Kumar, MD

Procalcitonin usefulness for the initiation of antibiotic treatment in intensive care unit patients
Layios N, Lambermont B, Canivet J-L, et al (Univ Hosp of Liege, Belgium)
Crit Care Med 40:2304-2309, 2012

Objectives.—To test the usefulness of procalcitonin serum level for the reduction of antibiotic consumption in intensive care unit patients.

Design.—Single-center, prospective, randomized controlled study.

Setting.—Five intensive care units from a tertiary teaching hospital.

Patients.—All consecutive adult patients hospitalized for > 48 hrs in the intensive care unit during a 9-month period.

Interventions.—Procalcitonin serum level was obtained for all consecutive patients suspected of developing infection either on admission or during intensive care unit stay. The use of antibiotics was more or less strongly discouraged or recommended according to the Muller classification. Patients were randomized into two groups: one using the procalcitonin results (procalcitonin group) and one being blinded to the procalcitonin results (control group). The primary end point was the reduction of antibiotic use expressed as a proportion of treatment days and of daily defined dose per 100 intensive care unit days using a procalcitonin-guided approach. Secondary end points included: a *posteriori* assessment of the accuracy of the infectious diagnosis when using procalcitonin in the intensive care unit and of the diagnostic concordance between the intensive care unit physician and the infectious-disease specialist.

Measurements and Main Results.—There were 258 patients in the procalcitonin group and 251 patients in the control group. A significantly higher amount of withheld treatment was observed in the procalcitonin group of patients classified by the intensive care unit clinicians as having possible infection. This, however, did not result in a reduction of antibiotic consumption. The treatment days represented $62.6 \pm 34.4\%$ and $57.7 \pm 34.4\%$ of the intensive care unit stays in the procalcitonin and control groups, respectively ($p = .11$). According to the infectious-disease specialist, 33.8% of the cases in which no infection was confirmed, had a procalcitonin value > 1 µg/L and 14.9% of the cases with confirmed infection had procalcitonin levels < 0.25 µg/L. The ability of procalcitonin to differentiate between certain or probable infection and possible or no infection, upon initiation of antibiotic treatment was low, as confirmed by the receiving operating curve analysis (area under the curve = 0.69). Finally, procalcitonin did not help improve concordance between the diagnostic confidence of the infectious-disease specialist and the ICU physician.

Conclusions.—Procalcitonin measuring for the initiation of antimicrobials did not appear to be helpful in a strategy aiming at decreasing the antibiotic consumption in intensive care unit patients.

▶ Procalcitonin has been advocated to be a useful marker for the presence of clinical infection. However, the optimal use of procalcitonin in critical illness is uncertain. The evidence for sequential assessment of this marker to support antimicrobial de-escalation is most accepted.[1] However, the use of procalcitonin to trigger initiation of antimicrobial therapy in potentially infected critically ill patients is controversial. This randomized but unblinded study found that procalcitonin assessment on suspicion of clinical infection in critically ill patients did not differentiate well between low and high probability infection. Not surprisingly, it was also not helpful in decreasing cumulative antibiotic consumption in the intensive care unit. A similar randomized study by Jensen and colleagues also failed to demonstrate a beneficial effect of procalcitonin on outcome when used as a driver of antimicrobial escalation (in addition to standard therapy) compared with standard therapy alone.[2] While the totality of available evidence supports the use of procalcitonin to drive appropriate antimicrobial de-escalation, its use to direct antimicrobial initiation and escalation is not advisable based on the current evidence.

A. Kumar, MD

References

1. Nobre V, Harbarth S, Graf JD, Rohner P, Pugin J. Use of procalcitonin to shorten antibiotic treatment duration in septic patients: a randomized trial. *Am J Respir Crit Care Med.* 2008;177:498-505.
2. Jensen JU, Hein L, Lundgren B, et al. Procalcitonin-guided interventions against infections to increase early appropriate antibiotics and improve survival in the intensive care unit: a randomized trial. *Crit Care Med.* 2011;39:2048-2058.

Limiting Severe Outcomes and Impact on Intensive Care Units of Moderate-Intermediate 2009 Pandemic Influenza: Role of Infectious Diseases Units

Carbonara S, Bruno G, Ciaula GD, et al (Univ of Bari, Italy)
PLoS One 7:e42940, 2012

Purpose.—The rate of severe outcomes of patients with 2009 pandemic (A/H1N1) influenza (2009pI) hospitalized in non-intensive care units (ICUs) has not been defined thus far. This study aims to assess the efficacy of the management of patients with influenza-like illness (ILI) of moderate intermediate severity in an infectious diseases unit (IDU) during the first wave of 2009pI and its influence on the burden of ICUs.

Methods.—All patients hospitalized from October 27, 2009, to February 5, 2010, with ILI were included in this prospective observational study. The IDU was organized and the staff was trained to provide intermediate care; patients were transferred to the ICU only if they required invasive ventilation, extracorporeal membrane oxygenation, or advanced cardiovascular support. Demographic data, clinical presentation, coexisting medical conditions, and laboratory and radiological findings were recorded and analyzed, as well as treatment and outcome data.

Results.—Overall, 108 patients (median age 36 years [IQR 27−54], 57.4% males) including 66.7% with ≥1 risk factor for severe influenza, 47.2% with confirmed 2009pI by RT-PCR and 63.9% with pneumonia, were enrolled in the study. All subjects received intravenous fluids and 83.3% were administered oseltamivir, 96.3% antibacterials, 19.4% oxygen therapy without ventilatory support, and 10.2% non-invasive ventilation. A total of 106 (98.1%) subjects were discharged after a 6-day median hospital stay [IQR 4−9]. Two patients (1.9%) were transferred to the ICU. There were no deaths.

Conclusions.—These results suggest that the aggressive treatment of patients with moderate intermediate severity 2009 pandemic ILI in non-ICU wards may result in a low rate of severe outcomes and brief hospitalization. IDUs, if properly organized for intermediate care, may efficiently provide correct disease management, in addition to complying with infection control requirements, thus reducing the burden of the pandemic on ICUs. Further studies are warranted to evaluate the outcome of patients with moderate intermediate 2009pI in different non-ICU settings.

▶ In 2009, pandemic H1N1 influenza (pH1N1) overwhelmed many intensive care units (ICUs) throughout the world. Between 14% and 27% of confirmed pH1N1 patients required admission to an ICU. As with septic shock, the delayed administration of antivirals (specifically oseltamivir) was associated with increased odds of being admitted to an ICU. Available data also suggest that rapid response teams and care in a high-dependency unit reduce adverse patient outcomes, including cardiac arrest and admission to the ICU.

In this study, Carbonara et al describe their experience with admitting patients with influenza-like illness to a high-acuity infectious disease unit during the 2009 influenza pandemic. This unit was able to provide intravenous fluids, noninvasive ventilator support, and low-dose vasopressors. It also had a 1/3 nurse-to-patient ratio and was able to provide continuous cardiorespiratory monitoring.

Of 108 patients admitted to this intermediate care unit (47.2% of whom tested positive for pH1N1 via polymerase chain reaction), there were no deaths and only 1.9% (2 patients) who required transfer to an ICU. This study is interesting in that it suggests that patients who are treated early and aggressively with antivirals, have continuous monitoring, and increased nursing care might help avoid clinical deterioration and admission to the ICU. It also suggests that these kinds of intermediate care units may represent an effective approach to increasing high-acuity patient capacity in the setting of natural disasters and epidemic events.

The concept of a high-dependency infectious disease unit may benefit patients with other potentially life-threatening conditions, including infections, not just influenza. Observing early clinical deterioration of patients with severe sepsis and intervening in an attempt to prevent organ failure may benefit patients and reduce the need for ICU admission and patient morbidity. This has everyday practical implications for resource management due to the paucity of critical care beds in most institutions and could be an invaluable resource when the next pandemic strikes. More data are required to determine if the resources required in starting an infectious disease high-dependency unit consistently reduce admission to the ICU and limit ICU costs.

A. Kumar, MD

Validation of a Clinical Score for Assessing the Risk of Resistant Pathogens in Patients With Pneumonia Presenting to the Emergency Department
Shorr AF, Zilberberg MD, Reichley R, et al (Washington Hosp Ctr, DC; EviMed Res Group, Goshen, MA; Barnes-Jewish Hosp, St Louis, MO; et al)
Clin Infect Dis 54:193-198, 2012

Background.—Resistant organisms (ROs) are increasingly implicated in pneumonia in patients presenting to the emergency department (ED). The concept of healthcare-associated pneumonia (HCAP) exists to help identify patients infected with ROs but may be overly broad. We sought to validate a previously developed score for determining the risk for an RO and to compare it with the HCAP definition.

Methods.—We evaluated adult patients admitted via the ED with bacterial pneumonia (January—December 2010). We defined methicillin-resistant *Staphylococcus aureus* (MRSA), *Pseudomonas aeruginosa*, and extended-spectrum β-lactamases as ROs. The risk score was as follows: 4, recent hospitalization; 3, nursing home; 2, chronic hemodialysis; 1, critically ill. We evaluated the screening value of the score and of HCAP by determining their areas under the receiver-operating characteristic (AUROC) curves for predicting ROs.

Results.—The cohort included 977 patients, and ROs were isolated in 46.7%. The most common organisms included MRSA (22.7%), *P. aeruginosa* (19.1%), and *Streptococcus pneumoniae* (19.1%). The risk score was higher in those with an RO (median score, 4 vs 1; $P < .001$). The AUROC for HCAP equaled 0.62 (*95%* confidence interval [CI], *.58—.65*) versus 0.71 (*95%* CI, *.66—.73*) for the risk score. As a screening test for ROs, a score > 0 had a high negative predictive value (84.5%) and could lead to fewer patients unnecessarily receiving broad-spectrum antibiotics.

Conclusions.—ROs are common in patients presenting to the ED with pneumonia. A simple clinical risk score performs moderately well at classifying patients regarding their risk for an RO.

▶ Many studies have found that initiation of inappropriate antimicrobial therapy that fails to cover the microbial pathogen in life-threatening infections, sepsis, and septic shock is associated with substantial reductions in clinical cure and survival. Assuming that standard antimicrobial guidelines are followed, the most common cause for initiation of microbially inappropriate therapy is the presence of unanticipated resistant organisms as the primary pathogen in these infections. This has been shown to be the case for both community-acquired and nosocomial pathogens.[1,2]

Most serious infections admitted from the emergency department are community-acquired. However, this does not mean that only typical community pathogens need to be covered in a patient presenting with life-threatening infection. Over the last several decades, a major shift in medical practice has occurred. The number of in-patient beds and lengths of stay per capita have decreased substantially. Patients who might formerly have been admitted for prolonged periods are now treated at home. Prolonged survival in the community setting of chronically immunocompromised patients with chronic organ failure (ie, cirrhosis, dialysis-dependent renal failure, malignancy) or immunosuppression (eg, HIV infection, organ transplant) at risk for infection with resistant organisms (in part caused by frequent contact with the health care system) is common.

For these reasons, the regular occurrence of inappropriate antimicrobial initiation in the emergency department persists. This study points out this fact but further shows that a more discriminating approach to assessment of risk factors for infection with resistant organisms can help reduce the frequency of antimicrobial prescription failures. Although the score the authors have developed is far from ideal, the approach is a valid one. Clinicians should be aware of the real risk of resistant organisms among the many immunocompromised patients with health care contact who are admitted through the emergency department with life-threatening infections. These patients who are said to have "healthcare associated infections" require antimicrobial therapy similar to that provided to those with nosocomial infections.

A. Kumar, MD

References

1. Capp R, Chang Y, Brown DF. Effective antibiotic treatment prescribed by emergency physicians in patients admitted to the intensive care unit with severe sepsis or septic shock: where is the gap? *J Emerg Med.* 2011;41:573-580.
2. Ibrahim EH, Sherman G, Ward S, Fraser VJ, Kollef MH. The influence of inadequate antimicrobial treatment of bloodstream infections on patient outcomes in the ICU setting. *Chest.* 2000;118:146-155.

Effect of Empirical Treatment With Moxifloxacin and Meropenem vs Meropenem on Sepsis-Related Organ Dysfunction in Patients With Severe Sepsis: A Randomized Trial

Brunkhorst FM, for the German Study Group Competence Network Sepsis (SepNet) (Friedrich-Schiller Univ, Jena, Germany; et al)
JAMA 307:2390-2399, 2012

Context.—Early appropriate antimicrobial therapy leads to lower mortality rates associated with severe sepsis. The role of empirical combination therapy comprising at least 2 antibiotics of different mechanisms remains controversial.

Objective.—To compare the effect of moxifloxacin and meropenem with the effect of meropenem alone on sepsis-related organ dysfunction.

Design, Setting, and Patients.—A randomized, open-label, parallel-group trial of 600 patients who fulfilled criteria for severe sepsis or septic shock (n = 298 for monotherapy and n = 302 for combination therapy). The trial was performed at 44 intensive care units in Germany from October 16, 2007, to March 23, 2010. The number of evaluable patients was 273 in the monotherapy group and 278 in the combination therapy group.

Interventions.—Intravenous meropenem (1 g every 8 hours) and moxifloxacin (400 mg every 24 hours) or meropenem alone. The intervention was recommended for 7 days and up to a maximum of 14 days after randomization or until discharge from the intensive care unit or death, whichever occurred first.

Main Outcome Measure.—Degree of organ failure (mean of daily total Sequential Organ Failure Assessment [SOFA] scores over 14 days; score range: 0-24 points with higher scores indicating worse organ failure); secondary outcome: 28-day and 90-day all-cause mortality. Survivors were followed up for 90 days.

Results.—Among 551 evaluable patients, there was no statistically significant difference in mean SOFA score between the meropenem and moxifloxacin group (8.3 points; 95% CI, 7.8-8.8 points) and the meropenem alone group (7.9 points; 95% CI, 7.5-8.4 points) (*P* =.36). The rates for 28-day and 90-day mortality also were not statistically significantly different. By day 28, there were 66 deaths (23.9%; 95% CI, 19.0%-29.4%) in the combination therapy group compared with 59 deaths (21.9%; 95% CI, 17.1%-27.4%) in the monotherapy group (*P* =.58). By day 90, there were 96 deaths (35.3%; 95% CI, 29.6%-41.3%) in the combination therapy group compared with 84 deaths (32.1%; 95% CI, 26.5%-38.1%) in the monotherapy group (*P* =.43).

Conclusion.—Among adult patients with severe sepsis, treatment with combined meropenem and moxifloxacin compared with meropenem alone did not result in less organ failure.

Trial Registration.—clinicaltrials.gov Identifier: NCT00534287.

▶ Although it is well accepted that early, pathogen-appropriate antimicrobial therapy improves outcome in life-threatening infections, sepsis, and septic shock, the potential role of combination therapy in these conditions is much more uncertain. Several recent studies, including a propensity-matched retrospective cohort study[1] and a meta-analysis/meta-regression analysis,[2] have suggested the utility of combination therapy in septic shock. In this context, combination therapy, defined as a minimum of 2 drugs of different antimicrobial classes active for a given pathogen, may yield improved outcome as a consequence of accelerated pathogen clearance (ie, synergy). This study, a randomized controlled trial, on the other hand, failed to demonstrate any advantage to combination therapy.

Although guidelines do support the use of combination therapy to broaden coverage in some scenarios to ensure that resistant pathogens are covered,[3] many of the most potent modern antimicrobials have an exceptional range of antimicrobial activity. Carbapenems, in particular, such as imipenem, meropenem, and doripenem, and extended-range β-lactam/β-lactamase inhibitors, such as piperacillin/tazobactam, exert strong activity against *Staphylococcus aureus*, strep species, and gram-negatives, including *Pseudomonas* and anaerobes. This potent activity may explain the divergent results of some of these studies.

The key issue may be the ability of combination therapy to augment bacterial clearance compared with monotherapy. Augmented bacterial clearance with combination therapy may only be clinically relevant when the beta-lactam component of combination therapy is less than maximally potent. The majority of pathogens causing septic shock are relatively sensitive to agents, such as extended spectrum penicillins and first- and second-generation cephalosporins, that often achieve submaximal bacterial clearing with 60% to 70% time above the minimal inhibitory concentration (T > MIC) of the pathogen in the plasma. Although this is adequate to improve survival for many serious infections, there is evidence to suggest that 100% T > MIC may result in more effective clearance. Use of high-potency carbapenems will generate a time > MIC of 100% and maximally rapid bacterial clearance for all but a few relatively resistant pathogens such as *Pseudomonas*. A second agent would not be expected to increase bacterial clearance (and correspondingly fail to improve outcome) in this circumstance. This insensitivity to combination therapy for regimens that included carbapenems was noted in our own analysis in the propensity study of combination therapy in septic shock mentioned earlier.[1]

Further study is clearly needed to address the question of under what circumstances combination therapy may be useful in sepsis and septic shock. It is important to understand that this article showed that the combination of a very potent and broad antimicrobial in a low-resistance environment with a second agent is not useful. This environment may be very different from the real world where minimal inhibitory concentrations are increasing and the use of less potent agents is common.

A. Kumar, MD

References

1. Kumar A, Zarychanski R, Light B, et al. Early combination antibiotic therapy yields improved survival compared with monotherapy in septic shock: a propensity-matched analysis. *Crit Care Med.* 2010;38:1773-1785.
2. Kumar A, Safdar N, Reddy S, Chateau D. A survival benefit of combination antibiotic therapy for serious infections associated with sepsis and septic shock is

contingent only on the risk of death: a meta-analytic/meta-regression study. *Crit Care Med.* 2010;38:1651-1664.

3. Dellinger RP, Levy MM, Carlet JM, et al; International Surviving Sepsis Campaign Guidelines Committee. Surviving Sepsis Campaign: international guidelines for management of severe sepsis and septic shock: 2008. *Crit Care Med.* 2008;36: 296-327.

The utility of procalcitonin in critically ill trauma patients

Sakran JV, Michetti CP, Sheridan MJ, et al (Inova Regional Trauma Ctr, Falls Church, VA)

J Trauma Acute Care Surg 73:413-418, 2012

Background.—Procalcitonin (PCT), the prohormone of calcitonin, has an early and highly specific increase in response to systemic bacterial infection. The objectives of this study were to determine the natural history of PCT for patients with critical illness and trauma, the utility of PCT as a marker of sepsis versus systemic inflammatory response syndrome (SIRS), and the association of PCT level with mortality.

Methods.—PCT assays were done on eligible patients with trauma admitted to the trauma intensive care unit (ICU) of a Level I trauma center from June 2009 to June 2010, at hours 0, 6, 12, 24, and daily until discharge from ICU or death. Patients were retrospectively diagnosed with SIRS or sepsis by researchers blinded to PCT results.

Results.—A total of 856 PCT levels from 102 patients were analyzed, with mean age of 49 years, 63% male, 89% blunt trauma, mean Injury

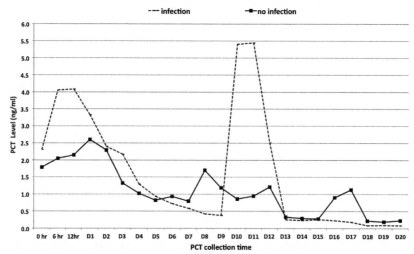

FIGURE 1.—Trend of PCT in patients with critical illness and trauma: infected (n = 33) versus noninfected (n = 47). Both groups (n = 80). (Reprinted from Sakran JV, Michetti CP, Sheridan MJ, et al. The utility of procalcitonin in critically ill trauma patients. *J Trauma Acute Care Surg.* 2012;73:413-418, with permission from Lippincott Williams & Wilkins.)

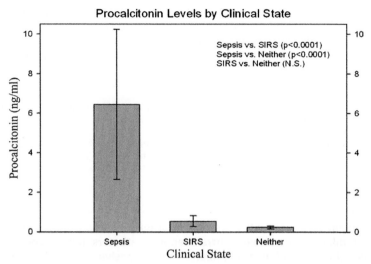

FIGURE 2.—Comparison of groups by PCT level (n = 80). (Reprinted from Sakran JV, Michetti CP, Sheridan MJ, et al. The utility of procalcitonin in critically ill trauma patients. *J Trauma Acute Care Surg.* 2012;73:413-418, with permission from Lippincott Williams & Wilkins.)

Severity Score of 21, and hospital mortality of 13%. PCT concentration for patients with sepsis, SIRS, and neither were evaluated. Mean PCT levels were higher for patients with sepsis versus SIRS ($p < 0.0001$). Patients with a PCT concentration of 5 ng/mL or higher had an increased mortality when compared with those with a PCT of less than 5 ng/mL in a univariate analysis (odds ratio, 3.65; 95% confidence interval, 1.03–12.9; $p = 0.04$). In a multivariate logistic analysis, PCT was found to be the only significant predictor for sepsis (odds ratio, 2.37; 95% confidence interval, 1.23–4.61, $p = 0.01$).

Conclusion.—PCT levels are significantly higher in ICU patients with trauma and sepsis and may help differentiate sepsis from SIRS in critical illness. An elevated PCT level was associated with increased mortality (Figs 1 and 2).

▶ Because of global changes, many inflammatory markers are of little use in early evaluation of the injured patient. This is particularly true for many of the molecular markers of hemostasis. These authors examine procalcitonin in injured patients as a laboratory tool to identify sepsis.[1] A significant relationship is identified. Within the confines of this work, it appears that procalcitonin may effectively distinguish sepsis in critical injury.

Clearly, these preliminary data warrant additional investigation. One obvious limitation of procalcitonin in the setting of injury is elevation in this marker in the initial 48 hours after trauma regardless of the presence of infection (Fig 1). After this time, however, procalcitonin may better identify the patient with a significant infectious complication (Fig 2). In addition, this is a small study without rigorous blinding. Trauma patients investigated are largely male and have suffered a blunt mechanism. The typical infection is pneumonia. A larger multicenter dataset is necessary to demonstrate broad application of procalcitonin to identify infection in injured patients.[2]

D. J. Dries, MSE, MD

References

1. Castelli GP, Pognani C, Cita M, Paladini R. Procalcitonin as a prognostic and diagnostic tool for septic complications after major trauma. *Crit Care Med.* 2009;37: 1845-1849.
2. Kopterides P, Siempos II, Tsangaris I, Tsantes A, Armaganidis A. Procalcitonin-guided algorithms of antibiotic therapy in the intensive care unit: a systematic review and meta-analysis of randomized controlled trials. *Crit Care Med.* 2010; 38:2229-2241.

Comparison of Oligon catheters and chlorhexidine-impregnated sponges with standard multilumen central venous catheters for prevention of associated colonization and infections in intensive care unit patients: A multicenter, randomized, controlled study
Arvaniti K, for the Catheter-Related Infections in ICU (CRI-ICU) Group ("Papageorgiou" General Hosp, Thessaloniki, Greece; et al)
Crit Care Med 40:420-429, 2012

Objective.—To evaluate silver-impregnated (Oligon) central venous catheters and chlorhexidine—gluconate-impregnated sponges for reducing catheter-related colonization and infection, nonbacteremic or bacteremic.

Design.—Multicenter, prospective, randomized, controlled study.

Setting.—Five general intensive care units in Greece.

Patients.—Intensive care unit patients requiring a multilumen central venous catheter between June 2006 and May 2008.

Interventions.—Patients were randomly assigned to receive a standard catheter (standard group), a standard catheter plus chlorhexidine—gluconate-impregnated sponge (chlorhexidine—gluconate-impregnated sponge group), or an Oligon catheter (Oligon group). Catheter colonization was defined as a positive quantitative tip culture ($\geq 10^3$ colony-forming units/mL), catheter-related infection was defined by the previous criterion plus clinical evidence of sepsis, and bacteremia catheter-related infection as catheter-related infection plus a positive peripheral blood culture with the same micro-organism as in the catheter tip.

Measurements and Main Results.—Data were obtained from 465 patients, 156 in the standard-group, 150 in the chlorhexidine—gluconate-impregnated sponge group, and 159 in the Oligon-group. Colonization occurred in 24 (15.4%) standard catheters, 21 (14%) in the chlorhexidine—gluconate-impregnated sponge group, and 25 (15.7%) in the Oligon catheters ($p = .35$) (20.9, 19.9, 21.8/1000 catheter-days, respectively). Catheter-related infections were recorded in nine (5.8%) standard catheters, six (4%) in the chlorhexidine—gluconate-impregnated sponge group, and

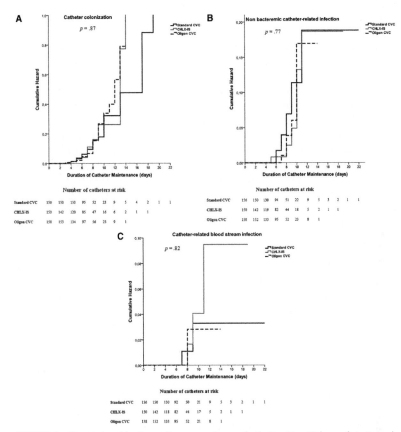

FIGURE 2.—Cumulative risk of central venous catheter colonization ($p = .87$ log-rank test), nonbacteremic central venous catheter-related infections ($p = .77$, log-rank test), central venous catheter related bloodstream infections ($p = .82$, log-rank test). A, Central venous catheter colonization. B, Nonbacteremic central venous catheter-related infections. C, Central venous catheter-related bloodstream infections. CVC, central venous catheter; CHLX-IS, chlolexidine—gluconate-impregnated sponge. (Reprinted from Arvaniti K, for the Catheter-Related Infections in ICU (CRI-ICU) Group. Comparison of Oligon catheters and chlorhexidine-impregnated sponges with standard multilumen central venous catheters for prevention of associated colonization and infections in intensive care unit patients: a multicenter, randomized, controlled study. *Crit Care Med*. 2012;40:420-429, with permission from the Society of Critical Care Medicine and Lippincott Williams & Wilkins.)

seven (4.4%) in the Oligon catheters ($p = .58$) (7.8/1,000, 5.7/1,000, 6.1/1,000 catheter-days, respectively). No difference was observed between the chlorhexidine—gluconate-impregnated sponge group and the standard group regarding catheter colonization (hazard ratio 1.21; 95% confidence interval 0.56–2.61; $p = .64$) and catheter-related infections (hazard ratio 0.65; 95% confidence interval 0.23–1.85; $p = .42$). The Oligon catheter did not reduce colonization or catheter-related infections when compared with the standard catheter (colonization: hazard ratio 1.0; 95% confidence interval 0.46–2.21; $p = .98$; catheter-related infection: hazard ratio 0.72; 95% confidence interval 0.27–1.95; $p = .52$). Seven patients (1.5%,

2.09/1,000 catheter-days) presented bacteremic catheter-related infections. Central venous catheters inserted either in the internal jugular or the femoral vein had greater risk to be colonized than catheters inserted in the subclavian vein (internal jugular vs. subclavian: hazard ratio 3.29; 95% confidence interval 1.26–8.61; $p = .01$; femoral vs. subclavian: hazard ratio 3.36; 95% confidence interval 1.17–9.65; $p = .02$). *Acinetobacter baumannii* was the predominant pathogen (37.1% episodes of colonization, 36.4% catheter-related infections, 57.1% bacteremic catheter-related infections).

Conclusion.—For short-term (median duration 7 days) central venous catheters in intensive care units with high prevalence of multiresistant Gram-negative bacteria, chlorhexidine-impregnated sponges and Oligon catheters as single preventive measures did not reduce catheter colonization or catheter-related infections. As a result of the limited amount of events, no conclusion could be reached regarding bacteremic catheter-related infections. The femoral site was the most frequently colonized insertion site in all types of catheters (Fig 2).

▶ This negative study demonstrates the safety of central venous catheters placed with appropriate technique in critically ill patients for at least the first week (Fig 2). This is consistent with epidemiologic data in my institution that document an increased incidence of catheter-related complications, particularly infectious, during the second week of insertion. As the authors in this article and the accompanying reference note,[1] most catheters are removed within the first 7 days. Thus, the risk of infectious complications is small.

An excellent review from the *New England Journal of Medicine* summarizes mechanical complications associated with central venous catheterization.[2] Overall, the femoral approach has the highest complication risk, and, as others have noted, the highest risk of contamination. The greatest mechanical risk with femoral catheterization is arterial puncture. The subclavian approach has a 3% to 5% risk of arterial puncture with a 1% to 3% risk of pneumothorax. The internal jugular approach has a small risk of pneumothorax, particularly with ultrasound and a small risk of hematoma relative to the other 2 approaches. Arterial puncture rates reported in this data are still relatively high, but improved results are noted with ultrasound guidance.

D. J. Dries, MSE, MD

References

1. McLaws ML, Burrell AR. Zero risk for central line-associated bloodstream infection: are we there yet? *Crit Care Med.* 2012;40:388-393.
2. McGee DC, Gould MK. Preventing complications of central venous catheterization. *N Engl J Med.* 2003;348:1123-1133.

Association between systemic corticosteroids and outcomes of intensive care unit—acquired pneumonia

Ranzani OT, Ferrer M, Esperatti M, et al (Universitat de Barcelona, Spain; et al)
Crit Care Med 40:2552-2561, 2012

Objective.—The use of corticosteroids is frequent in critically-ill patients. However, little information is available on their effects in patients with intensive care unit—acquired pneumonia. We assessed patients' characteristics, microbial etiology, inflammatory response, and outcomes of previous corticosteroid use in patients with intensive care unit—acquired pneumonia.

Design.—Prospective observational study.

Setting.—Intensive care units of a university teaching hospital.

Patients.—Three hundred sixteen patients with intensive care unit—acquired pneumonia. Patients were divided according to previous systemic steroid use at onset of pneumonia.

Interventions.—None.

Measurements and Main Results.—Survival at 28 days was analyzed using Cox regression, with adjustment for the propensity for receiving

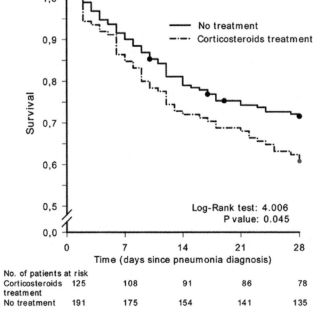

FIGURE 2.—Kaplan—Meier curves showing the 28-day survival of patients with intensive care unit—acquired pneumonia with and without previous systemic corticosteroids treatment. *Solid line*, no treatment group; *dashed line*, corticosteroid treatment group. (Reprinted from Ranzani OT, Ferrer M, Esperatti M, et al. Association between systemic corticosteroids and outcomes of intensive care unit—acquired pneumonia. *Crit Care Med.* 2012;40:2552-2561, with permission from the Society of Critical Care Medicine and Lippincott Williams & Wilkins.)

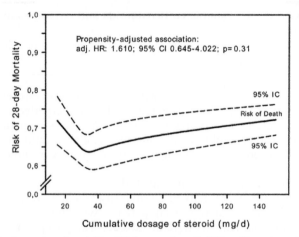

FIGURE 3.—Propensity-adjusted risk of 28-day mortality with 95% confidence interval (*CI*) by cumulative dosage of corticosteroid treatment at the time of pneumonia diagnosis for the 125 patients with previous corticosteroids. *Adj. HR*, adjusted hazard ratio. *Solid lines*, adj. HR; *dashed lines*, point-wise 95% CI. (Reprinted from Ranzani OT, Ferrer M, Esperatti M, et al. Association between systemic corticosteroids and outcomes of intensive care unit–acquired pneumonia. *Crit Care Med.* 2012;40:2552-2561, with permission from the Society of Critical Care Medicine and Lippincott Williams & Wilkins.)

steroid therapy. One hundred twenty-five (40%) patients were receiving steroids at onset of pneumonia. Despite similar baseline clinical severity, steroid treatment was associated with decreased 28-day survival (adjusted hazard ratio for propensity score and mortality predictors 2.503; 95% confidence interval 1.176–5.330; $p = .017$) and decreased systemic inflammatory response. In *post hoc* analyses, steroid treatment had an impact on survival in patients with nonventilator intensive care unit–acquired pneumonia, those with lower baseline severity and organ dysfunction, and those without etiologic diagnosis or bacteremia. The cumulative dosage of corticosteroids had no significant effect on the risk of death, but bacterial burden upon diagnosis was higher in patients receiving steroid therapy.

Conclusions.—In critically-ill patients, systemic corticosteroids should be used very cautiously because this treatment is strongly associated with increased risk of death in patients with intensive care unit–acquired pneumonia, particularly in the absence of established indications and in patients with lower baseline severity. Decreased inflammatory response may result in delayed clinical suspicion of intensive care unit–acquired pneumonia and higher bacterial count (Figs 2 and 3, Table 7).

▶ This study was conducted in 1 large university hospital where rounds were made by investigators to screen patients for admission over a 4-year period. Patients were enrolled in the trial if admitted to the intensive care unit (ICU) with clinical suspicion of ICU-acquired pneumonia. Immunosuppressed patients were excluded. Patients were followed for the impact of corticosteroid therapy on

TABLE 7.—Serum Levels of Inflammatory Biomarkers[a]

	No Treatment	Corticosteroid Treatment	p
C-reactive protein day 1, mg/dL	15.6 [8.0−23.7]	10.2 [4.4−21.0]	.002
C-reactive protein day 3, mg/dL	12.5 [6.8−20.1]	7.5 [2.4−16.1]	<.001
Procalcitonin day 1, ng/mL	0.45 [0.18−1.57]	0.30 [0.08−1.30]	.024
Procalcitonin day 3, ng/mL	0.38 [0.15−1.01]	0.21 [0.08−0.85]	.041
Midregional proadrenomedullin day 1, nmol/L	1.38 [0.43−2.33]	1.10 [0.34−1.95]	.19
Midregional proadrenomedullin day 3, nmol/L	1.39 [0.54−2.46]	0.96 [0.38−1.69]	.092
IL-6 day 1, pg/mL	192 [84−492]	94 [24−239]	<.001
IL-6 day 3, pg/mL	104 [54−275]	56 [13−149]	.006
IL-8 day 1, pg/mL	104 [63−205]	79 [52−162]	.10
IL-8 day 3, pg/mL	85 [42−168]	79 [45−162]	.96
Tumor necrosis factor-α day 1, pg/mL	9 [5−16]	6 [4−9]	.003
Tumor necrosis factor-α day 3, pg/mL	9 [6−14]	6 [4−11]	.003

[a]At onset of pneumonia, C-reactive protein was assessed in 296 patients, and procalcitonin, midregional proadrenomedullin, and other cytokines in 190 patients. On the third day after pneumonia diagnosis, serum levels of C-reactive protein were evaluated in 278 patients, and the other biomarkers were evaluated in 158 patients.

complications and mortality. Administration of corticosteroids was not controlled. Investigators were careful to ensure that study patients received at least the equivalent of 20 mg of methylprednisolone daily.

The majority of these patients were admitted with altered level of consciousness, hypoxemic respiratory failure, or for postoperative care. Coronary and trauma patients were infrequently enrolled.

As a whole, administration of corticosteroids was associated with increasing mortality (Fig 2). This was not a dose-dependent response (Fig 3). Increased mortality also corresponded with diminished levels of a variety of serum biomarkers (Table 7).

It is important to note that patients with most severe insults manifest by high sequential organ failure assessment scores or acute respiratory distress syndrome criteria did not have an increased risk of mortality with corticosteroid use. Although no explanation is offered, it seems possible that in the patient group with exaggerated inflammatory response, attenuation of systemic inflammation may be beneficial. It appears that patients with lesser severity insults did not benefit from steroid administration regardless of indication.[1,2]

In patients with less dramatic inflammatory response, the authors suggest that the antiinflammatory effect of steroids may be associated with delayed recognition of pneumonia and a longer hospital course. Epidemiology from patients receiving steroid therapy also suggests an increased incidence of opportunistic organisms including fungal pneumonia, *Aspergillus*, and *Pseudomonas aeruginosa*.

D. J. Dries, MSE, MD

References

1. Minneci PC, Deans KJ, Eichacker PQ, Natanson C. The effects of steroids during sepsis depend on dose and severity of illness: an updated meta-analysis. *Clin Microbiol Infect.* 2009;15:308-318.
2. Eichacker PQ, Parent C, Kalil A, et al. Risk and the efficacy of antiinflammatory agents: retrospective and confirmatory studies of sepsis. *Am J Respir Crit Care Med.* 2002;166:1197-1205.

Infections Caused by Multidrug Resistant Organisms Are Not Associated with Overall, All-Cause Mortality in the Surgical Intensive Care Unit: The 20,000 Foot View

Rosenberger LH, LaPar DJ, Sawyer RG (Univ of Virginia Health System, Charlottesville)

J Am Coll Surg 214:747-755, 2012

Background.—Resistant pathogens are increasingly common in the ICU, with controversy regarding their relationship to outcomes. We hypothesized that an increasing number of infections with resistant pathogens in our surgical ICU would not be associated with increased overall mortality. *Study Design.*—All ICU-acquired infections were prospectively identified between January 1, 2000 and December 31, 2009 in a single surgical ICU. Crude in-hospital, all-cause mortality data were obtained using a prospectively collected ICU database. Trends in rates were compared using linear regression.

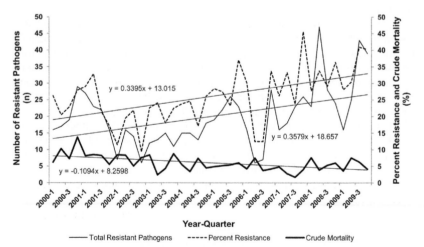

FIGURE 4.—ICU resistant pathogens, percent resistance, and crude mortality. (Reprinted from Rosenberger LH, LaPar DJ, Sawyer RG. Infections caused by multidrug resistant organisms are not associated with overall, all-cause mortality in the surgical intensive care unit: the 20,000 foot view. *J Am Coll Surg.* 2012;214:747-755, Copyright 2012, with permission from the American College of Surgeons.)

Results.—A total of 799 resistant pathogens were identified (257 gram-positive, 542 gram-negative) from a total of 3,024 isolated pathogens associated with 2,439 ICU-acquired infections. The most frequently identified resistant gram-positive and -negative pathogens (defined as resistant to at least 1 major class of antimicrobials) were methicillin-resistant *Staphylococcus aureus* and *Pseudomonas aeruginosa*, respectively. Pathogens were most commonly isolated from the lung, blood, and urine. The crude mortality rate declined steadily from 2000 to 2009 (9.4% to 5.4%; equation for trend $y = -0.11x + 8.26$). Linear regression analysis of quarterly rates revealed a significant divergence in trends between increasing total resistant infections (equation for trend $y = 0.34x + 13.02$) and percentage resistant infections (equation for trend $y = 0.36x + 18.66$) when compared with a decreasing mortality ($p = 0.0003$, $p < 0.0001$, respectively).

Conclusions.—Despite a steady rise in the proportion of resistant bacterial infections in the ICU, crude mortality rates have decreased over time. The rates of resistant infections do not appear to be a significant factor in overall mortality in our surgical ICU patients (Fig 4).

▶ This article reports carefully collected retrospective data from a large surgical critical care practice. It suffers limitations of the blend of administrative and clinical data.[1] Nonetheless, it highlights how intensive care unit (ICU) mortality has stabilized or improved despite a greater burden of pathology and pathogens (Fig 4).

The authors claim to have a prospective dataset but report in the manuscript that charts are reviewed on an episodic basis. I am also concerned that admission criteria and utilization of ICU resources may have changed during the years of this trial. We are given no information about how the pattern of ICU utilization has been affected. In our institution, palliative care teams play a greater role in determining propriety of admission to ICU and patients who have care withdrawn while in ICU. These 2 interventions could play a significant role in the results obtained.

In the discussion, the authors highlight many of the advances in critical care over the past several years. I agree with these observations. Thus, there are a number of cofounders that have not been reported here.

D. J. Dries, MSE, MD

Reference

1. Koch CG, Li L, Hixson E, Tang A, Phillips S, Henderson JM. What are the real rates of postoperative complications: elucidating inconsistencies between administrative and clinical data sources. *J Am Coll Surg.* 2012;214:798-805.

5 Postoperative Management

Cardiovascular Surgery

Pilot Implementation of a Perioperative Protocol to Guide Operating Room—to—Intensive Care Unit Patient Handoffs
Petrovic MA, Aboumatar H, Baumgartner WA, et al (Johns Hopkins Univ School of Medicine, Baltimore, MD; et al)
J Cardiothorac Vasc Anesth 26:11-16, 2012

Objectives.—Perioperative handoffs are a particularly highrisk period given patients' postprocedural physiology, their physical transport through the hospital, and the triad transfer of personnel, information, and technology. The authors piloted a new perioperative handoff process to guide patient transfers from the cardiac operating room (OR) to the cardiac surgical intensive care unit (CSICU). The aim of the study was to evaluate the impact of a standardized handoff process on patient care and provider satisfaction.

Design.—A prospective, unblinded intervention study.

Setting.—A CSICU in a teaching hospital.

Participants.—Two hundred thirty-eight health care practitioners during the transfer of care of 60 patients.

Interventions.—The implementation of a standardized handoff protocol and checklist.

Measurements and Main Results.—After the protocol's implementation, the presence of all handoff core team members at the bedside increased from 0% at baseline to 68% after intervention. The percentage of missed information in the surgery report decreased from 26% to 16% ($p = 0.03$), but the percentage of missed information in the anesthesia report showed no significant change (19% to 17%, $p > 0.05$). Handoff satisfaction scores among intensive care unit (ICU) nurses increased from 61% to 81%. On average, the duration of handoff increased by 1 minute.

Conclusions.—A standardized handoff protocol that guides the transfer of care from the OR team to the CSICU team can reduce the risk of missed information and improve satisfaction among perioperative providers.

▶ Communication breakdowns continue to be highlighted as important contributors to sentinel events. Transitions of care create potential gaps in information flow that can significantly impact the care of patients, a fact especially true for the complex cardiac surgical patient. Presented here are 2 examples of perioperative handover protocols in cardiac surgery. The first by Petrovic et al is in an adult patient population, and the second by Agarwal et al[1] focuses on the pediatric cardiac patient. Both studies showed improvements in information transfer.

Both studies implemented a standardized reporting protocol in the intensive care unit (ICU) that included a checklist of key elements. Petrovic et al used checklists that were unique for each of the care providers: surgeon, anesthesiologist, and ICU nurse. These checklists included broad categories of key elements compared with the more proscriptive checklist used by Agarwal et al. In both instances, all team members were present. The Johns Hopkins team (Petrovic) explicitly stated in training that all members would be present and specified the order in which the information and technology were to be transferred. In addition, the transferring team was to identify their greatest patient safety concerns to the receiving team. Agarwal's Vanderbilt team had similar specifications but broadened its handoff process to include a call from the operating room (OR) to the pediatric ICU to give a preliminary verbal report that would set the stage for the face-to-face report. A key element shared by both: opportunity for questions by the receiving team.

Although both of these protocols noted improvements in the transfer of information, and Agarwal et al showed improvements in 24-hour outcomes, questions remain about what constitutes the optimal handoff protocol from the OR to the ICU and other postoperative destinations and how it should be implemented. Centers that consider adopting a protocol should ensure it is adapted to their local practice—to make it their own—and assess the results with an eye to both the positive changes or improvements and unintended consequences. Future studies should include one or more measures that quantify the impact of the handover process with respect to longer-term outcomes, because these matter most to patients and families.

E. A. Martinez, MD, MHS

Reference

1. Agarwal HS, Saville BR, Slayton JM, et al. Standardized postoperative handover process improves outcomes in the intensive care unit: a model for operational sustainability and improved team performance*. *Crit Care Med.* 2012;40: 2109-2115.

Comparative Effectiveness of Preventative Therapy for Venous Thromboembolism After Coronary Artery Bypass Graft Surgery

Kulik A, Rassen JA, Myers J, et al (Brigham and Women's Hosp, Boston, MA)
Circ Cardiovasc Interv 5:590-596, 2012

Background.—Controversy exists regarding the optimal preventative therapy for venous thromboembolism (VTE) after coronary artery bypass graft (CABG) surgery. We sought to compare the effectiveness and safety of the most commonly used regimens.

Methods and Results.—We assembled a cohort of 92 699 patients who underwent CABG between 2004 and 2008, using the Premier database. Patients were categorized by method of VTE prevention initiated within 48 hours of surgery, including no preventative therapy (n = 55 400), mechanical preventative therapy (n = 21 162), subcutaneous unfractionated or low-molecular-weight heparin (n = 10 718), subcutaneous fondaparinux (n = 88), and concurrent mechanical-chemical therapy (n = 5331). The incidence of VTE and major bleeding events within 6 weeks of CABG were compared, using multivariable and propensity score adjustment. The overall incidence of VTE for the entire cohort was 0.74%, and the incidence of major bleeding was 1.43%. VTE and bleeding events occurred with similar incidence in each of the patient categories (VTE: 0.70%, 0.79%, 0.81%, 1.14%, and 0.73%; major bleeding: 1.36%, 1.45%, 1.69%, 3.41%, 1.50%; no prevention, mechanical prevention, subcutaneous heparin, subcutaneous fondaparinux, concurrent mechanical-chemical prevention, respectively). Compared with receiving no prevention, the use of mechanical prevention or subcutaneous heparin did not significantly reduce the risk of VTE or change the risk of major bleeding (P = NS).

Conclusions.—Venous thromboembolism occurs infrequently after CABG. Compared with the use of no prevention, the administration of chemical or mechanical preventative therapies to CABG patients does not appreciably lower the risk of VTE. These data provide support for the

TABLE 3.—Risk of Venous Thromboembolism With Preventative Therapy Compared With the Use of No Prevention

	Unadjusted HR (95% CI)	Adjusted HR (95% CI)*	Adjusted HR (95% CI) Plus Propensity Score[†]	Estimated Risk Difference (95% CI)[‡]
TED or SCD	1.12 (0.93, 1.34)	1.16 (0.96, 1.39)	1.14 (0.90, 1.43)	0.02% (−0.06%, 0.11%)
Heparin or LMWH	1.15 (0.91, 1.45)	1.07 (0.84, 1.35)	0.89 (0.68, 1.16)	0.01% (−0.07%, 0.09%)

HR indicates hazard ratio; CI, confidence interval; TED, thromboembolic deterrent stockings; SCD, sequential compression devices; and LMWH, low-molecular-weight heparin.
*Multivariable adjustment.
[†]Multivariable adjustment with high-dimensional propensity score.
[‡]Estimates of absolute risk difference determined from Cox proportional hazard models using reference covariate values.

TABLE 4.—Risk of Bleeding With Preventative Therapy Compared With the Use of No Prevention

	Unadjusted HR (95% CI)	Adjusted HR (95% CI)*	Adjusted HR (95% CI) Plus Propensity Score†	Estimated Risk Difference (95% CI)‡
TED or SCD	0.88 (0.77, 1.00)	0.90 (0.79, 1.03)	0.95 (0.81, 1.11)	−0.18% (−0.81%, 0.44%)
Heparin or LMWH	0.95 (0.80, 1.11)	1.01 (0.86, 1.19)	1.04 (0.87, 1.24)	0.02% (−0.67%, 0.72%)

HR indicates hazard ratio; CI, confidence interval; TED, thromboembolic deterrent stockings; SCD, sequential compression devices; and LMWH, low-molecular-weight heparin.
*Multivariable adjustment.
†Multivariable adjustment with high-dimensional propensity score.
‡Estimates of absolute risk difference determined from Cox proportional hazard models using reference covariate values.

common practice of administering no VTE preventative therapy after CABG, used for nearly 60% of patients within this cohort (Tables 3 and 4).

▶ The prevention of deep venous thromboembolism (DVT) and pulmonary embolism (PE) is a national quality metric. In fact, this diagnosis is included in the Centers for Medicare Services nonpayment list for certain orthopedic procedures. Although cardiac surgery is not included in this nonpayment group, it remains an important complication and is associated with increased morbidity and mortality. In cardiac surgery, chemical prevention has been somewhat controversial. Many practitioners believe that because their patients are on heparin during bypass, they are not at risk of developing a DVT or PE. Furthermore, they are very concerned about an increased risk of bleeding in this patient population, for whom surgical bleeding can result in cardiac tamponade, putting the patient at significant risk.

In this article by Kulik and colleagues, the authors retrospectively evaluate the safety of the multiple regimens of DVT/PE prevention in a cohort comprising more than 92 000 patients who underwent coronary artery bypass grafting (CABG). The regimens evaluated were: (1) no preventive therapy, (2) mechanical preventive therapy that included thromboembolic-deterrent socks (TEDs) and sequential or intermittent pneumatic compression device (SCD), (3) subcutaneous (subQ) unfractionated or low-molecular-weight heparin, (4) subQ fondaparinux, and (5) combined mechanical-chemical (medication) therapy. They report that there is no benefit in using any preventive measures (Table 3) and that there is no increased risk of bleeding (Table 4) with any of the chemical preventive measures except with the potential exception of fondaparinux. The authors conclude by stating that "the data support the common practice of administering no venous thromboembolism preventative therapy after CABG, used for nearly 60% of patients within this cohort."

Although the cohort was large and the statistical methods employed were robust, the results should be considered carefully. Because of its retrospective nature, the clinical criteria used to make the treatment decisions regarding chemical prophylaxis are not known, and there is no measure of whether TEDs and SCDs were actually used on patients the majority of the time. There are data that although orders may be written for such devices, they are not actually used according to the orders. In addition, it is unclear what protocols for early ambulation (which is well known to reduce DVT/TE risk) might have been used across this cohort. It seems prudent to consider these data and the individual patient and institutional characteristics given the complexity of the operation and the vulnerability of the patients when making decisions about perioperative DVT/PE prophylaxis.

E. A. Martinez, MD, MHS

Variability in Surgeons' Perioperative Practices May Influence the Incidence of Low-Output Failure After Coronary Artery Bypass Grafting Surgery
Likosky DS, for the Northern New England Cardiovascular Disease Study Group (Dartmouth-Hitchcock Med Ctr, Lebanon, NH)
Circ Cardiovasc Qual Outcomes 5:638-644, 2012

Background.—Postoperative low-output failure (LOF) is an important contributor to morbidity and mortality after coronary artery bypass grafting surgery. We sought to understand which pre- and intra-operative factors contribute to postoperative LOF and to what degree the surgeon may influence rates of LOF.

Methods and Results.—We identified 11 838 patients undergoing nonemergent, isolated coronary artery bypass grafting surgery using cardiopulmonary bypass by 32 surgeons at 8 centers in northern New England from 2001 to 2009. Our cohort included patients with preoperative ejection fractions > 40%. Patients with preoperative intraaortic balloon pumps were excluded. LOF was defined as the need for ≥ 2 inotropes at 48 hours, an intra- or post-operative intraaortic balloon pumps, or return to cardiopulmonary bypass (for hemodynamic reasons). Case volume varied across the 32 surgeons (limits, 80—766; median, 344). The overall rate of LOF was 4.3% (return to cardiopulmonary bypass, 2.6%; intraaortic balloon pumps, 1.0%; inotrope usage, 0.8%; combination, 1.0%). The predicted risk of LOF did not differ across surgeons, $P = 0.79$, and the observed rates varied from 1.1% to 10.2%, $P < 0.001$. Patients operated by low-rate surgeons had shorter clamp and bypass times, antegrade cardioplegia, longer maximum intervals between cardioplegia doses, lower cardioplegia volume per anastomosis or minute of ischemic time, and less hot-shot use. Patients operated on by higher LOF surgeons had higher rates of postoperative acute kidney injury.

Conclusions.—Rates of LOF significantly varied across surgeons and could not be explained solely by patient case mix, suggesting that variability in perioperative practices influences risk of LOF (Fig 2).

▶ The prevalence and complexity of cardiac surgical care, coupled with public reporting of cardiac surgical outcomes, has sustained a similarly intense focus on quality improvement efforts related to cardiac surgery. The Northern New

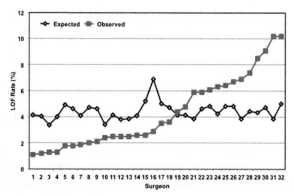

FIGURE 2.—Observed (red line and squares) vs expected (black line and diamonds) risk of low cardiac output (low-output failure [LOF]) among 32 regional surgeons. For interpretation of the references to color in this figure legend, the reader is referred to web version of this article. (Reprinted from Likosky DS, for the Northern New England Cardiovascular Disease Study Group. Variability in surgeons' perioperative practices may influence the incidence of low-output failure after coronary artery bypass grafting surgery. *Circ Cardiovasc Qual Outcomes*. 2012;5:638-644, © 2012, with permission from American Heart Association, Inc.)

England Cardiovascular Study Group has been studying variations in care delivery and driving quality improvements since the early 1990s.[1] This collaborative uses outcome data to identify variations in care and to inform continuous quality improvement initiatives among cardiac surgical centers in Northern New England. This study by Likosky et al is another affirmation of their outstanding work.

In this article, the researchers sought to better understand what influences postoperative low output failure (LOF), known to be a significant contributor to morbidity and mortality after coronary artery bypass grafting surgery. For this study, patients were defined as having LOF if they had 1 of the following: the need for ≥ 2 inotropes at 48 hours, an intra- or postoperative intra-aortic balloon pump or return to cardiopulmonary bypass. They analyzed data collected prospectively on all patients, including: patient demographics, comorbidities, cardiac anatomy and function, number and type of occluded vessels, and cardiac history. They found that the expected rate of LOF did not differ between surgeons, but observed that there was significant variation in mortality rates among the entire cohort (1.1–10.2%, $P < .001$; Fig 2). In further analysis, they identified that surgeons with low LOF rates tended to have shorter cross-clamp and bypass times, used antegrade cardioplegia, had longer intervals between cardioplegia doses, lower cardioplegia volume per anastomosis, and less hot-shot use. This study's important contribution is its evaluation of intraoperative factors in addition to patient characteristics—intraoperative factors and management decisions might be amenable to change, whereas patient vulnerabilities typically are not.

Because of its observational nature, a cause-and-effect relationship cannot be presumed and the relationships are associations. Furthermore, the authors were unable to pinpoint the relative contribution of each of these practices to the outcome. However, it informs future studies that should begin to parse these questions. In addition, this study represents an important trend using outcome research to identify variations in care that contribute to variations in outcome, and in so doing begin identifying best practices which advance our ability to deliver safe and effective care.

E. A. Martinez, MD, MHS

Reference

1. O'Connor GT, Plume SK, Olmstead EM, et al. A regional intervention to improve the hospital mortality associated with coronary artery bypass graft surgery. The Northern New England Cardiovascular Disease Study Group. *JAMA*. 1996;275: 841-846.

Temporary biventricular pacing decreases the vasoactive-inotropic score after cardiac surgery: A substudy of a randomized clinical trial
Nguyen HV, Havalad V, Aponte-Patel L, et al (Columbia Univ College of Physicians and Surgeons, NY; Columbia Univ, NY)
J Thorac Cardiovasc Surg 2012 [Epub ahead of print]

Objective.—Vasoactive medications improve hemodynamics after cardiac surgery but are associated with high metabolic and arrhythmic burdens. The vasoactive-inotropic score was developed to quantify vasoactive and inotropic support after cardiac surgery in pediatric patients but may be useful in adults as well. Accordingly, we examined the time course of this score in a substudy of the Biventricular Pacing After Cardiac Surgery trial. We hypothesized that the score would be lower in patients randomized to biventricular pacing.

Methods.—Fifty patients selected for increased risk of left ventricular dysfunction after cardiac surgery and randomized to temporary biventricular pacing or standard of care (no pacing) after cardiopulmonary bypass were studied in a clinical trial between April 2007 and June 2011. Vasoactive agents were assessed after cardiopulmonary bypass, after sternal closure, and 0 to 7 hours after admission to the intensive care unit.

Results.—Over the initial 3 collection points after cardiopulmonary bypass (mean duration, 131 minutes), the mean vasoactive-inotropic score decreased in the biventricular pacing group from 12.0 ± 1.5 to 10.5 ± 2.0 and increased in the standard of care group from 12.5 ± 1.9 to 15.5 ± 2.9. By using a linear mixed-effects model, the slopes of the time courses were significantly different ($P = .02$) and remained so for the first hour in the intensive care unit. However, the difference was no longer significant beyond this point ($P = .26$).

Conclusions.—The vasoactive-inotropic score decreases in patients undergoing temporary biventricular pacing in the early postoperative period. Future studies are required to assess the impact of this effect on arrhythmogenesis, morbidity, mortality, and hospital costs (Fig 1).

▶ Biventricular (BiV) pacing has become a mainstay of therapy among patients with chronic heart failure. Typically reserved for patients with ejection fractions less than or equal to 35%, the goal of such therapy is to better synchronize

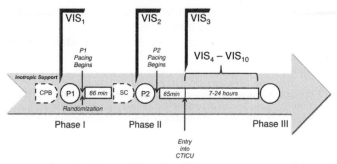

FIGURE 1.—Time course of BiPACS protocol. During phase I, after weaning from CPB, the protocol maximizing cardiac output was determined. This protocol was designated P1. Patients were randomized after phase I into the BiVP or SOC arm. Patients in the BiVP arm were paced under P1 until phase II. During phase II, after sternal closure, the protocol maximizing mean arterial pressure was determined and designated P2. Pacing was then resumed using P2 in the BiVP arm until phase III optimization, at which point the study period was concluded. VIS was calculated before randomization (VIS$_1$), before phase II (VIS$_2$), on relocation from the operating room to the ICU (VIS$_3$), and hourly when the patient was in the ICU (VIS$_4$-VIS$_{10}$). *VIS*, Vasoactiveinotropic score; *CPB*, cardiopulmonary bypass; *SC*, sternal closure; *CTICU*, cardiothoracic intensive care unit. (Reprinted from the Journal of Thoracic and Cardiovascular Surgery. Nguyen HV, Havalad V, Aponte-Patel L, et al. Temporary biventricular pacing decreases the vasoactive-inotropic score after cardiac surgery: a substudy of a randomized clinical trial. *J Thorac Cardiovasc Surg* 2012; [Epub ahead of print], Copyright 2012, with permission from The American Association for Thoracic Surgery.)

ventricular contractions. The technique has been shown to improve symptoms for patients with heart failure and improve intraoperative cardiac output after coming off bypass.[1] Thus, the logical next step is to evaluate whether this practice might improve cardiac output in the perioperative phase and thus reduce the need for inotropic support. If BiV improves cardiac output perioperatively, 2 potential benefits include: (1) improved synchronization in the perioperative period when the myocardium may be stunned and (2) reduced reliance on vasoactive or inotropic agents, both of which add an important metabolic load to the myocardium.

Using the vasoactive-inotropic score (VIS),[2,3] Nguyen et al evaluated whether the use of postoperative BiV reduced the need for vasoactive and/or inotropic agents in the context of the overall surgery outcome. The VIS assigns a point value to each of the medications normalized to a weight-based dosing. To optimize the pacing, the authors developed a protocol for commencing the BiV (Fig 1). The VIS score for the standard of care (SOC) group increased shortly after intensive care unit (ICU) admission and was significantly different from the time between separation from bypass through the first hour in the ICU (out to 2 hours following an optimization of the BiV pacing) but not beyond that time (up to 7 hours postoperatively).

Although this analysis represents an important starting point, the limited observation time (7 hours postoperatively) limits the assessment of longer term potential benefits, and perhaps a full appreciation of the true impact of BiV pacing. The relatively lower VIS score for the BiV-paced patients "for 2 hours after the last optimization" suggests that if they continued to optimize the BiV pacing by evaluating the atrioventricular and interventricular delay, greater impact may have been demonstrated. The authors suggest that future studies should evaluate the impact of various lengths of BiV pacing, and its impact on short- and long-term outcomes.

E. A. Martinez, MD, MHS

References

1. Wang DY, Richmond ME, Quinn TA, et al. Optimized temporary biventricular pacing acutely improves intraoperative cardiac output after weaning from cardiopulmonary bypass: a substudy of a randomized clinical trial. *J Thorac Cardiovasc Surg.* 2012;141:1002-1008, 1008.e1.
2. Gaies MG, Gurney JG, Yen AH, et al. Vasoactive-inotropic score as a predictor of morbidity and mortality in infants after cardiopulmonary bypass. *Pediatr Crit Care Med.* 2010;11:234-238.
3. Wernovsky G, Wypij D, Jonas RA, et al. Postoperative course and hemodynamic profile after the arterial switch operation in neonates and infants. A comparison of low-flow cardiopulmonary bypass and circulatory arrest. *Circulation.* 1995;92: 2226-2235.

Standardized postoperative handover process improves outcomes in the intensive care unit: A model for operational sustainability and improved team performance
Agarwal HS, Saville BR, Slayton JM, et al (Monroe Carell Jr Children's Hosp at Vanderbilt, Nashville, TN; Vanderbilt Univ Med Ctr, Nashville, TN)
Crit Care Med 40:2109-2115, 2012

Objective.—To determine whether structured handover tool from operating room to pediatric cardiac intensive care unit following cardiac surgery is associated with a reduction in the loss of information transfer and an improvement in the quality of communication exchange. In addition, whether this tool is associated with a decrease in postoperative complications and an improvement in patient outcomes in the first 24 hrs of pediatric cardiac intensive care unit stay.

Design.—Prospective observational clinical study.

Setting.—Pediatric cardiac intensive care unit of an academic medical center.

Patients.—Pediatric cardiac surgery patients over a 3-yr period. Evaluation of communication and patients studied for two time periods: verbal handover (July 2007—June 2009) and structured handover (July 2009—June 2010).

Interventions.—None.

Measurements and Main Results.—Two anonymous surveys administered to the entire clinical team of the pediatric cardiac intensive care unit evaluated loss of information transfer for each of the two handover processes. Quality of structured handover tool was evaluated by Likert scale (1—5) responses in the second survey. Patient complications including cardiopulmonary resuscitation, mediastinal reexploration, placement on extracorporeal membrane oxygenation, development of severe metabolic

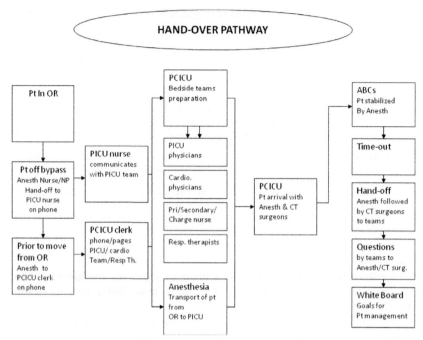

FIGURE 1.—Structured process for pediatric cardiac surgery patient (*Pt*) transfer from the operating room (*OR*) to the pediatric cardiac intensive care unit (*PCICU*). Step 1 involves phone communication between OR and *PCICU*; Step 2 involves face-to-face report on arrival in the PCICU. *ABC:* A, airway; *B*, breathing; *C*, circulation established and stable before beginning the handover process in the PCICU. *Anesth*, anesthesia; *NP*, nurse practitioner; *Cardio*, cardiology; *Resp Th.*, respiratory therapist; *Pri*, primary bedside nurse; *Resp.*, respiratory; *CT*, cardio-thoracic. (Reprinted from Agarwal HS, Saville BR, Slayton JM, et al. Standardized postoperative handover process improves outcomes in the intensive care unit: a model for operational sustainability and improved team performance. *Crit Care Med.* 2012;40:2109-2115, with permission from the Society of Critical Care Medicine and Lippincott Williams & Wilkins.)

acidosis, and number of early extubations in the first 24-hr pediatric cardiac intensive care unit stay were compared for the two time periods. Survey results showed the general opinion that the structured handover tool was of excellent quality to enhance communication (Likert scale: 4.4 ± 0.7). In addition, the tool was associated with a significant reduction ($p < .001$) in loss of information for every category of patient clinical care including patient, preoperative, anesthesia, operative, and postoperative details and laboratory values. Patient data revealed significant decrease ($p < .05$) for three of the four major complications studied and a significant increase ($p < .04$) in the number of early extubations following introduction of our standardized handover tool.

Conclusions.—In this setting, a standardized handover tool is associated with a decrease in the loss of patient information, an improvement in the quality of communication during postoperative transfer, a decrease in postoperative complications, and an improvement in 24-hr patient outcomes (Fig 1).

▶ Communication breakdowns continue to be highlighted as important contributors to sentinel events. Transitions of care create potential gaps in information flow that can significantly impact the care of patients, a fact especially true for the complex cardiac surgical patient. Presented here are 2 examples of perioperative handover protocols in cardiac surgery. The first by Petrovic et al[1] is in an adult patient population, and the second by Agarwal et al focuses on the pediatric cardiac patient. Both studies found improvements in information transfer.

Both studies implemented a standardized reporting protocol in the intensive care unit (ICU) that included a checklist of key elements. Petrovic, et al,[1] used checklists that were unique for each of the care providers: surgeon, anesthesiologist, and ICU nurse. These checklists included broad categories of key elements compared with the more proscriptive checklist used by Agarwal et al. In both instances, all team members were present. The Johns Hopkins team (Petrovic) explicitly stated in training that all members would be present and specified the order in which the information and technology were to be transferred. In addition, the transferring team was to identify their greatest patient safety concerns to the receiving team. Agarwal's Vanderbilt team had similar specifications but broadened its handoff process to include a call from the operating room (OR) to the pediatric ICU to give a preliminary verbal report that would set the stage for the face-to-face report (Fig 1). A key element shared by both: opportunity for questions by the receiving team.

Although both of these protocols noted improvements in the transfer of information, and Agarwal et al showed improvements in 24-hour outcomes, questions remain about what constitutes the optimal handoff protocol from the OR to the ICU and other postoperative destinations and how it should be implemented. Centers that consider adopting a protocol should ensure it is adapted to their local practice—to make it their own—and assess the results with an eye to both the positive changes or improvements and unintended consequences. Future studies should include one or more measures that quantify the impact of the handover process with respect to longer-term outcomes, because these matter most to patients and families.

E. A. Martinez, MD, MHS

Reference

1. Petrovic MA, Aboumatar H, Baumgartner WA, et al. Pilot implementation of a perioperative protocol to guide operating room-to-intensive care unit patient handoffs. *J Cardiothorac Vasc Anesth.* 2012;26:11-16.

Institutional Factors Beyond Procedural Volume Significantly Impact Center Variability in Outcomes After Orthotopic Heart Transplantation
Kilic A, Weiss ES, Yuh DD, et al (The Johns Hopkins Hosp, Baltimore, MD; Yale School of Medicine, New Haven, CT)
Ann Surg 256:616-623, 2012

Objective.—To evaluate the contribution of institutional volume and other unmeasured institutional factors beyond volume to the between-center variability in outcomes after orthotopic heart transplantation (OHT).

Background.—It is unclear if institutional factors beyond volume have a significant impact on OHT outcomes.

Methods.—The United Network for Organ Sharing registry was used to identify OHTs performed between 2000 and 2010. Separate mixed-effect logistic regression models were constructed, with the primary endpoint being post-OHT mortality. Model A included only individual centers, model B added validated recipient and donor risk indices as well as the year of transplantation, and model C added institutional volume as a continuous variable to model B. The reduction in between-center variability in mortality between models B and C was used to define the contribution of institutional volume. Kaplan-Meier survival curves were also compared after stratifying patients into equal-size tertiles based on center volume.

Results.—A total of 119 centers performed OHT in 19,156 patients. After adjusting for transplantation year and differences in recipient and donor risk, decreasing center volume was associated with an increased risk of 1-year mortality (*P* < 0.001). However, procedural volume only accounted for 16.7% of the variability in mortality between centers, and significant between-center variability persisted after adjusting for institutional volume (*P* < 0.001). In Kaplan-Meier analysis, there was significant variability in 1-year survival between centers within each volume category: low-volume

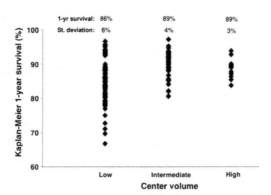

FIGURE 2.—Variability in Kaplan-Meier 1-year survival between individual centers stratified by institutional volume. Each diamond represents an individual center. (Reprinted from Kilic A, Weiss ES, Yuh DD, et al. Institutional factors beyond procedural volume significantly impact center variability in outcomes after orthotopic heart transplantation. *Ann Surg.* 2012;256:616-623, © 2012 Southeastern Surgical Congress.)

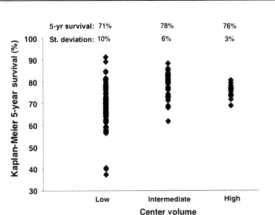

FIGURE 3.—Variability in Kaplan-Meier 5-year survival between individual centers stratified by institutional volume. Each diamond represents an individual center. (Reprinted from Kilic A, Weiss ES, Yuh DD,
et al. Institutional factors beyond procedural volume significantly impact center variability in outcomes
after orthotopic heart transplantation. *Ann Surg.* 2012;256:616-623, © 2012 Southeastern Surgical
Congress.)

(66.7%—96.6%), intermediate-volume (80.7%—97.3%), and high-volume
(83.8%—93.9%). These trends were also observed with 5-year mortality.

Conclusions.—This large-cohort analysis demonstrates that although
institutional volume is a significant predictor of post-OHT outcomes,
there are other unmeasured institutional factors that contribute substantially
to the between-center variability in outcomes. Institutional volume should
therefore not be the sole indicator of "center quality" in OHT (Figs 2 and
3, Table 1).

▶ The volume-outcome relationship in cardiac surgery has been a topic of
debate for decades.[1] While early data supported an inverse relationship between
volume and mortality, more recent studies have suggested otherwise. In this
study, the authors evaluate whether there is a volume-outcome relationship in
heart transplantation.

The authors also evaluate institutional volume and other unmeasured institutional factors that may contribute to differences in outcomes for patients undergoing orthotopic heart transplantation. In a cohort of more than 19 000 patients
from 119 centers, Kilic and colleagues assessed the impact of center volume in
addition to a year of transplantation and patient risk factors that are included in
the Mortality Prediction After Cardiac Transplantation score on outcomes. This
score incorporates 50 patient variables (Table 1) derived from the United
Network for Organ Sharing Database to do the analysis.

Using mixed-effect logistic regression models, the authors show that volume
does have an impact on 1- and 5-year mortality rates among patients who have
undergone orthotropic heart transplantation. However, they note that volume
only explains up to 17% of the variability, and that even within centers
having a similar caseload, there is important variation in outcomes (Figs 2 and 3).

TABLE 1.—Index for Mortality Prediction After Cardiac Transplantation Recipient Risk Score

Recipient Variable	Points Assigned
Age ≥60 years	3
Serum bilirubin (mg/dL)	
0–0.99	0
1–1.99	1
2–3.99	3
≥4	4
Creatinine clearance (mL/min)	
≥50	0
30–49	2
<30	5
Dialysis between listing and transplant	4
Female sex	3
Heart failure etiology	
Idiopathic	0
Ischemic	2
Congenital	5
Other	1
Recent infection	3
Intraaortic balloon pump	3
Mechanical ventilation before transplant	5
Race	
White	0
African American	3
Hispanic	0
Other	0
Temporary circulatory support*	7
Ventricular assist device	
Older generation pulsatile	3
Newer generation continuous[†]	5
HeartMate II	0
Total points possible	50

*Temporary circulatory support includes extracorporeal membrane oxygenation and extracorporeal ventricular assist device support.
[†]Excluding HeartMate II.

This study highlights that while the adage "practice makes perfect" contributes somewhat to improved outcomes, there are other important factors that account for a large degree of variation. It is important for future research to begin identifying common themes about the structures and processes of care that appear to impact outcomes the most and then assess whether implementation of these processes in poor performing centers can improve outcomes. Clearly, work remains with respect to identifying true predictors of reliable and safe cardiac surgery performance and broadening their implementation.

E. A. Martinez, MD, MHS

Reference

1. Birkmeyer JD, Dimick JB. Potential benefits of the new Leapfrog standards: effect of process and outcomes measures. *Surgery.* 2004;135:569-575.

Advanced care nurse practitioners can safely provide sole resident cover for level three patients: impact on outcomes, cost and work patterns in a cardiac surgery programme

Skinner H, Skoyles J, Redfearn S, et al (Nottingham Univ Hosps, UK)
Eur J Cardiothorac Surg 43:19-22, 2013

Objectives.—There are significant pressures on resident medical rotas on intensive care. We have evaluated the safety and feasibility of nurse practitioners (NPs) delivering first-line care on an intensive care unit with all doctors becoming non-resident. Previously, resident doctors on a 1:8 full-shift rota supported by NPs delivered first-line care to patients after cardiac surgery. Subsequently, junior doctors changed to a 1:5 non-resident rota and NPs onto a 1:7 full-shift rota provided first-line care.

Methods.—A single centre before-and-after service evaluation on cardiac intensive care. Key measures for improvement: mortality rates, surgical trainee attendance in theatre and cost before and after the change. After-hour calls by NPs to doctors and subsequent actions were also audited after the change.

Results.—The overall mortality rates in the 12 months before the change were 2.8 and 2.2% in the 12 months after ($P = 0.43$). The median [range] logistic EuroSCORE was 5.3 [0.9−84] before and 5.0 [0.9−85] after the change ($P = 0.16$). After accounting for the risk profile, the odds ratio for death after the change relative to before was 0.83, 95% confidence interval 0.41−1.69. Before the change, a surgical trainee attended theatre 467 of 702 (68%) cases. This increased to 539 of 677 (80%) cases after the change ($P < 0.001$). The annual cost of staffing the junior doctor and NP programme before the change was £933,344 and £764,691 after. In the year after the change, 192 after-hour calls were made to doctors. In 57% of cases telephone advice sufficed and doctors attended in 43%.

Conclusions.—With adequate training and appropriate support, resident NPs can provide a safe, sustainable alternative to traditional staffing models of cardiac intensive care. Training opportunities for junior surgeons increased and costs were reduced (Table 1).

▶ Alternative staffing plans became an imperative for the Trent Cardiac Center in the United Kingdom following changes in resident hours, a reduction in applicants for residency, and implementation of the European Working Time Directive

TABLE 1.—Patient Risk and Outcomes

	May 2009 to April 2010	May 2010 to April 2011	P-value
Open heart procedures	702	678	
Logistic EuroSCORE	5.3 [0.9−84]	5.0 [0.9−85]	0.16
Mortality	2.8%	2.2%	0.43

Logistic EuroSCOREs are median [range]; P-value for Mann−Whitney test. Mortality rates; P-value for χ^2 test.

with its restrictive immigration laws for doctors from outside of the European Union. The intensive care unit (ICU) was an area of particular focus for the Trent Center given that staffing pressures had forced the facility, like most others, to rely on physician extenders to fill important roles. Given that staffing patterns and management paradigms are an important structural component of the quality of care delivery in the ICU, the specific impact of staffing decisions were evaluated at the Trent Center ICU.

The literature suggests that physician[1] and nurse staffing levels and organization[2] are substantively related to quality of care in the ICU. Following the staffing changes discussed in this study, the Trent Center Board undertook the task of evaluating what, if any, impact there was to patient care by transitioning from predominantly physician coverage to nurse practitioners (NPs) as first-line caregivers. The measures of success reviewed were: no change in mortality, appropriate management of cardiac arrest, and no undue delay in notifying physicians. In addition, a sustainability measure evaluated how engaged the residents remained in learning, even though they were less responsible as front-line caregivers overnight. Following the implementation of the program, the investigators reported that mortality decreased, although not significantly, from 2.8% to 2.2%, cardiac arrests were managed well, and consults were called appropriately (Table 1).

The authors highlight key aspects of the program that contributed to its success, yet that also make this model challenging to replicate. Five of the seven NPs who started with this program had more than 3 years' experience, a relatively unusual luxury given that it takes approximately 2 to 3 years to train an NP. Finally, as a pre—post study with inherent limitations because of its observational nature, the authors suggest that similar programmatic changes should be evaluated locally. Skinner et al should be applauded for developing a robust assessment of the impact of their intervention. In our response to external requirements to increase efficiency and achieve quality improvement goals, we must be ever-vigilant for the introduction of unintended consequences which do more harm than good.

E. A. Martinez, MD, MHS

References

1. Pronovost PJ, Angus DC, Dorman T, Robinson KA, Dremsizov TT, Young TL. Physician staffing patterns and clinical outcomes in critically ill patients: a systematic review. *JAMA.* 2002;288:2151-2162.
2. Dimick JB, Swoboda SM, Pronovost PJ, Lipsett PA. Effect of nurse-to-patient ratio in the intensive care unit on pulmonary complications and resource use after hepatectomy. *Am J Crit Care.* 2001;10:376-382.

Frequency, characteristics, and outcomes of pediatric patients readmitted to the cardiac critical care unit

Bastero-Miñón P, Russell JL, Humpl T (Univ of Toronto, Ontario, Canada)
Intensive Care Med 38:1352-1357, 2012

Purpose.—To describe the characteristics and outcomes of patients readmitted to a pediatric cardiac critical care unit (CCCU) from the ward within 72 h of their first discharge.

Methods.—This was a retrospective analysis of data collected on patients admitted to the CCCU between January 1, 2000 and January 31, 2007. The setting was an 18-bed pediatric CCCU in a tertiary care university hospital. No interventions were performed.

Results.—Among the 4,625 patients admitted to the CCCU, 112 (2.4 %) were readmitted from the ward within 72 h of their discharge. The most common cause for readmission was respiratory symptoms (42.9 %). Significant changes in the chest X-ray prior to discharge were identified retrospectively in 12.5% of these patients. Cardiovascular symptoms were similarly frequent (40.2%) among these patients. Nine (8%) of the patients died during the readmission period, a rate which is considerably higher than the overall CCCU mortality rate (3.8%) in the same period of time.

Conclusions.—Respiratory reasons are the most common cause for early CCCU readmission among pediatric cardiac patients. The readmitted patients have higher rates of death compared to the overall pediatric cardiac critical care population. The development of objective predischarge scores might help planning appropriately for discharge to the ward and avoid readmission to the CCU (Table 1).

▶ Intensive care unit (ICU) readmission during the same hospitalization has been shown to be associated with increased morbidity and mortality.[1] Bastero-Miñón et al sought to identify the risks associated with readmission to a pediatric cardiac critical care unit (CCCU) at a tertiary center and profiled the patients who required readmission. Patients admitted to this ICU between 2000 and 2007 presented varied diagnoses, and for the purposes of analysis and risk identification, the authors grouped them according to single-ventricle physiology, biventricular physiology, and nonstructural heart disease.

TABLE 1.—Main Characteristic of the Entire Patient Population and the Readmitted Cohort

	All Patients	Readmitted Patients
n	4,625	112
Biventricular physiology	3,427 (74.1%)	67 (59.8%)
Single ventricle physiology	83 (18.0%)	34 (30.4%)
Non-structural heart disease	365 (7.9 %)	11 (9.8%)
Gender (male)	2,735 (59%)	59 (53%)
Median age (range)	2.8 years (1 day–18.3 years)	0.3 years (1 day–16 years)
Median length of stay in CCCU (first admission)	2.4 days (3 h–221 days)	3.9 days (19 h–112 days)

Of the cohort of 4625 patients readmitted, 112 met the inclusion criteria of 72 hours following discharge. Of these, 30% had single-ventricle physiology, 60% biventricular, and 10% non-structural heart disease (Table 1). The most common precipitator for readmission was respiratory symptoms followed by cardiac symptoms. Of those who were readmitted, 58% required reintubation and mechanical ventilation, 30.4% required noninvasive mechanical ventilation, 46.4% required inotropic support, and 0.9% required extracorporeal membrane oxygenation. The mortality rate for these readmitted patients was 8% (compared with 3.8% in the remainder of the CCCU cohort).

For 71.4% (n = 82) of the readmitted patients, the last X-ray before discharge demonstrated a change, either minor (defined as small areas of atelectasis, trivial pleural effusions, and changes in association with the underlying cardiac defect) or significant (defined as bilateral atelectasis, bilateral pleural effusions, and/or progressive pulmonary edema). The authors also note that the most common CCCU discharge day among those readmitted was a Friday. Discharge decisions were made at the discretion of the attending staff. Because this is a retrospective study, there are likely unmeasured confounders that may have contributed to the decision to discharge a patient. It is not uncommon in many centers that when space becomes an issue, patients may be transferred out somewhat prematurely to accommodate the day's surgical cases.

The authors highlight the risks of readmission and propose several areas for further research, such as standardized discharge criteria, the impact of discharge on Fridays with respect to weekend staffing on the receiving floors, and the utility of a handover protocol identifying aspects of care that may need close follow-up (eg, a repeat chest X-ray) within the next 24 to 48 hours. Exploring decisions about transfer will offer greater insights into the opportunities to reduce readmissions and their associated morbidity and mortality.

E. A. Martinez, MD, MHS

Reference

1. Rosenberg AL, Watts C. Patients readmitted to ICUs: a systematic review of risk factors and outcomes. *Chest.* 2000;118:492-502.

Blood Transfusion and the Risk of Acute Kidney Injury After Transcatheter Aortic Valve Implantation

Nuis R-J, Rodés-Cabau J, Sinning J-M, et al (Erasmus Med Ctr, Rotterdam, Netherlands; Quebec Heart and Lung Inst, Canada; Univ Hosp Bonn, Germany; et al)
Circ Cardiovasc Interv 5:680-688, 2012

Background.—Blood transfusion is associated with acute kidney injury (AKI) after transcatheter aortic valve implantation (TAVI). We sought to elucidate in more detail the relation between blood transfusion and AKI and its effects on short- and long-term mortality.

Methods and Results.—Nine hundred ninety-five patients with aortic stenosis underwent TAVI with the Medtronic CoreValve or the Edwards Valve in 7 centers. AKI was defined by the Valve Academic Research Consortium (absolute increase in serum creatinine ≥ 0.3 mg/dL [≥ 26.4 μmol/L] or ≥ 50% increase ≤ 72 hours). Logistic and Cox regression was used for predictor and survival analysis. AKI occurred in 20.7% (n = 206). The number of units of blood transfusion ≤ 24 hours was the strongest predictor of AKI (≥ 5 units, OR, 4.81 [1.45−15.95], 3−4 units, OR, 3.05 [1.24−7.53], 1−2 units, OR, 1.47 [0.98−2.22]) followed by peripheral vascular disease (OR, 1.48 [1.05−2.10]), history of heart failure (OR, 1.43 [1.01−2.03]), leucocyte count ≤ 72 hours after TAVI (OR, 1.05 [1.02−1.09]) and European System for Cardiac Operative Risk Evaluation (EuroSCORE; OR, 1.02 [1.00−1.03]). Potential triggers of blood transfusion such as baseline anemia, bleeding-vascular complications, and perioperative blood loss were not identified as predictors. AKI and life-threatening bleeding were independent predictors of 30-day mortality (OR, 3.15 [1.56−6.38], OR,

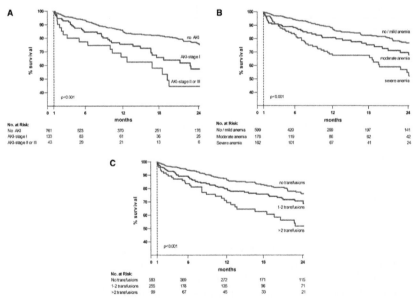

FIGURE 3.—Time-to-event curves for selected risk factors in patients who survived the first 30 days after transcatheter aortic valve implantation (TAVI) (landmark analysis). Event rates were calculated with the use of Kaplan—Meier methods and compared with the use of the log-rank test. A, Time-to-event curves for patients without acute kidney injury (AKI), AKI-stage I and with AKI-stage II or III after TAVI. B, Time-to-event curves for patients without transfusions, 1−2 transfusions and with >2 transfusions ≤72 h after TAVI. C, Time-to-event curves for patients with no and various degrees of baseline anemia. Baseline anemia was defined as Hb <13 g/dL in men and <12 g/dL in women[23]; mild anemia 12.0 to 12.99 g/dL in men and 11.30 to 11.99 g/dL in women, moderate anemia 10.80 to 11.99 g/dL in men and 10.23 to 11.29 g/dL in women, and severe anemia <10.80 g/dL in men and <10.23 g/dL in women. Hb indicates hemoglobin. *Editor's Note*: Please refer to original journal article for full references. (Reprinted from Nuis R-J, Rodés-Cabau J, Sinning J-M, et al. Blood transfusion and the risk of acute kidney injury after transcatheter aortic valve implantation. *Circ Cardiovasc Interv.* 2012;5:680-688, with permission from American Heart Association, Inc.)

TABLE 3.—Independent Predictors of AKI After TAVI

Variable	OR (95% CI)	P Value
RBC transfusion ≤24 h		
None	Reference	0.003
1−2 units	1.47 (0.98−2.22)	0.064
3−4 units	3.05 (1.24−7.53)	0.015
≥5 units	4.81 (1.45−15.95)	0.010
Peripheral vascular disease	1.48 (1.05−2.10)	0.026
Congestive heart failure	1.43 (1.01−2.03)	0.042
Maximum leucocyte count ≤72 h (per 10^9 cells/L increase)	1.05 (1.02−1.09)	0.001
Logistic EuroSCORE (per % increase)	1.02 (1.00−1.03)	0.006

AKI indicates acute kidney injury; TAVI, transcatheter aortic valve implantation; RBC, red blood cell.

TABLE 5.—Independent Predictors of Mortality >30 Days After Transcatheter Aortic Valve Implantation

Variable	HR (95% CI)	P Value
RBC transfusion ≤72 h		
None	Reference	0.004
1−2 units	1.32 (0.94−1.86)	0.11
3−4 units	2.03 (1.26−3.24)	0.003
≥5 units	2.54 (1.34−4.81)	0.004
Baseline anemia		
None	Reference	0.005
Mild	0.85 (0.54−1.34)	0.48
Moderate	1.49 (1.01−2.20)	0.043
Severe	1.75 (1.18−2.60)	0.005
Acute kidney injury	1.57 (1.13−2.17)	0.007
Peripheral vascular disease	1.69 (1.25−2.30)	0.001
Congestive heart failure	1.62 (1.16−2.26)	0.004
Male sex	1.53 (1.14−2.06)	0.005
Atrial fibrillation	1.46 (1.06−1.99)	0.019

RBC denotes red blood cell.

6.65 [2.28−19.44], respectively), whereas transfusion (≥ 3 units), baseline anemia, and AKI predicted mortality beyond 30 days.

Conclusions.—AKI occurred in 21% of the patients after TAVI. The number of blood transfusions but not the indication of transfusion predicted AKI. AKI was a predictor of both short- and long-term mortality, whereas blood transfusion predicted long-term mortality. These findings indicate that outcome of TAVI may be improved by more restrictive use of blood transfusions (Fig 3, Tables 3 and 5).

▶ Over the last decade, the data have increasingly suggested that blood transfusions have a detrimental effect on outcomes for patients undergoing cardiac surgery.[1,2] The recent literature has also noted an increase in minimally invasive surgical procedures, many of which have shown equal or better outcomes than with more invasive approaches. The transcatheter aortic valve implantation procedure is one such example of a much less invasive valve replacement surgery. However, many of the patients who are candidates for this procedure are in a high risk group at baseline. For this vulnerable population, the risk of acute kidney injury (AKI) is a particular concern, as it affects 12% to 57% of these patients, and AKI is associated with a 2- to 6-fold increased risk of death. In addition, some data have suggested that transfusions increase the risk of AKI.

To better understand the relationships between transfusions, AKI, and outcomes, the authors performed a retrospective analysis among 995 patients to quantify the association between blood transfusions (number of units and anemia as an indicator for transfusion) and AKI, and, finally, outcomes. They found a significant association between red blood cell (RBC) transfusions and the incidence of AKI (Table 3) and that both RBCs transfused and AKI were independent predictors of mortality (Table 5). Finally, the authors found that transfusion (> 2 units packed red blood cells), baseline anemia, and AKI each predicted 30-day mortality (Fig 3).

This article leaves us with some important questions about risks associated with transfusion and how to better define appropriate transfusion triggers. It would seem that avoiding transfusions would be prudent in this patient population, as has been shown in other perioperative and intensive care unit studies. However, 2 key issues remain: (1) identify the appropriate transfusion triggers, which should guide transfusion therapy, and (2) identify the unintended consequences of more restrictive transfusion guidelines in this group of very high-risk patients.

E. A. Martinez, MD, MHS

References

1. Koch CG, Li L, Duncan AI, et al. Morbidity and mortality risk associated with red blood cell and blood-component transfusion in isolated coronary artery bypass grafting. *Crit Care Med.* 2006;34:1608-1616.
2. Koch CG, Khandwala F, Li L, Estafanous FG, Loop FD, Blackstone EH. Persistent effect of red cell transfusion on health-related quality of life after cardiac surgery. *Ann Thorac Surg.* 2006;82:13-20.

In Vivo Molecular Imaging of Murine Embryonic Stem Cells Delivered to a Burn Wound Surface via Integra® Scaffolding
Hamrahi VF, Goverman J, Jung W, et al (Massachusetts General Hosp, Boston; et al)
J Burn Care Res 33:e49-e54, 2012

It has been demonstrated that restoration of function to compromised tissue can be accomplished by transplantation of bone marrow stem cells and/or embryonic stem cells (ESCs). One limitation to this approach has been the lack of noninvasive techniques to longitudinally monitor stem cell attachment and proliferation. Recently, murine ESC lines that express green fluorescent protein (GFP), luciferase (LV), and herpes simplex thymidine kinase (HVTK) were developed for detection of actively growing cells in vivo by imaging. In this study, the authors investigated the use of these ESC lines in a burned mouse model using Integra® as a delivery scaffolding/matrix. Two different cell lines were used: one expressing GFP and LV and the other expressing GFP, LV, and HVTK. Burn wounds were produced by application of a brass block (2 × 2 cm kept in boiling water before application) to the dorsal surface of SV129 mice for 10 seconds. Twenty-four hours after injury, Integra® with adherent stem cells was engrafted onto a burn wound immediately after excision of eschar. The stem cells were monitored in vivo by measuring bioluminescence with a charge-coupled device camera and immunocytochemistry of excised tissue. Bioluminescence progressively increased in intensity over the time course of the study, and GFP-positive cells growing into the Integra® were detected. These studies demonstrate the feasibility of using Integra® as a scaffolding, or matrix, for the delivery of stem cells to burn wounds as well as the utility of bioluminescence for monitoring in vivo cellular tracking of stably transfected ESC cells.

▶ Although not a human study, this is a work that has great potential in the very near future to impact burn patients on a large scale. Integra® is a dermal regeneration template that has been commercially available for several decades. After the full-thickness burn wound is treated with excisional debridement, Integra is placed on the wound. After neovascularization occurs (weeks later) the patient then undergoes subsequent split-thickness skin grafting. Cosmesis and eventual wound contracture due to burn scarring is improved with the use of Integra; however, the process is lengthy and costly, the need for multiple surgical procedures remains, and all the attendant problems of large donor sites remain. Using the Integra as a scaffolding for stem cells is a fantastic interim solution to the problems of full-thickness burns requiring excision and skin grafting. Although in its infancy, the concept of impregnating a dermal matrix will move along, gain momentum, and, hopefully, at some time in the not-so-distant future, burn patients will be able to experience reconstructed skin, complete with skin appendages, that much more closely mirrors their skin in its preburned state. This work is way too important to become mired in religious or legal wrangling. Look for continued work on the subject from this laboratory, where Integra began.

B. A. Latenser, MD, FACS

Miscellaneous

Association Between Hospital Intraoperative Blood Transfusion Practices for Surgical Blood Loss and Hospital Surgical Mortality Rates
Wu W-C, Trivedi A, Friedmann PD, et al (Brown Univ, Providence, RI; et al)
Ann Surg 255:708-714, 2012

Objective.—Blood loss during surgery is an important operative complication in patients undergoing major noncardiac surgery and may increase postoperative morbidity and mortality. Variations in the delivery of operative blood transfusions to treat blood loss depend not only on the patient and surgery characteristics but also on the hospital transfusion practices, and may explain differences in the hospitals' postoperative outcomes. We determine the relationship between hospital-level rates of intraoperative blood transfusion and 30-day mortality among older patients with significant intraoperative blood loss.

Methods.—Among 46,608 operative patients aged 65 years or older whose estimated blood loss was 500 mL or greater in 122 Veterans Affairs (VA) hospitals during years 1997 to 2004, we examined the relationship between hospital-level transfusion rates and adjusted 30-day postoperative mortality rates using linear regression modeling.

Results.—Hospital-level rates of intraoperative blood transfusion for older surgical patients with significant blood loss varied from 10% to 92%. Hospitals in the highest tertile for the rate of intraoperative transfusion had the highest number of patients with 500 mL or more surgical blood loss and lowest risk-adjusted 30-day surgical mortality. For every 10% increase in the rate of intraoperative blood transfusion, there was a 0.7% (95% CI: 0.3%−1.1%) decrease in the hospital's adjusted 30-day postoperative mortality for these high-risk patients.

Conclusions.—Large variation exists in hospitals' intraoperative blood transfusion practices for older patients with significant surgical blood loss. Hospitals with higher transfusion rates for patients with significant surgical blood loss have lower adjusted 30-day mortality for these patients. Hospital intraoperative blood transfusion practices may be a promising surgical quality indicator.

▶ This study reviews the extensive Veterans Administration (VA) Quality Assurance database. Remarkably, more aggressive transfusion practices are associated with improved outcome. Although multiple authors have described the risk associated with transfusion, these data seem to parallel that in the trauma literature of mortality and morbidity benefit in patients with significant blood loss who are transfused aggressively.[1]

Although the data available from the VA system provide an attractive tool for studies such as this, it is important to note, as the authors discuss, that the study sample is mostly male. In addition, this is largely univariate analysis. Differences in institution practice beside blood transfusion are not accounted for. However, the extensive dataset provides 1 additional cause to consider aggressive blood product use in higher risk patients with an identified risk of significant blood loss.

Although transfusion is needless in the resuscitated patient without symptomatic anemia or critical oxygen transport compromise, we have little rigid guidance in the perioperative setting.[2-4] This work suggests a more aggressive approach to transplantation in high-risk groups with significant blood loss.

D. J. Dries, MSE, MD

References

1. Dries DJ. The contemporary role of blood products and components used in trauma resuscitation. *Scand J Trauma Resusc Emerg Med.* 2010;18:63.
2. American Society of Anesthesiologists Task Force on Perioperative Blood Transfusion and Adjuvant Therapies. Practice guidelines for perioperative blood transfusion and adjuvant therapies: an updated report by the American Society of Anesthesiologists Task Force on Perioperative Blood Transfusion and Adjuvant Therapies. *Anesthesiology.* 2006;105:198-208.
3. Practice guidelines for blood component therapy: a report by the American Society of Anesthesiologists Task Force on Blood Component Therapy. *Anesthesiology.* 1996;84:732-747.
4. Gramm J, Smith S, Gamelli RL, Dries DJ. Effect of transfusion on oxygen transport in critically ill patients. *Shock.* 1996;5:190-193.

Acute abdomen in pregnancy requiring surgical management: a 20-case series
Unal A, Sayharman SE, Ozel L, et al (Haydarpasa Numune Training and Res Hosp, Istanbul, Turkey)
Eur J Obstet Gynecol Reprod Biol 159:87-90, 2011

Objectives.—The obstetrician often has a difficult task in diagnosing and managing the acute abdomen in pregnancy. A reluctance to operate during pregnancy adds unnecessary delay, which may increase morbidity for both mother and fetus. In this study, we present our experience in pregnant patients with acute abdomen.

Study Design.—Pregnant patients with acute abdomen requiring surgical exploration were enrolled from 2007 to 2010. Demographics, gestational age, symptoms, fetal loss, preterm delivery, imaging studies, operative results, postoperative complications and histopathologic evaluations were recorded. Ultrasound (US) and magnetic resonance (MR) imaging studies were evaluated. Data analyses were performed with Microsoft Excel and statistical evaluations were done by using Student's *t*-test.

Results.—There were 20 patients with a mean age of 32 years. The rate of emergency surgery was seen to be significantly higher in the second trimester ($p < 0.05$). Most common symptoms were abdominal pain (100%) and nausea (80%). US was done in all patients while MR imaging was used in 30%. However, US findings were consistent with surgical findings in only 55%, while MR was successful in assigning the correct diagnosis in 83.3%. Appendicitis and adhesive small bowel obstruction were the most common etiologies causing acute abdomen (30% and 15%, respectively). All patients tolerated surgery well, and postoperative complications included wound infection, 10%, preterm labor, 5%, and prolonged paralytic ileus, 5%. One patient died from advanced gastric carcinoma and the only fetal death was seen in this case.

Conclusions.—Prompt diagnosis and appropriate therapy are crucial in pregnant with acute abdomen. The use of US may be limited and CT is not desirable due to fetal irradiation. MR has thus become increasingly popular in the evaluation of such patients. Adhesive small bowel obstruction should be kept in mind as an important etiology.

▶ There are several important points in this clinical series. Magnetic resonance imaging (MRI) is clearly becoming the imaging modality of choice in pregnant patients with abdominal pain. Appendicitis is still the most common cause of acute abdomen in pregnancy, in part because of the age of patients involved.[1,2] However, bowel obstruction, particularly in the setting of previous cesarean section, is also a possibility. Laparoscopy may be successfully used in the first 2 trimesters, as has been done in this series. Clinical reports suggest that laparoscopy may also be done successfully in the third trimester, though most surgeons are reluctant to use this surgical approach.

The intensivist encountering acute abdomen in pregnancy should consider standard resuscitation techniques, reassured that the likelihood of premature labor is small. MRI, if available, should be an early diagnostic modality consideration.

D. J. Dries, MSE, MD

References

1. Choi JJ, Mustafa R, Lynn ET, Divino CM. Appendectomy during pregnancy: follow-up of progeny. *J Am Coll Surg.* 2011;213:627-632.
2. Pedrosa I, Lafornara M, Pandharipande PV, Goldsmith JD, Rofsky NM. Pregnant patients suspected of having acute appendicitis: effect of MR imaging on negative laparotomy rate and appendiceal perforation rate. *Radiology.* 2009;250:749-757.

Postoperative Complications in Patients With Obstructive Sleep Apnea
Kaw R, Pasupuleti V, Walker E, et al (Cleveland Clinic, OH)
Chest 141:436-441, 2012

Background.—Unrecognized obstructive sleep apnea (OSA) is associated with unfavorable perio-perative outcomes among patients undergoing noncardiac surgery (NCS).

Methods.—The study population was chosen from 39,771 patients who underwent internal medicine preoperative assessment between January 2002 and December 2006. Patients undergoing NCS within 3 years of polysomnography (PSG) were considered for the study, whereas those < 18 years of age, with a history of upper airway surgery, or who had had minor surgery under local or regional anesthesia were excluded. Patients with an apnea-hypopnea index (AHI) ≥ 5 were defined as OSA and those with an AHI < 5 as control subjects. For adjusting baseline differences in age, sex, race, BMI, type of anesthesia, American Society of Anesthesiology class, and medical comorbidities, the patients were classified into five quintiles according to a propensity score.

Results.—Out of a total of 1,759 patients who underwent both PSG and NCS, 471 met the study criteria. Of these, 282 patients had OSA, and the remaining 189 served as control subjects. The presence of OSA was associated with a higher incidence of postoperative hypoxemia (OR, 7.9; $P = .009$), overall complications (OR, 6.9; $P = .003$), and ICU transfer (OR, 4.43; $P = .069$), and a longer hospital length of stay (LOS), (OR, 1.65; $P = .049$). Neither an AHI nor use of continuous positive airway pressure at home before surgery was associated with postoperative complications ($P = .3$ and $P = .75$, respectively) or LOS ($P = .97$ and $P = .21$, respectively).

Conclusions.—Patients with OSA are at higher risk of postoperative hypoxemia, ICU transfers, and longer hospital stay (Tables 1 and 3).

▶ Much is written about sleep apnea and its related pathophysiology.[1,2] This is an extremely popular diagnosis in the perioperative period. However, I have not seen many studies in which a large number of patients with this problem was surveyed.

This work comes from the extensive clinical experience of the Cleveland Clinic. In a retrospective review of patients screened and scored using an apnea-hypopnea index, a significant increase in resource consumption was identified. Remarkably, the incidence of complications we might expect such as atrial fibrillation, myocardial infarction, congestive heart failure, and reintubation was no different between the patients with obstructive sleep apnea (OSA) and those without.[3,4] However, the overall risk of operative complications was higher in patients with a higher apnea-hypopnea index (Table 3).

TABLE 1.—Baseline Characteristics of Patients With and Without OSA

Variables	AHI ≥ 5 (n = 282)	AHI < 5 (n = 189)	P Value	Propensity-Adjusted P Value[a]
Age, mean ± SD, y	55.9 ± 12.2	46.3 ± 14.3	< .0001	0.68
Female	156 (55.3)	152 (80.4)	< .0001	0.74
White	198 (70.2)	145 (76.7)	.12	0.63
BMI, mean ± SD, kg/m²	38.3 ± 11.1	33.0 ± 9.5	< .0001	0.78
Anesthesia				
General	225 (80.9)	152 (82.6)	.65	0.35
Others[b]	53 (19.1)	32 (17.4)		
ASA risk category 1-2	110 (39.1)	124 (66.0)	< .0001	0.42
Comorbidity ≥ 1	230 (81.8)	104 (55.0)	< .0001	0.99
Hypertension	183 (64.9)	63 (33.3)	< .0001	0.36
Diabetes	74 (26.3)	19 (10.0)	< .0001	0.29
Asthma	51 (18.1)	38 (20.1)	.6	0.24
CAD	43 (15.2)	12 (6.4)	.003	0.29
COPD	33 (11.7)	7 (3.7)	.002	0.50
Smoking history[c]	85 (30.1)	38 (20.1)	.02	0.78
Surgical risk category			.03	0.42
1: High	5 (1.8)	1 (0.5)		
2: Intermediate	250 (88.6)	155 (82.0)		
3: Low	27 (9.6)	33 (17.5)		
AHI, median (interquartile range)	27 (15-49)	2.1 (0.8-3.2)		

Data are presented as No. (%) unless indicated otherwise. AHI = apnea-hypopnea index; ASA = American Society of Anesthesiologists; CAD = coronary artery disease; OSA = obstructive sleep apnea.
[a]Propensity model includes the first seven baseline characteristics and their interactions.
[b]Spinal anesthesia, local anesthesia, epidural block, and paravertebral block.
[c]Current or previous smoker.

TABLE 3.—Postoperative Complications/Outcomes Among Patients With and Without OSA

Complications	AHI ≥ 5 (n = 282)	AHI < 5 (n = 189)	Propensity-Adjusted OR	Propensity-Adjusted *P* Value[a]
Atrial fibrillation	3 (1.1)	0	...	...
Myocardial infarction	2 (0.7)	0	...	...
Delirium	9 (3.4)	0	...	...
Congestive heart failure	3 (1.1)	0	...	...
Postoperative hypoxemia	35 (12.4)	4 (2.1)	7.9	.009
Respiratory failure[b]	14 (4.9)	4 (2.1)	4.3	...
Reintubation[b]	4 (1.4)	1 (0.5)	9.2	...
ICU transfer	19 (6.7)	3 (1.6)	5.7	.049
Any complication	40 (14.2)	5 (2.6)	6.9	.003
LOS > 2 d	135 (48.2)	53 (28.0)	1.65	.049
Overall LOS, median (interquartile range)	2 (0-4)	1 (0-3)	....	...

Data are presented as No. (% of AHI group) unless indicate otherwise. LOS = length of stay. See Table 1 legend for expansion of other abbreviation.
[a]Propensity model includes the first seven baseline characteristics and their interactions.
[b]JMP software will not compute a correct *P* value when numbers in the comparison group are small.

While multivariate analysis was used to eliminate the impact of these variables, it is important to note that patients with OSA had higher ASA risk, more frequent hypertension, diabetes, asthma, coronary artery disease, and chronic obstructive pulmonary disease (Table 1).

Limitations of this study should be noted. First, and perhaps most important, is its retrospective nature. Second, the majority of operations were of intermittent severity. It is possible that a large number of high-complexity operative procedures could have unmasked additional complications related to OSA. There was no pattern of anesthetic or type of clinical practice favored in this patient review.

I recommend this article for the survey data, carefully reviewed. Optimal care, for an underrecognized risk of surgery, remains unclear.

D. J. Dries, MSE, MD

References

1. Eckert DJ, Malhotra A. Pathophysiology of adult obstructive sleep apnea. *Proc Am Thorac Soc.* 2008;5:144-153.
2. Punjabi NM. The epidemiology of adult obstructive sleep apnea. *Proc Am Thorac Soc.* 2008;5:136-143.
3. Gozal D, Kheirandish-Gozal L. Cardiovascular morbidity in obstructive sleep apnea: oxidative stress, inflammation, and much more. *Am J Respir Crit Care Med.* 2008;177:369-375.
4. Pedrosa RP, Drager LF, Genta PR, et al. Obstructive sleep apnea is common and independently associated with atrial fibrillation in patients with hypertrophic cardiomyopathy. *Chest.* 2010;137:1078-1084.

Haloperidol prophylaxis decreases delirium incidence in elderly patients after noncardiac surgery: A randomized controlled trial

Wang W, Li H-L, Wang D-X, et al (Peking Univ First Hosp, Beijing, China; Peking Univ Third Hosp, Beijing, China)
Crit Care Med 40:731-739, 2012

Objectives.—To evaluate the efficacy and safety of short-term low-dose intravenous haloperidol for delirium prevention in critically ill elderly patients after noncardiac surgery.

Design.—Prospective, randomized, double-blind, and placebo-controlled trial in two centers.

Setting.—Intensive care units of two large tertiary teaching hospitals.

Patients.—Four hundred fifty-seven patients 65 yrs or older who were admitted to the intensive care unit after noncardiac surgery.

Intervention.—Haloperidol (0.5 mg intravenous bolus injection followed by continuous infusion at a rate of 0.1 mg/h for 12 hrs; n = 229) or placebo (n = 228) was randomly administered from intensive care unit admission.

Measures.—The primary end point was the incidence of delirium within the first 7 days after surgery. Secondary end points included time to onset of delirium, number of delirium-free days, length of intensive care unit stay, all-cause 28-day mortality, and adverse events. Delirium was assessed using the confusion assessment method for the intensive care unit.

Results.—The incidence of delirium during the first 7 days after surgery was 15.3% (35/229) in the haloperidol group and 23.2% (53/228) in the control group ($p = .031$). The mean time to onset of delirium and the mean number of delirium-free days were significantly longer (6.2 days [95% confidence interval 5.9–6.4] vs. 5.7 days [95% confidence interval 5.4–6.0]; $p = .021$; and 6.8 ± 0.5 days vs. 6.7 ± 0.8 days; $p = .027$, respectively), whereas the median length of intensive care unit stay was significantly shorter (21.3 hrs [95% confidence interval 20.3–22.2] vs. 23.0 hrs [95% confidence interval 20.9–25.1]; $p = .024$) in the haloperidol group than in the control group. There was no significant difference with regard to all-cause 28-day mortality between the two groups (0.9% [2/229] vs. 2.6% [6/228]; $p = .175$). No drug-related side effects were documented.

Conclusions.—For elderly patients admitted to intensive care unit after noncardiac surgery, short-term prophylactic administration of low-dose intravenous haloperidol significantly decreased the incidence of postoperative delirium. The therapy was well-tolerated (Fig 2).

▶ This trial examines prophylactic infusion of haloperidol, the only antipsychotic widely used to manage perioperative delirium in an elderly patient population, the majority of whom had abdominal operations and had short intensive care unit (ICU) stays (Fig 2).[1,2] Obviously, the impact of such a study might be increased if carried out in a critically ill patient population with a long ICU duration, such as severely injured patients or patients receiving multiple operative procedures. QTC interval was monitored, and the majority of patients were

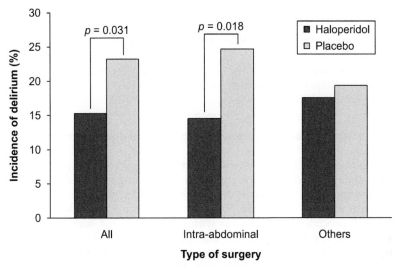

FIGURE 2.—Incidence of postoperative delirium by type of surgery. The incidence of postoperative delirium was significantly lower in the haloperidol group than in the placebo group in all patients and in those undergoing intra-abdominal surgery. (Reprinted from Wang W, Li H-L, Wang D-X, et al. Haloperidol prophylaxis decreases delirium incidence in elderly patients after noncardiac surgery: a randomized controlled trial. *Crit Care Med.* 2012;40:731-739, with permission from the Society of Critical Care Medicine and Lippincott Williams & Wilkins.)

tolerant of medication. The likelihood of switching off of haloperidol due to prolonged QTC interval was small.

The authors were careful to titrate sedation in these patients and examine this population for delirium rigorously. Not surprisingly, the incidence of delirium in this carefully studied group was lower than is typically reported. In part, I believe this is because of the relatively short ICU stay required by this patient population.[3,4] We are told nothing of pain management strategies or the type of operative procedures performed beyond body region.

The authors have gone further than any group to date to report results of a large patient group receiving prophylactic antipsychotics to reduce the incidence of perioperative delirium. The next step in such trials must include patients with longer ICU stays, a wider range of procedures, and a specific protocol for pain management.

D. J. Dries, MSE, MD

References

1. Inouye SK. Delirium in older persons. *N Engl J Med.* 2006;354:1157-1165.
2. Demeure MJ, Fain MJ. The elderly surgical patient and postoperative delirium. *J Am Coll Surg.* 2006;203:752-757.
3. Ely EW, Truman B, Shintani A, et al. Monitoring sedation status over time in ICU patients: reliability and validity of the Richmond Agitation-Sedation Scale (RASS). *JAMA.* 2003;289:2983-2991.
4. Ely EW, Inouye SK, Bernard GR, et al. Delirium in mechanically ventilated patients: validity and reliability of the confusion assessment method for the intensive care unit (CAM-ICU). *JAMA.* 2001;286:2703-2710.

Other

Rates and patterns of death after surgery in the United States, 1996 and 2006

Semel ME, Lipsitz SR, Funk LM, et al (Harvard School of Public Health, Boston, MA; Brigham and Women's Hosp, Boston, MA)

Surgery 151:171-182, 2012

Background.—Nationwide rates and patterns of death after surgery are unknown.

Methods.—Using the Nationwide Inpatient Sample, we compared deaths within 30 days of admission for patients undergoing surgery in 1996 and 2006. International Classification of Diseases codes were used to identify 2,520 procedures for analysis. We examined the inpatient 30-day death rate for all procedures, procedures with the most deaths, high-risk cardiovascular and cancer procedures, and patients who suffered a recorded complication. We used logistic regression modeling to adjust 1996 mortality rates to the age and gender distributions for patients undergoing surgery in 2006.

Results.—In 1996, there were 12,573,331 admissions with a surgical procedure (95% confidence interval [CI], 12,560,171−12,586,491) and 224,111 inpatient deaths within 30 days of admission (95% CI, 221,912−226,310). In 2006, there were 14,333,993 admissions with a surgical procedure (95% CI, 14,320,983−14,347,002) and 189,690 deaths (95% CI, 187,802−191,578). Inpatient 30-day mortality declined from 1.68% in 1996 to 1.32% in 2006 ($P < .001$). Of the 21 procedures with the most deaths in 1996, 15 had significant declines in adjusted mortality in 2006. Among these 15 procedures, 8 had significant declines in operative volume. The inpatient 30-day mortality rate for patients who suffered a complication decreased from 12.10% to 9.84% ($P < .001$).

Conclusion.—Nationwide reporting on surgical mortality suggests that the number of inpatient deaths within 30 days of surgery has declined. Additional research to determine the underlying causes for decreased mortality is warranted (Tables 3 and 5).

▶ In this article by Semel and colleagues, a national administrative database is used to identify trends in surgical procedures, complications, and mortality during the period 1996−2006. They report an increase in the overall number of surgical procedures and an overall reduction in mortality from 1.68% to 1.32% ($P < .001$). Of interest, of the 21 procedures with the most deaths in 1996, 15 demonstrated improvements in the risk-adjusted mortality rate; the overall volume of cases declined for 8 of these procedures. Also encouraging was the apparent reduction in 30-day mortality rates among patients at increased risk of poorer outcomes (Table 3B Appendix). Consistent with the established literature, such patients tended to be those in the lowest income quartile, those undergoing emergent procedures, patients with Medicare or Medicaid, and

TABLE 3B APPENDIX.—Admissions, Deaths, and the Rate of Death Within 30 Days of Admission for Inpatient Surgical Procedures, 1996 and 2006

	No. of Admissions with a Procedure		No. of Inpatient Deaths within 30 Days of Admission		Rate of Death within 30 Days of Admission		Adjusted Mortality Rate*		P Value†
	1996	2006	1996	2006	1996	2006	1996	2006	
Distribution of household income quartiles									
First	3,767,806	3,591,118	72,443	53,285	1.92%	1.48%	1.76%	—	<.001
Second	2,499,056	3,592,077	46,123	48,286	1.85%	1.34%	1.76%		<.001
Third	1,873,565	3,523,707	33,051	43,892	1.76%	1.25%	1.67%		<.001
Fourth	3,806,739	3,313,693	61,724	39,333	1.62%	1.19%	1.60%		<.001
Admission type									
Emergency	3,258,322	4,189,584	118,425	109,661	3.63%	2.62%	3.65%	—	<.001
Urgent	2,377,327	2,250,597	49,325	32,626	2.07%	1.45%	1.83%		.002
Elective	4,318,344	5,379,765	30,232	26,038	0.70%	0.48%	0.67%		<.001
Other	1,108,766	1,154,442	1,060	2,882	0.05%	0.06%	0.05%		.553
Charlson comorbidity index									
0	7,229,401	7,589,931	29,697	23,484	0.41%	0.31%	0.36%	—	.073
1	2,176,022	2,708,860	46,621	34,596	2.14%	1.28%	1.99%		<.001
2	1,512,129	1,809,170	47,915	37,679	3.17%	2.08%	3.03%		<.001
3	654,351	914,999	31,700	29,939	4.84%	3.27%	4.73%		<.001
≥4	1,001,428	1,311,034	68,178	63,992	6.81%	4.88%	6.94%		<.001
Payer									
Medicare	4,669,166	5,212,651	155,998	127,826	3.34%	2.45%	3.4%	—	<.001
Medicaid	1,489,829	2,037,761	14,841	14,752	1.00%	0.72%	1.01%		<.001
Private	5,385,109	5,877,714	41,382	34,297	0.77%	0.58%	0.72%		<.001
Self-pay	484,064	587,814	7,823	7,573	1.62%	1.29%	1.68%		.623
No charge	12,391	64,848	161	479	1.30%	0.74%	1.85%		.070
Other	480,604	531,754	3,458	4,496	0.72%	0.85%	0.71%		.149

*Death rate adjusted to the 2006 age and gender distribution.
†P value is for the age- and gender-adjusted rate of death within 30 days of admission in 1996 compared to the 2006 rate of death within 30 days of admission.

TABLE 5.—Comparing Failure to Rescue Rates Between 1996 and 2006 for Patients Who Underwent a Surgical Procedure (95% CIs)

	Complications by Coding Rules*		No. of Inpatient Deaths within 30 Days of Admission		FTR Rate (%)		Adjusted FTR Rate† (%)		P Value‡
	1996	2006	1996	2006	1996	2006	1996	2006	
Sepsis	66,102	127,203	12,750	17,846	19.29 (18.48–20.12)	14.03 (13.40–14.68)	18.69 (17.81–19.61)	—	<.001
Hospital-acquired pneumonia	169,431	204,253	14,627	14,993	8.63 (8.07–9.23)	7.34 (6.93–7.77)	8.54 (7.93–9.19)	—	<.001
DVT/PE	39,649	36,602	3,474	1,986	8.76 (8.08–9.50)	5.43 (4.90–6.00)	8.69 (7.97–9.49)	—	<.001
Shock or cardiac arrest	19,475	20,306	10,583	8,965	54.34 (52.36–56.31)	44.15 (42.07–46.26)	53.82 (51.72–56.02)	—	<.001
Upper GI bleeding	18,257	18,874	1,839	1,295	10.07 (9.04–11.21)	6.86 (6.03–7.79)	9.96 (8.82–11.24)	—	<.001
Overall	292,612	373,364	35,918	36,755	12.28 (11.76–12.80)	9.84 (9.43–10.28)	12.10 (11.54–12.68)	—	<.001

CI, Confidence interval; DVT, deep vein thrombosis; FTR, failure to rescue; GI, gastrointestinal; PE, pulmonary embolism.
Editor's Note: Please refer to original journal article for full references.
*Coding rules are from Needleman et al.[25]
†FTR adjusted to the 2006 age and gender distribution.
‡P values are for the comparison of the 2006 FTR rate to the 1996 adjusted FTR rate.

patients with the highest Charlson index. The 30-day mortality rate also declined for patients who experienced a complication (Table 5).

Although this study gives us insights into the trends of mortality, several limitations should be noted. The authors acknowledged the limitations of an administrative database and that coding for complications may not be accurate. However, they point out that their findings with regard to rates of failure to rescue are similar to other contemporary studies. Another shortcoming of the analysis is that the National Inpatient Sample does not allow for linkage across multiple admissions; thus the potential exists that patients who were discharged and died during a readmission would not be captured in this analysis.

Nevertheless, the findings from this study suggest that perhaps care has improved over the decade covered. It remains unclear, however, what changes contributed to this difference. Insights into the contributors to the lower rates and improved management of patients with complications will be important to elucidate in future studies. This is the information that we need to further drive improvements in outcomes for surgical patients.

E. A. Martinez, MD, MHS

Physical Fitness in People After Burn Injury: A Systematic Review
Disseldorp LM, Nieuwenhuis MK, Van Baar ME, et al (Univ of Groningen, The Netherlands; Martini Hosp, Groningen, The Netherlands; Maasstad Hosp, Rotterdam, The Netherlands)
Arch Phys Med Rehabil 92:1501-1510, 2011

Objective.—To gain insight into the physical fitness of people after burn injury compared with healthy subjects, and to present an overview of the effectiveness of exercise training programs in improving physical fitness in people after burn injury.

Data Sources.—Electronic databases EMBASE, PubMed, and Web of Science were searched for relevant publications. Additionally, references from retrieved publications were checked.

Study Selection.—The review includes studies that provide quantitative data from objective measures of physical fitness of both the intervention group and the control group.

Data Extraction.—Characteristics of each study such as study design, institution, and intervention are reported, as well as mean ages and burn sizes of the subjects. Results are divided into 5 components of physical fitness—muscular strength, muscular endurance, body composition, cardiorespiratory endurance, and flexibility—and reported for each component separately.

Data Synthesis.—Eleven studies met the inclusion criteria, and their methodological quality was assessed using the PEDro score and a modified Sackett scale. Six studies were used for the comparison of physical fitness in burned and nonburned subjects, and 9 studies for evaluating the effectiveness of exercise training programs.

Conclusions.—Physical fitness is affected in people with extensive burns, and exercise training programs can bring on relevant improvements in all components. However, because of the great similarities in the subjects and protocols used in the included studies, the current knowledge is incomplete. Future research should include people of all ages with a broad range of burn sizes, for both short-term and long-term outcomes.

▶ The authors evaluated English-language scholarly works to determine physical fitness in people after burn injury. Using criteria designed to eliminate any studies that did not have internal control groups, the authors were left with only 11 studies from 3 burn centers. One center contributed 9 of the 11 studies, and that center evaluated the same patient population in all their studies: young children with burns greater than 40% total body surface area burned. In testing strength and flexibility, the knee joint in the dominant leg was always studied. Although the title of this work is intriguing, the data available to the authors are monochromatic. It really represents the data from the Galveston Shriner's Burn Hospital and their evaluation and outcomes of severely burned children. Most burned children in the United States are not treated at a Shriner's Hospital nor do they have massive burn injuries. The findings represented here are not generalizable to the vast majority of burn survivors in North America. The paucity of data relevant to most burn care practitioners should encourage the authors or other interested parties to use a venue such as the European Burns Association or the Burn Science Advisory Panel of the American Burn Association to investigate the question. These data are lacking but could change the approach to postdischarge outpatient burn care.

B. A. Latenser, MD, FACS

Outcomes and Predictors in Burn Rehabilitation
Tan W-H, Goldstein R, Gerrard P, et al (Spaulding Rehabilitation Hosp, Boston, MA)
J Burn Care Res 33:110-117, 2012

Advances in burn care in recent decades have resulted in a growing population of burn survivors and an increased need for inpatient rehabilitation. Burn survivors who require inpatient rehabilitation typically experience severe and complicated injuries. The purpose of this study is to examine burn rehabilitation outcomes and their predictor variables. Data are obtained from the Uniform Data System for Medical Rehabilitation from 2002 to 2007. Inclusion criterion is primary diagnosis of burn injury. Predictor variables include demographic, medical, and facility data. Outcome measures are length of stay efficiency, FIM® gain, community discharge, and FIM® discharge of at least 78. Linear and logistic regression analyses are used to determine significant predictors of outcomes. There are 2920 patients who meet inclusion criteria. The mean age of the population is 51 years, 33% of the population is female, 73% is Caucasian, and 40%

are married. The median TBSA decile is 20 to 29%. The population exhibits a mean FIM® gain of 28 and length of stay efficiency of 2.1. A majority of the population is discharged to the community (76%) and has a FIM® discharge of at least 78 (81%). Significant predictors of outcomes in burn rehabilitation include age, FIM® admission, onset days, employment status, and marital status. Inpatient rehabilitation is critical to community reintegration of burn survivors. Survivors who are young, married, employed, and higher functioning at the time of admission to rehabilitation demonstrate the best outcomes. This research will help assess the rehabilitation potential of burn survivors and inform resource allocation.

▶ Of the 9000 burn patients discharged from an in-patient rehabilitation hospital after an acute injury, only about one third met study entry criteria: age greater than 18 years and diagnosis of burn injury. The patient population seems to be representative of the adult patient population admitted to North American burn centers. The most intriguing finding is the relatively small burn size (20% to 29% total body surface area [TBSA] burned) compared to the post-injury day (day 45) when the patients are admitted to a rehabilitation facility. Classical dogma is that each 1% of TBSA will require 1 hospital day, and that this measure is linearly related to TBSA. In the past decade, we have come to appreciate that for burns less than 40% TBSA, that length of stay may not be required. Smoothly running burn centers may demonstrate 0.6 days per percentage of TBSA burned for smaller burns, but greater than 50% TBSA burns may require 1.5 to 2.0 days per percentage of TBSA burned before being ready for discharge to an in-patient rehabilitation facility. These authors found 1.55 to 2.25 days per percentage of TBSA burned required prior to inpatient rehabilitation, longer than the anticipated 1 day for every percentage of TBSA, as found in a recent review of 52 000 patients in the American Burn Association's National Burn Repository.[1] The obvious question now becomes: What makes these patients different from the average burn patient? It is intriguing to speculate that perhaps these patients are the ones with more comorbidities, those who have difficult-to-heal wounds, with all the reasons behind that (obesity, diabetes, smoking, peripheral vascular disease, malnutrition, being immunocompromised), inhalation injury, electrical injury, or psychiatric diagnoses. Some studies have indicated that patients injured on the job will require longer to return to work than those injured in their leisure time with the same injury. It is intriguing to speculate on, and would be interesting to know, the impact of some of these data based on these findings.

B. A. Latenser, MD, FACS

Reference

1. Johnson LS, Shupp JW, Pavlovich AR, Pezzullo JC, Jeng JC, Jordan MH. Hospital length of stay—does 1% TBSA really equal 1 day? *J Burn Care Res.* 2011;32: 13-19.

6 Sepsis/Septic Shock

Prognostic Value of Incremental Lactate Elevations in Emergency Department Patients With Suspected Infection
Puskarich MA, Kline JA, Summers RL, et al (Univ of Mississippi Med Ctr, Jackson; Carolinas Med Ctr, Charlotte, NC)
Acad Emerg Med 19:983-985, 2012

Objectives.—Previous studies have confirmed the prognostic significance of lactate concentrations categorized into groups (low, intermediate, high) among emergency department (ED) patients with suspected infection. Although the relationship between lactate concentrations categorized into groups and mortality appears to be linear, the relationship between lactate as a continuous measurement and mortality is uncertain. This study sought to evaluate the association between blood lactate concentrations along an incremental continuum up to a maximum value of 20 mmol/L and mortality.

Methods.—This was a retrospective cohort analysis of adult ED patients with suspected infection from a large urban ED during 2007—2010. Inclusion criteria were suspected infection evidenced by administration of antibiotics in the ED and measurement of whole blood lactate in the ED. The primary outcome was in-hospital mortality. Logistic and polynomial regression were used to model the relationship between lactate concentration and mortality.

Results.—A total of 2,596 patients met inclusion criteria and were analyzed. The initial median lactate concentration was 2.1 mmol/L (interquartile range [IQR] = 1.3 to 3.3 mmol/L) and the overall mortality rate was 14.4%. In the cohort, 459 patients (17.6%) had initial lactate levels > 4 mmol/L. Mortality continued to rise across the continuum of incremental elevations, from 6% for lactate < 1.0 mmol/L up to 39% for lactate 19—20 mmol/L. Polynomial regression analysis showed a strong curvilinear correlation between lactate and mortality ($R = 0.72, p < 0.0001$).

Conclusions.—In ED patients with suspected infection, we found a curvilinear relationship between incremental elevations in lactate concentration and mortality. These data support the use of lactate as a continuous variable rather than a categorical variable for prognostic purposes.

▶ Previous studies have shown that increased serum lactate correlates with increased mortality. However, these studies all used categorical lactates (eg, normal, low, intermediate, high). This study questioned whether lactate as a continuous variable (it is after all) correlated with mortality in patients with suspected infection. Patients admitted to the hospital from the emergency department were included if they had suspected infection (antibiotics given in the emergency department) and a lactate measurement obtained. More than 2500 patients were enrolled and they seemed to represent a typical sepsis cohort based on length of stay, comorbidities, and mortality. The authors found definite correlations between incremental increases of lactate and incremental increases in mortality. They developed a regression model/equation that fit their data quite well. In other words, with a given lactate, their equation could predict mortality. This study was well done by a group of researchers with a good track record. Pay attention to lactate in patients with suspected infection: the higher it is, the more likely the patient in front of you is going to die.

M. D. Zwank, MD

Can changes in arterial pressure be used to detect changes in cardiac index during fluid challenge in patients with septic shock?
Pierrakos C, Velissaris D, Scolletta S, et al (Erasme Univ Hosp, Brussels, Belgium)
Intensive Care Med 38:422-428, 2012

Purpose.—Response to fluid challenge is often defined as an increase in cardiac index (CI) of more than 10–15%. However, in clinical practice CI values are often not available. We evaluated whether changes in mean arterial pressure (MAP) correlate with changes in CI after fluid challenge in patients with septic shock.

Methods.—This was an observational study in which we reviewed prospectively collected data from 51 septic shock patients in whom complete hemodynamic measurements had been obtained before and after a fluid challenge with 1,000 ml crystalloid (Hartman's solution) or 500 ml colloid (hydroxyethyl starch 6%). CI was measured using thermodilution. Patients were divided into two groups (responders and nonresponders) according to their change in CI (responders: %CI > 10%) after the fluid challenge. Statistical analysis was performed using a two-way analysis of variance test followed by a Student's t test with adjustment for multiple comparisons. Pearson's correlation and receiver operating characteristic curve analysis were also used.

Results.—Mean patient age was 67 ± 17 years and mean Sequential Organ Failure Assessment (SOFA) upon admittance to the intensive care unit was 10 ± 3. In the 25 responders, MAP increased from 69 ± 9 to 77 ± 9 mmHg, pulse pressure (PP) increased from 59 ± 15 to 67 ± 16, and CI increased from 2.8 ± 0.8 to 3.4 ± 0.9 L/min/m^2 (all $p < 0.001$). There were no significant correlations between the changes in MAP, PP, and CI.

Conclusions.—Changes in MAP do not reliably track changes in CI after fluid challenge in patients with septic shock and, consequently, should be interpreted carefully when evaluating the response to fluid challenge in such patients.

▶ Accurate, dynamic markers of fluid responsiveness in shock are highly sought after but often remain illusive. In a prospective observational study, Pierrakos et al assessed whether changes in arterial pressure could predict fluid responsiveness of 51 septic shock patients by determining the percentage of change in cardiac index (CI) via the thermodilution method. Half of the patients were determined to be fluid responders as defined by a greater than 10% increase in CI after fluid challenge with 1 L crystalloid or 500 mL colloid bolus. While pulse pressure and mean arterial pressure (MAP) significantly increased in responders when challenged with a fluid bolus, there was no significant correlation with CI. The lack of correlation between changes in arterial pressure and cardiac index should caution the intensivist that an increase in MAP after volume expansion does not necessarily improve hemodynamic status. In other words, augmentation of MAP with a fluid challenge does not accurately identify fluid responsiveness in septic shock patients.

E. Damuth, MD

Multiplex polymerase chain reaction pathogen detection in patients with suspected septicemia after trauma, emergency, and burn surgery

Tran NK, Wisner DH, Albertson TE, et al (Univ of California, Davis)
Surgery 151:456-463, 2012

Background.—The goal of this study is to determine the clinical value of multiplex polymerase chain reaction (PCR) study for enhancing pathogen detection in patients with suspected septicemia after trauma, emergency, and burn surgery. PCR-based pathogen detection quickly reveals occult bloodstream infections in these high-risk patients and may accelerate the initiation of targeted antimicrobial therapy.

Methods.—We conducted a prospective observational study comparing results for 30 trauma and emergency surgery patients to 20 burn patients. Whole-blood samples collected with routine blood cultures (BCs) were tested using a new multiplex, PCR-based, pathogen detection system. PCR results were compared to culture data.

Results.—PCR detected rapidly more pathogens than culture methods. Acute Physiology and Chronic Health Evaluation II (APACHE II), Sequential Organ Failure Assessment (SOFA), and Multiple Organ Dysfunction (MODS) scores were greater in PCR-positive versus PCR-negative trauma and emergency surgery patients ($P \leq .033$). Negative PCR results (odds ratio, 0.194; 95% confidence interval, 0.045−0.840; $P = .028$) acted as an independent predictor of survival for the combined surgical patient population.

Conclusion.—PCR detected the presence of pathogens more frequently than blood culture. These PCR results were reported faster than blood culture results. Severity scores were significantly greater in PCR-positive trauma and emergency surgery patients. The lack of pathogen DNA as determined by PCR served as a significant predictor of survival in the combined patient population. PCR testing independent of traditional prompts for culturing may have clinical value in burn patients. These results warrant further investigation through interventional trials.

▶ Trauma, emergency, and burn surgery patients are at a particularly high risk of septicemia secondary to their disease states. As a result, immediate empiric antibiotic treatment is necessary to improve mortality.[1] However, with increasing resistant pathogens, aggressive de-escalation is important as well.

In this prospective, observational study, patients displaying signs and symptoms of sepsis had blood cultures and blood samples run through polymerase chain reaction (PCR). Arbitrated case reviews were performed to determine if appropriate antibiotic regimens were dispensed, given first blood culture results alone and then PCR results. PCR had a markedly increased turnaround time (5.9 h vs 25.3 h). Additionally, PCR was positive in 11 cases, whereas blood cultures were either negative or failed to identify pathogen species. Arbitrated case review found antimicrobial therapy was inadequate relative to PCR results in 29% PCR-positive patients. PCR was found to have more pathogen detection events, even in serial samples while patients were on concurrent antimicrobial therapy. A negative PCR was found to be an independent predictor of survival.

While this practice is cost prohibitive and not approved by the US Food and Drug Administration, PCR can be a very powerful tool in early pathogen detection in sepsis. It can also serve as a predictor for mortality. According to the authors, it does have its limitations: it is dependent on the assay to detect specific pathogens, genetic polymorphisms, and whole blood sample matrix effects.

C. Cho, MD

S. Zanotti, MD

Reference

1. MacArthur RD, Miller M, Albertson T, et al. Adequacy of early empiric antibiotic treatment and survival in severe sepsis: experience from the MONARCS trial. *Clin Infect Dis*. 2004;38:284-288.

Advances in Mesenchymal Stem Cell Research in Sepsis
Wannemuehler TJ, Manukyan MC, Brewster BD, et al (Indiana Univ School of Medicine, Indianapolis)
J Surg Res 173:113-126, 2012

Background.—Sepsis remains a source of morbidity and mortality in the postoperative patient despite appropriate resuscitative and antimicrobial approaches. Recent research has focused upon additional interventions such as exogenous cell-based therapy. Mesenchymal stem cells (MSCs) exhibit multiple beneficial properties through their capacity for homing, attenuating the inflammatory response, modulating immune cells, and promoting tissue healing. Recent animal trials have provided evidence that MSCs may be useful therapeutic adjuncts.

Materials and Methods.—A directed search of recent medical literature was performed utilizing PubMed to examine the pathophysiology of sepsis, mechanisms of mesenchymal stem cell interaction with host cells, sepsis animal models, and recent trials utilizing stem cells in sepsis.

Results.—MSCs continue to show promise in the treatment of sepsis by their intrinsic ability to home to injured tissue, secrete paracrine signals to limit systemic and local inflammation, decrease apoptosis in threatened tissues, stimulate neoangiogenesis, activate resident stem cells, beneficially modulate immune cells, and exhibit direct antimicrobial activity. These effects are associated with reduced organ dysfunction and improved survival in animal models.

Conclusion.—Research utilizing animal models of sepsis has provided a greater understanding of the beneficial properties of MSCs. Their capacity to home to sites of injury and use paracrine mechanisms to change the local environment to ultimately improve organ function and survival make MSCs attractive in the treatment of sepsis. Future studies are needed to further evaluate the complex interactions between MSCs and host tissues.

▶ Sepsis holds a mortality rate of 28.6% and costs $16.7 billion nationally. As such, immediate, effective treatment for a septic patient is vital. Interest in mesenchymal stem cells (derived from bone marrow, adipose, placenta, and umbilical cord) has been applied in the treatment of sepsis for its multiple abilities, which is reviewed in this article.

Mesenchymal stem cells have the ability to home to injured tissues, partly from interacting with host cytokines. They also have paracrine signaling effects to promote tissue regeneration, prevent tissue loss, and improve tissue function via its anti-inflammatory, antiapoptotic, nonangiogenic activation of resident stem cell and immunomodulatory capabilities. Although in vivo studies mesenchymal cells also had antimicrobial effects, vitro models revealed they could not. Thus, they likely require host cell stimulation and signaling to do so. In animal studies, stem cell treatment of sepsis has shown reduced levels of proinflammatory cytokines (interleukin-1, tumor necrosis factor-α, interleukin-6), decreased organ injury, and increased organ function. Additionally, stem cells can improve bacterial clearance through increased macrophage phagocytic activity. More importantly, septic animals treated with stem cells had a significantly improved survival rate.

In conclusion, mesenchymal stem cells administration is a promising treatment for sepsis through its multiple effects on the host's immune system, organ tissue, and function. Although there are no clinical trials as of yet, continued research in the animal model is crucial.

S. Zanotti, MD

A multicenter trial to compare blood culture with polymerase chain reaction in severe human sepsis

Bloos F, Hinder F, Becker K, et al (Univ Hosp Jena, Germany; Univ Hosp Münster, Germany)
Intensive Care Med 36:241-247, 2010

Objective.—To assess the presence of microbial DNA in the blood by polymerase chain reaction (PCR) and its association with disease severity and markers of inflammation in severe sepsis and to compare the performance of PCR with blood culture (BC).

Design.—Prospective multicentric controlled observational study.

Setting.—Three surgical intensive care units in university centers and large teaching hospitals.

Patients.—One hundred forty-two patients with severe sepsis and 63 surgical controls.

Interventions.—Presence of microbial DNA was assessed by multiplex PCR upon enrollment, and each time a BC was obtained.

Measurements and Main Results.—Controls had both approximately 4% positive PCRs and BCs. In severe sepsis, 34.7% of PCRs were positive compared to 16.5% of BCs ($P < 0.001$). Consistently, 70.3% of BCs had a corresponding PCR result, while only 21.4% of PCR results were confirmed by BC. Compared to patients with negative PCRs at enrollment, those testing positive had higher organ dysfunction scores [SOFA, median (25th–75th percentile) 12 (7–15) vs. 9 (7–11); $P = 0.023$] and a trend toward higher mortality (PCR negative 25.3%; PCR positive 39.1%; $P = 0.115$).

Conclusions.—In septic patients, concordance between BC and PCR is moderate. However, PCR-based pathogen detection correlated with disease severity even if the BC remained negative, suggesting that presence of microbial DNA in the bloodstream is a significant event. The clinical utility to facilitate treatment decisions warrants investigation.

▶ Sepsis is one of the most important causes of morbidity and mortality in critically ill patients. The administration of early appropriate antibiotics is a cornerstone of sepsis therapy. Studies have shown that mortality is increased with delays in initiating antibiotics that cover the culprit pathogen in sepsis. This has led to an increase in the use of initial empiric antibiotic regimens with broad coverage. Without proper de-escalation, the increased use of broad-spectrum antibiotics will lead to increased antibiotic resistance. Unfortunately, negative blood cultures are a common occurrence in sepsis. This makes modification of antibiotic regimes and diagnosis of infection difficult.

Many experts have proposed that culture-independent molecular biology–based diagnostic tests, such as real-time polymerase chain reaction (PCR), could overcome some of the limitations cultures present and be more useful in the management of sepsis. In this intriguing prospective multicenter study, the authors assessed the diagnostic utility of culture-independent PCR-based detection of pathogens compared with blood cultures (BC) in sepsis. The study basically found that concordance between BC and PCR was moderate in septic patients. There were more positive PCRs with negative BCs. However, negative PCRs were still common, making it unlikely that at present a negative PCR could be used to rule out infection and/or stop antibiotics. An additional finding of great interest was the correlation of a positive PCR (presence of microbial DNA in the bloodstream) with increased severity and poor outcomes. This finding suggests that the presence of bacteria DNA (even with negative blood cultures) is an important clinical finding and may warrant further investigation regarding its value to guide therapeutic interventions.

S. Zanotti, MD

Diagnostic value of positron emission tomography combined with computed tomography for evaluating patients with septic shock of unknown origin
Kluge S, Braune S, Nierhaus A, et al (Univ Med Ctr Hamburg-Eppendorf, Germany)
J Crit Care 27:316.e1-316.e7, 2012

Purpose.—[18]F-fluorodeoxyglucose (FDG) positron emission tomography (PET) combined with computed tomography (CT) is a promising new tool for the identification of infectious foci. The aim of our work was to evaluate the diagnostic value of FDG-PET/CT in critically ill patients with septic shock of unknown origin.

Methods.—We performed a single-center, 6-year retrospective evaluation of the value of FDG-PET/CT in critically ill patients with severe sepsis or septic shock of unknown origin.

Results.—Eighteen patients underwent FDG-PET/CT. Microbiological tests (blood culture, urine, and respiratory secretions), chest x-rays, CT scans, and transesophageal echocardiography were performed on all patients before FDG-PET/CT scanning. Pathologic FDG accumulation could be demonstrated in 14 of 18 FDG-PET/CT scans. On a per-patient basis, 11 were "true positive," 3 were "false positive," 4 were true negative, and there were no false negatives. In 6 cases, the results of the PET/CT scan had direct therapeutic consequences (surgery, 2; pacemaker removal, 2; initiation of antibiotic therapy, 1; and prolonged antibiotic therapy, 1); 12 (66%) of the 18 patients survived to hospital discharge.

Conclusions.—The FDG-PET/CT is a valuable tool for the localization of infectious foci in critically ill patients with severe sepsis/septic shock in whom conventional diagnostic methods fail to detect these foci. Prospective studies with more patients are warranted to further evaluate the diagnostic accuracy and feasibility of this diagnostic tool in critically ill patients with severe sepsis.

▶ Positron emission tomography/computed tomography (PET/CT) is well established in the arena of oncologic imaging and evaluation of chronic infections. Its potential role in evaluating acute infections and patients with severe sepsis and septic shock is undetermined. Simons et al (2010) previously investigated the role of PET/CT in mechanically ventilated intensive care unit (ICU) patients.[1] This study presents a novel application of an established modality to evaluate for acute infections in the setting of severe sepsis and septic shock. This was a retrospective observational study in all adult ICU patients over a 6-year period with severe sepsis or septic shock with an unknown source who underwent PET/CT evaluation. The results of PET/CT were compared with a final diagnosis that was made using all clinical information excluding the PET/CT findings. In 5 cases (27%), PET/CT was essential for diagnosis in the following cases: pseudomembranous colitis, infected bypass graft, infected inferior vena cava thrombus, infected pacemaker, and cervical abscess. In 6 cases (33%), PET/CT results altered patient management. The survival rate for this group of patients was 66%. Most of the patients in this study were evaluated for persistent fever or suspected septic emboli. This study did not specify severe sepsis or septic shock as indications. In 14% of patients, the PET/CT results altered management. The limitations of the current study were the retrospective design and the small study population. A major drawback of PET/CT in the critical care setting is the time required for the exam, the expense, and availability as an inpatient. PET/CT evaluation may serve as an important adjunct for diagnosis of sources of severe sepsis or septic shock when other modalities (clinical, microbiologic, and anatomic imaging) have proven unrevealing. Further validation of this modality in sepsis in a prospective randomized trial would determine if a survival benefit exists.

A. F. Miller, MD

S. Zanotti, MD

Reference

1. Simons KS, Pickkers P, Bleeker-Rovers CP, Oyen WJ, van der Hoeven JG. F-18-fluorodeoxyglucose positron emission tomography combined with CT in critically ill patients with suspected infection. *Intensive Care Med.* 2010;36:504-511.

Early goal-directed therapy (EGDT) for severe sepsis/septic shock: which components of treatment are more difficult to implement in a community-based emergency department?
O'Neill R, Morales J, Jule M (Genesys Regional Med Ctr, Grand Blanc, MI)
J Emerg Med 42:503-510, 2012

Background.—Early goal-directed therapy (EGDT) has been shown to reduce mortality in patients with severe sepsis/septic shock, however, implementation of this protocol in the emergency department (ED) is sometimes difficult.

Objectives.—We evaluated our sepsis protocol to determine which EGDT elements were more difficult to implement in our community-based ED.

Methods.—This was a non-concurrent cohort study of adult patients entered into a sepsis protocol at a single community hospital from July 2008 to March 2009. Charts were reviewed for the following process measures: a predefined crystalloid bolus, antibiotic administration, central venous catheter insertion, central venous pressure measurement, arterial line insertion, vasopressor utilization, central venous oxygen saturation measurement, and use of a standardized order set. We also compared the individual component adherence with survival to hospital discharge.

Results.—A total of 98 patients presented over a 9-month period. Measures with the highest adherence were vasopressor administration (79%; 95% confidence interval [CI] 69—89%) and antibiotic use (78%; 95% CI 68—85%). Measures with the lowest adherence included arterial line placement (42%; 95% CI 32—52%), central venous pressure measurement (27%; 95% CI 18—36%), and central venous oxygen saturation measurement (15%; 95% CI 7—23%). Fifty-seven patients survived to hospital discharge (Mortality: 33%). The only element of EDGT to demonstrate a statistical significance in patients surviving to hospital discharge was the crystalloid bolus (79% vs. 46%) (respiratory rate [RR] = 1.76, 95% CI 1.11—2.58).

Conclusion.—In our community hospital, arterial line placement, central venous pressure measurement, and central venous oxygen saturation measurement were the most difficult elements of EGDT to implement. Patients who survived to hospital discharge were more likely to receive the crystalloid bolus.

▶ It has been more than a decade since the publication of the landmark early goal-directed therapy (EGDT) study by Rivers et al.[1] This study showed a significant improvement in mortality in patients with severe sepsis-induced hypoperfusion treated with EGDT. Despite the questions that remain unanswered and concerns with specific aspects of the trial, EGDT has been widely recommended by various guidelines, such as the Surviving Sepsis Guidelines.[2] In this study, the investigators sought to evaluate the adherence of specific elements of the EGDT protocol in a community emergency department (ED). The authors report that arterial line placement, central venous pressure measurement, and central venous oxygen saturation measurement were the most difficult elements of EGDT to implement. The authors also report that the patients who survived to hospital discharge were more likely to receive the crystalloid bolus (2 L in the first hour) as prescribed in their protocol. Although this study does not provide answers to which aspects of EGDT work in decreasing survival, it does shed important light on some of the barriers that still persist in the implementation of these protocols in community EDs. Currently, there are 3 large multicenter studies evaluating different aspects of EGDT and resuscitation of patients with severe sepsis/septic shock. The results of these ongoing trials may help define the best way forward.

S. Zanotti, MD

References

1. Rivers E, Nguyen B, Havstad S, et al. Early goal-directed therapy in the treatment of severe sepsis and septic shock. *N Engl J Med.* 2001;345:1368-1377.
2. Dellinger RP, Levy MM, Carlet JM, et al. Surviving Sepsis Campaign: international guidelines for management of severe sepsis and septic shock: 2008. *Crit Care Med.* 2008;36:296-327.

Antibiotic strategies in severe nosocomial sepsis: Why do we not de-escalate more often?
Heenen S, Jacobs F, Vincent J-L (Erasme Hosp, Brussels, Belgium)
Crit Care Med 40:1404-1409, 2012

Objectives.—To assess the use of antibiotic de-escalation in patients with hospital-acquired severe sepsis in an academic setting.

Design.—We reviewed all episodes of severe sepsis treated over a 1-yr period in the department of intensive care. Antimicrobial therapy was considered as appropriate when the antimicrobial had in vitro activity against the causative microorganisms. According to the therapeutic strategy in the 5 days after the start of antimicrobial therapy, we classified patients into four groups: de-escalation (interruption of an antimicrobial agent or change of antibiotic to one with a narrower spectrum); no change in antibiotherapy; escalation (addition of a new antimicrobial agent or change in antibiotic to one with a broader spectrum); and mixed changes.

Setting.—A 35-bed medico-surgical intensive care department in which antibiotic strategies are reviewed by infectious disease specialists three times per week.

Patients.—One hundred sixty-nine patients with 216 episodes of severe sepsis attributable to a hospital-acquired infection who required broad-spectrum β-lactam antibiotics alone or in association with other anti-infectious agents.

Measurements and Main Results.—The major sources of infection were the lungs (44%) and abdomen (38%). Microbiological data were available in 167 of the 216 episodes (77%). Initial antimicrobial therapy was inappropriate in 27 episodes (16% of culture-positive episodes). De-escalation was applied in 93 episodes (43%), escalation was applied in 22 episodes (10%), mixed changes were applied in 24 (11%) episodes, and there was no change in empirical antibiotic therapy in 77 (36%) episodes. In these 77 episodes, the reasons given for maintaining the initial antimicrobial therapy included the sensitivity pattern of the causative organisms and previous antibiotic therapy. The number of episodes when the chance to de-escalate may have been missed was small (4 episodes [5%]).

Conclusion.—Even in a highly focused environment with close collaboration among intensivists and infectious disease specialists, de-escalation may actually be possible in <50% of cases.

▶ Early appropriate antibiotics are a cornerstone in the treatment of patients with severe sepsis and septic shock. Studies have found that both delays in initiation and the use of inappropriate empiric antibiotics (defined as antibiotics that do not cover organisms recovered later in cultures) are associated with increased morbidity and mortality. This finding has led to recommendations supporting the use of broad-spectrum antibiotics as the initial regimen in critically ill patients with the goal of assuring appropriate coverage. However, utilization of broad-spectrum antibiotics can also increase antibiotic pressure and facilitate the emergence of resistant bacteria, already a significant problem in most intensive care units (ICUs). Rapid de-escalation is recommended to decrease the risk for increased antibiotic resistance. In this very interesting study, the authors assessed how de-escalation is applied in patients with hospital-acquired severe sepsis in an academic ICU. In this study, most infections were in the lungs and abdomen. De-escalation was applied in 43% of the cases, and initial antibiotics were inappropriate in 16% of culture-positive cases. De-escalation was not associated with increased morbidity and mortality. It is important to recognize that the results of this study may not be applicable to ICUs with different patterns of antibiotic resistance or different set-ups. However, in an academic environment with close collaboration with infection diseases, de-escalation was possible in less than 50% of cases of severe nosocomial sepsis. Clinicians can learn from this study and continue to push for de-escalation as soon as possible.

S. Zanotti, MD

Etomidate is associated with mortality and adrenal insufficiency in sepsis: A meta-analysis
Chan CM, Mitchell AL, Shorr AF (Washington Hosp Ctr, DC; Univ of Maryland Med Ctr, Baltimore)
Crit Care Med 40:2945-2953, 2012

Objective.—To evaluate the effects of single-dose etomidate on the adrenal axis and mortality in patients with severe sepsis and septic shock.

Design.—A systematic review of randomized controlled trials and observational studies with meta-analysis.

Setting.—Literature search of EMBASE, Medline, Cochrane Database, and Evidence-Based Medical Reviews.

Subjects.—Sepsis patients who received etomidate for rapid sequence intubation.

Interventions.—None.

Measurements and Main Results.—We conducted a systematic review of randomized controlled trials and observational studies with meta-analysis assessing the effects of etomidate on adrenal insufficiency and all-cause mortality published between January 1950 and February 2012. We only

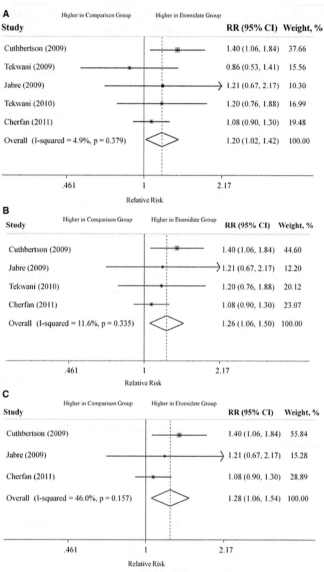

FIGURE 2.—*A*, Pooled relative risks (*RRs*) for all-cause mortality: all studies. *B*, Pooled RR for mortality: randomized controlled trials. *C*, Pooled RR for mortality: 28-day mortality rates only. *CI*, confidence interval. (Reprinted from Chan CM, Mitchell AL, Shorr AF. Etomidate is associated with mortality and adrenal insufficiency in sepsis: a meta-analysis. *Crit Care Med.* 2012;40:2945-2953, with permission from the Society of Critical Care Medicine and Lippincott Williams and Wilkins.)

examined studies including septic patients. All-cause mortality served as our primary end point, whereas the prevalence of adrenal insufficiency was our secondary end point. Adrenal insufficiency was determined using a cosyntropin stimulation test in all studies. We used a random effects model for analysis; heterogeneity was assessed with the I^2 statistic. Publication bias was evaluated with Begg's test. Five studies were identified that assessed mortality in those who received etomidate. A total of 865 subjects were included. Subjects who received etomidate were more likely to die (pooled relative risk 1.20; 95% confidence interval 1.02−1.42; Q statistic, 4.20; I^2 statistic, 4.9%). Seven studies addressed the development of adrenal suppression associated with the administration of etomidate; 1,303 subjects were included. Etomidate administration increased the likelihood of developing adrenal insufficiency (pooled relative risk 1.33; 95% confidence interval 1.22−1.46; Q statistic, 10.7; I2 statistic, 43.9%).

Conclusions.—Administration of etomidate for rapid sequence intubation is associated with higher rates of adrenal insufficiency and mortality in patients with sepsis (Fig 2).

▶ Etomidate was initially developed as a continuous infusion drug for sedation. It was later shown to cause prolonged adrenal insufficiency and its use for prolonged sedation was abandoned. However, some of its characteristics, mainly its rapid onset/offset of action and its favorable hemodynamic profile, made it an attractive candidate for rapid sequence intubation. In this context, clinicians started using a single dose of etomidate as part of their rapid sequence intubation. Concerns of the potential effects on adrenal function lead to several studies that once again documented suppression of adrenal function with administration of etomidate. The potential perils of this effect were particularly concerning in patients with severe sepsis and septic shock because of their increased risk of adrenal dysfunction from their underlying disease. The lack of studies showing a clear association between etomidate administration to increased mortality in sepsis led to an ongoing debate on the topic. This systematic review and meta-analysis evaluated the hypothesis that the use of etomidate during rapid sequence intubation increases the risk of death and induces adrenal insufficiency in patients with sepsis. The study showed a clear association between the administration of a single dose of etomidate and increased mortality (Fig 2). It also showed that etomidate effectively produces adrenal insufficiency as measured by cosyntropin stimulation testing in patients with sepsis. The results of this study should serve as a strong indicator of the need for clinicians to carefully weigh the benefits/risks of using etomidate as a part of their rapid sequence intubation protocol. Furthermore, it serves as a great basis for a randomized controlled study to further examine this issue.

S. Zanotti, MD

Severe Sepsis and Septic Shock in Pregnancy

Barton JR, Sibai BM (Central Baptist Hosp, Lexington, KY; Univ of Texas Health Science Ctr, Houston)
Obstet Gynecol 120:689-706, 2012

Pregnancies complicated by severe sepsis and septic shock are associated with increased rates of preterm labor, fetal infection, and preterm delivery. Sepsis onset in pregnancy can be insidious, and patients may appear deceptively well before rapidly deteriorating with the development of septic shock, multiple organ dysfunction syndrome, or death. The outcome and survivability in severe sepsis and septic shock in pregnancy are improved with early detection, prompt recognition of the source of infection, and targeted therapy. This improvement can be achieved by formulating a stepwise approach that consists of early provision of time-sensitive interventions such as: aggressive hydration (20 mL/kg of normal saline over the first hour), initiation of appropriate empiric intravenous antibiotics (gentamicin, clindamycin, and penicillin) within 1 hour of diagnosis, central hemodynamic monitoring, and the involvement of infectious disease specialists and critical care specialists familiar with the physiologic changes in pregnancy. Thorough physical examination and imaging techniques or empiric exploratory laparotomy are suggested to identify the septic source. Even with appropriate antibiotic therapy, patients may continue to deteriorate unless septic foci (ie, abscess, necrotic tissue) are surgically excised. The decision for delivery in the setting of antepartum severe sepsis or septic shock can be challenging but must be based on gestational age, maternal status, and fetal status. The natural inclination is to proceed with emergent delivery for a concerning fetal status, but it is imperative to stabilize the mother first, because in doing so the fetal status will likewise improve. Prevention Aggressive treatment of sepsis can be expected to reduce the progression to severe sepsis and septic shock and prevention strategies can include preoperative skin preparations and prophylactic antibiotic therapy as well as appropriate immunizations (Fig 4).

▶ Sepsis is one of the leading causes of morbidity and mortality in critically ill patients. Pregnancy is associated with specific risk factors predisposing pregnant patients to develop sepsis. Furthermore, when pregnant patients develop severe sepsis or septic shock, they are at risk for increased morbidity and mortality. Caring for critically ill pregnant patients poses a number of challenges for the intensivist. First, there is the added stress of caring for more than 1 life at the same time (mother and fetus). Concerns for using drugs, procedures, or diagnostic tests that are potentially harmful for the fetus are a constant in these cases. Second, pregnancy is associated with significant physiological changes that need to be considered by the intensivist, especially when providing organ support and evaluating hemodynamics. Finally, there are certain conditions that are unique to pregnancy that can compound the clinical picture in a pregnant patient with severe sepsis or septic shock. In this comprehensive review, Barton and Sibai thoroughly discuss relevant aspects of caring for pregnant patients with

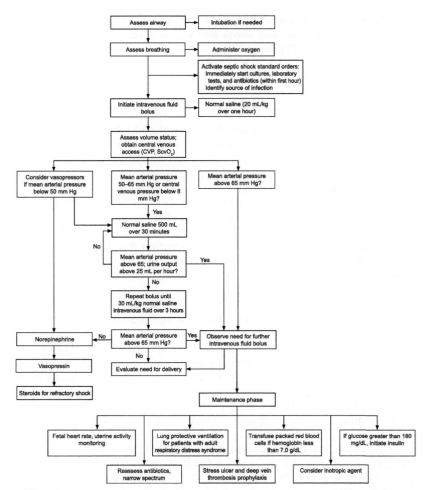

FIGURE 4.—An algorithm of management for septic shock in pregnancy. Data from: Rivers E, Nguyen B, Havstad S, Ressler J, Muzzin A, Knoblich B, et al. Early goal-directed therapy in the treatment of severe sepsis and septic shock. *N Engl J Med* 2001;345:1368—77. CVP, central venous pressure; ScvO₂, central venous oxygen saturation. (Reprinted from Barton JR, Sibai BM. Severe sepsis and septic shock in pregnancy. *Obstet Gynecol.* 2012;120:689-706, with permission from The American College of Obstetricians and Gynecologists.)

severe sepsis and septic shock. One of the most valuable aspects of this review is the algorithm presented for overall management (Fig 4). The paucity or lack of studies in this particular population makes review articles such as this one very valuable for practicing physicians.

S. Zanotti, MD

The effectiveness of hypertonic saline and pentoxifylline (HTS–PTX) resuscitation in haemorrhagic shock and sepsis tissue injury: Comparison with LR, HES, and LR–PTX treatments

Kim HJ, Lee KH (Bucheon Hosp of Soonchunhyang Univ, South Korea; Wonju Christian Hosp of Yonsei Univ, South Korea)
Injury 43:1271-1276, 2012

Purpose.—To compare lung and liver injury and laboratory results in haemorrhagic shock and sepsis models treated with combinations of lactated Ringer's solution (LR), 7.5% hypertonic saline (HTS), hydroxyethyl starch (HES), and pentoxifylline (PTX).

Methods.—Male Sprague-Dawley rats (200–290 g) were assigned randomly to one of four treatment groups (n = 16 per group): (1) LR; (2) HES; (3) LR–PTX; and (4) HTS–PTX. Each group was subdivided into (1) haemorrhagic shock (n = 8) and (2) sepsis (n = 8) model groups. A venous catheter was used to inject resuscitation fluids, and an arterial catheter was used to withdraw blood and monitor mean arterial pressure (MAP). Lung and liver histology, bronchoalveolar lavage (BAL) fluid, and cytokine levels were evaluated.

Results.—The mean lung injury score was 1.7. At 24 h after treatment, the total leucocyte count in the BAL fluid was significantly ($p < 0.05$) higher with LR treatment ($10 \times 10^6 \pm 0.8$) than with other treatments in the sepsis model groups (HES, $6 \times 10^6 \pm 1.2$; LR–PTX, $5 \times 10^6 \pm 1.5$; HTS–PTX, $5 \times 10^6 \pm 0.6$). The higher total leucocyte count after LR treatment was attributable to a greater increase in the number of neutrophils ($17 \pm 1.5\%$) compared with increases after the other treatments (HES, $6 \pm 0.8\%$; LR–PTX, $10 \pm 1.3\%$; HTS–PTX, $5 \pm 0.4\%$). In the sepsis model groups, the total hepatic injury score was also significantly ($p < 0.05$) higher with LR treatment (9.9 ± 0.5) than with the other treatments (HES, 6.7 ± 0.8; LR–PTX, 5.6 ± 0.7; HTS–PTX, 3.1 ± 0.9). This also occurred in the shock model (LR, 10.6 ± 2.1; HES, 5.8 ± 0.9; LR–PTX, 7.3 ± 0.9; HTS–PTX, 3.5 ± 0.9). As compared with LR treatment, HTS–PTX resuscitation resulted in a 49% decrease in TNF-α, 29% decrease in IL-1β, and 58% decrease in IL-6 in the shock model at 24 h ($p < 0.05$), and the respective decreases were 45, 24, and 35% in the sepsis model ($p < 0.05$).

Conclusion.—HTS–PTX was superior to HES, LR–PTX, and LR for treating shock and sepsis, and LR–PTX and HES gave better results than LR therapy alone.

▶ Sepsis and hemorrhagic shock are both pathologies that require large resuscitative efforts; however, even with adequate resuscitation these can result in large fluid volumes. Additionally, the resuscitative fluid of choice (usually lactated Ringer's solution) can lead to proinflammatory states, exacerbating an already inflammatory pathology. As such, the authors looked into a fluid that would reduce fluid volume as well as decrease inflammatory effects. Pentoxifylline, a nonspecific phosphodiesterase inhibitor, was found to decrease neutrophil activation and decrease organ injury; thus, it would provide an anti-inflammatory effect opposite that of lactated Ringer's solution alone. Other fluids that have been studied are hydroxyethyl starch, which decreased pulmonary microvascular permeability in one study, and hypertonic saline. Hypertonic saline has the benefit of requiring minimum fluid for increased intravascular volume expansion (therefore improved organ perfusion) as well as immunomodulatory effects via decreases in neutrophil accumulation and cytokine release.[1]

Rats were assigned to 4 different resuscitative fluids: lactated Ringer's (LR), Hydroxyethyl starch (HES), lactated Ringer's and pentoxifylline (LR-PTX), and hypertonic saline and pentoxifylline (HTS-PTX). They underwent either hemorrhagic shock or sepsis through intratracheal lipopolysaccharide adminis-tration. Parameters observed were histology of the lung, particularly macrophage and neutrophil accumulation, as well as alveolar hemorrhage and edema. A bronchial lavage was performed for neutrophil and total leukocyte count. Histologic hepatic pathology was examined along with alanine aminotransferase levels. Finally, inflammatory cytokines tumor necrosis factor-alpha (TNF-α), interleukin-beta (IL-1β), and IL-6 were studied between the 4 resuscitative groups.

In the septic shock and hemorrhagic shock models, HTS-PTX performed significantly better than lactated Ringer's solution alone with decreased inflam-matory effects, organ damage, and edema. It also appeared superior to HES in the hemorrhagic shock model.

This study has very promising implications in sepsis and hemorrhagic shock resuscitative efforts. From a fluid status standpoint, the consequences of massive fluid resuscitation can be just as morbid as the diseases themselves—for example, abdominal compartment syndrome, and pulmonary edema. Using hypertonic saline has a 2-fold benefit of reducing fluid requirements as well as its anti-inflammatory effects. Combining these attributes with pentoxifylline, which is also anti-inflammatory and reduces organ injury, can produce a more ideal resuscitative fluid.

S. Zanotti, MD

Reference

1. Oliveira RP, Velasco I, Soriano FG, Friedman G. Clinical review: hypertonic saline resuscitation in sepsis. *Crit Care.* 2002;6:418-423.

Transfusion of packed red blood cells is not associated with improved central venous oxygen saturation or organ function in patients with septic shock
Fuller BM, Gajera M, Schorr C, et al (Washington Univ School of Medicine, St Louis, MO; Cooper Univ Hosp, Camden, NJ)
J Emerg Med 43:593-598, 2012

Background.—The exact role of packed red blood cell (PRBC) transfu-sion in the setting of early resuscitation in septic shock is unknown.

Study Objective.—To evaluate whether PRBC transfusion is associated with improved central venous oxygen saturation ($ScvO_2$) or organ function in patients with severe sepsis and septic shock receiving early goal-directed therapy (EGDT).

Methods.—Retrospective cohort study (n = 93) of patients presenting with severe sepsis or septic shock treated with EGDT.

Results.—Thirty-four of 93 patients received at least one PRBC transfusion. The $ScvO_2$ goal > 70% was achieved in 71.9% of the PRBC group and 66.1% of the no-PRBC group ($p = 0.30$). There was no difference in the change in Sequential Organ Failure Assessment (SOFA) score within the first 24 h in the PRBC group vs. the no-PRBC group (8.6−8.3 vs 5.8−5.6, $p = 0.85$), time to achievement of central venous pressure > 8 mm Hg (732 min vs. 465 min, $p = 0.14$), or the use of norepinephrine to maintain mean arterial pressure > 65 mm Hg (81.3% vs. 83.8%, $p = 0.77$).

Conclusions.—In this study, the transfusion of PRBC was not associated with improved cellular oxygenation, as demonstrated by a lack of improved achievement of $ScvO_2 > 70\%$. Also, the transfusion of PRBC was not associated with improved organ function or improved achievement of the other goals of EGDT. Further studies are needed to determine the impact of transfusion of PRBC within the context of early resuscitation of patients with septic shock.

▶ Packed red blood cell (PRBC) transfusion is a common practice in the intensive care unit. Despite evidence linking PRBC transfusion to adverse clinical outcomes, significant controversy exists over its use in early goal-directed therapy (EGDT) sepsis resuscitation. After achieving adequate volume status and mean arterial pressure, the EGDT protocol recommends considering PRBC transfusion for patients with persistent central venous oxygen saturation ($ScvO_2$) less than 70% and hematocrit less than 30%. The PRBC transfusion is part of a bundle approach to improve global tissue hypoxia. In this retrospective study, the effect of PRBC transfusion on $ScvO_2$ and organ function was evaluated. Data were collected on 93 patients with severe sepsis and septic shock. All were treated with EGDT protocol. The PRBC group consisted of 34 patients who received an average of 4.56 units of PRBC transfusion per patient. The units were ordered during the first 6 hours and administered within the first 24 hours of the start of resuscitation. The primary outcome of $ScvO_2$ greater than 70% was achieved in 71.9% of the PRBC group and 66.1% of the non-PRBC group.

The secondary outcome included improvement in Sequential Organ Failure Assessment (SOFA) scores. Both results did not reach statistical significance.

The EGDT bundle is a complex approach with multiple components, which includes PRBC transfusion. What makes this study interesting is that both the transfused arm and nontransfused arm were resuscitated using the EGDT protocol. This allowed controlling of different factors and evaluating PRBC transfusion as a single variable between the 2 groups.

The results of the study are even more interesting. On one hand, they are consistent with previous data suggesting that physiologic indicators may not necessarily identify patients that are likely to benefit from PRBC transfusion. This is attributed to the changes occurring at the cellular level during PRBC storage. Stored PRBCs seem to lose functional and structural capability to improve tissue oxygen deficit. On the other hand, these study results are in major conflict with those of the Rivers et al[1] trial. Rivers et al showed significant improvement in $ScvO_2$ after transfusion and decreased mortality when used as a part of the EGDT protocol in the emergency department (ED) within 6 hours of the sepsis diagnosis. This difference could be in part secondary to the timing of transfusion. Sixty-four percent of the patients in the Rivers et al trial received their transfusions in the first 6 hours in the ED. In this study, although PRBC transfusions were ordered in ED, the time of administration was not clear. The timing of transfusion could be an important factor in determining benefit. The other limitation could be the small sample size. This might have contributed to the insignificant improvement in the $ScvO_2$ and SOFA scores.

This study raises concerns regarding basic physiologic principles that involve red cell changes and oxygen delivery and consumption. It can serve as hypothesis for larger prospective trials that should take into account potential modifiers such as the age of the stored PRBCs and the timing of transfusion.

Z. Kobeissi, MD

Reference

1. Rivers E, Nguyen B, Havstad MA, et al. Early goal-directed therapy in the treatment of severe sepsis and septic shock. *N Engl J Med.* 2001;345:1368-1377.

Dopamine versus norepinephrine in the treatment of septic shock: A meta-analysis

De Backer D, Aldecoa C, Njimi H, et al (Université Libre de Bruxelles, Brussels, Belgium; Rio Hortega Univ Hosp, Valladolid, Spain)
Crit Care Med 40:725-730, 2012

Objectives.—There has long-been controversy about the possible superiority of norepinephrine compared to dopamine in the treatment of shock. The objective was to evaluate the effects of norepinephrine and dopamine on outcome and adverse events in patients with septic shock.

Data Sources.—A systematic search of the MEDLINE, Embase, Scopus, and CENTRAL databases, and of Google Scholar, up to June 30, 2011.

Study Selection and Data Extraction.—All studies providing information on the outcome of patients with septic shock treated with dopamine compared to norepinephrine were included. Observational and randomized trials were analyzed separately. Because time of outcome assessment varied among trials, we evaluated 28-day mortality or closest estimate. Heterogeneity among trials was assessed using the Cochrane Q homogeneity test.

A Forest plot was constructed and the aggregate relative risk of death was computed. Potential publication bias was evaluated using funnel plots.

Methods and Main Results.—We retrieved five observational (1,360 patients) and six randomized (1,408 patients) trials, totaling 2,768 patients (1,474 who received norepinephrine and 1,294 who received dopamine). In observational studies, among which there was significant heterogeneity ($p < .001$), there was no difference in mortality (relative risk, 1.09; confidence interval, 0.84–1.41; $p = .72$). A sensitivity analysis identified one trial as being responsible for the heterogeneity; after exclusion of that trial, no heterogeneity was observed and dopamine administration was associated with an increased risk of death (relative risk, 1.23; confidence interval, 1.05–1.43; $p < .01$). In randomized trials, for which no heterogeneity or publication bias was detected ($p = .77$), dopamine was associated with an increased risk of death (relative risk, 1.12; confidence interval, 1.01–1.20; $p = .035$). In the two trials that reported arrhythmias, these were more frequent with dopamine than with norepinephrine (relative risk, 2.34; confidence interval, 1.46–3.77; $p = .001$).

Conclusions.—In patients with septic shock, dopamine administration is associated with greater mortality and a higher incidence of arrhythmic events compared to norepinephrine administration.

▶ Investigation of the optimal vasopressor for the management of septic shock has generated considerable controversy. The 2008 Surviving Sepsis Campaign (SSC) guidelines recommend the use of norepinephrine or dopamine as first-line in septic shock. However, dopamine has more recently been associated with increased mortality in several observational trials. Prior meta-analyses were underpowered to demonstrate superiority, but the recent publication of large, randomized, clinical trials has added a significant volume of outcome data comparing the 2 vasopressors. De Backer et al performed a meta-analysis through June 2011 incorporating 5 observational and 6 randomized trials assessing short-term mortality in septic shock patients treated with norepinephrine versus dopamine. Analysis of all trials found no mortality difference in the presence of significant heterogeneity. Exclusion of one trial eliminated heterogeneity and showed increased mortality with use of dopamine compared with norepinephrine (relative risk, 1.23). In addition, the number of arrhythmic events was significantly greater in patients treated with dopamine versus those treated with norepinephrine. While the results of the meta-analysis were heavily influenced by the large size of the Sepsis Occurrence in Acutely Ill Patients randomized trial, exclusion of this trial produces similar mortality risk with wider confidence intervals. Therefore, the authors' conclusions are consistent with the growing body of evidence that dopamine is associated with greater risk of death and arrhythmias than norepinephrine in the treatment of septic shock. Moreover, this has led to the modification of the current 2013 SSC guidelines to downgrade the recommendation for dopamine as a first-line alternative to norepinephrine, specifying its use only in select patients at low risk of tachyarrhythmias.

E. Damuth, MD

S. Zanotti, MD

Red blood cell transfusions are associated with lower mortality in patients with severe sepsis and septic shock: A propensity-matched analysis
Park DW, Chun B-C, Kwon S-S, et al (Korea Univ College of Medicine, Ansan; Korea Univ College of Medicine, Seoul; et al)
Crit Care Med 40:3140-3145, 2012

Objectives.—To evaluate the effects of transfusions in patients with severe sepsis and septic shock on mortality.
Design.—Propensity-matched analysis of a prospective observational database (April 2005 to February 2009).
Setting.—Twenty-two medical and surgical intensive care units in 12 teaching hospitals in Korea.
Patients.—One thousand fifty-four patients with community-acquired severe sepsis and septic shock.
Interventions.—None.
Measurements and Main Results.—Of the 1,054 patients, 407 (38.6%) received a blood transfusion. The mean pretransfusion hemoglobin level was 7.7 ± 1.2 g/dL. Transfused patients had higher 28-day and in-hospital mortality rates (32.7% vs. 17.3%; $p < .001$, 41.3% vs. 20.3%; $p < .001$, respectively) and a longer duration of hospital stay (21 [interquartile range, 10−35] vs. 13 [interquartile range, 8−24] days; $p < .001$), but were more severely ill at admission (lower systolic blood pressure, higher Acute Physiology and Chronic Health Evaluation II score, and Sequential Organ Failure Assessment score at admission). In 152 pairs matched according to the propensity score depending on patient transfusion status, transfused patients had a lower risk of 7-day (9.2% vs. 27.0%; $p < .001$), 28-day (24.3% vs. 38.8%; $p = .007$), and in-hospital mortality rates (31.6% vs. 42.8%; $p = .044$). After adjusting for blood transfusion as a time-dependent variable in multivariable analysis, blood transfusion was independently associated with lower risk of 7-day (hazard ratio 0.42, 95% confidence interval 0.19−0.50, $p = .026$), 28-day (hazard ratio 0.43, 95% confidence interval 0.29−0.62, $p < .001$), and in-hospital mortality (hazard ratio 0.51, 95% confidence interval 0.39−0.69, $p < .001$).
Conclusions.—In this observational study of patients with community-acquired severe sepsis and septic shock, red blood cell transfusions were associated with lower risk of mortality.

▶ After the Transfusion Requirements in Critical Care trial, an extensive body of data has accumulated showing that packed red blood cell (PRBC) transfusion in critically ill patients should be meticulously weighed between risks and benefits. The early goal-directed therapy resuscitation approach recommends transfusion of PRBC to maintain hematocrit level greater than 30% if mixed central venous O_2 saturation ($ScvO_2$) is less than 70%. This reignited the debate about the specific indications for transfusion in the intensive care settings.

In this study, the authors evaluated the effects of red blood cell transfusions on mortality in patients with severe sepsis and septic shock. A multicenter observational study was conducted evaluating 1054 patients using the Korean sepsis registry from April 2005 to February 2009. A total of 407 (38.6%) of these patients received a blood transfusion. From the demographics, the transfused group was sicker as noted from a higher Charlson's index score, APACHE II score, and Sequential Organ Failure Assessment score. Transfused patients had both higher mortality and longer duration of hospital stays. The authors performed a propensity-matched analysis that included 152 patients from each group. Transfused patients had lower risk of 7-day, 28-day, and in-hospital mortality. The authors concluded that blood transfusions may be associated with survival benefit and can be used in the critical care setting.

This conclusion should be approached with caution, as there are a few points worthy of discussion.

1. The characteristics of the propensity-matched patients show the nontransfused group is sicker than the total number of nontransfused patients. The transfused patients in the propensity-matched group are less sick than the group of all transfused patients. In addition to acuity differences among the groups, the indication for transfusion is not reported. This raises the question of selection bias. Because the hemoglobin in the nontransfused arm was not measured, it is not clear whether the hemoglobin in this group reached a critical level below which patients needed to be transfused.

2. The median hemoglobin level for all transfused patients was less than 7.7 g/dL. It would have been interesting to see the actual hemoglobin value in the propensity-matched arm. This raises the question whether there is a lower cutoff point below which transfusion could be beneficial.

3. Furthermore, outcomes in severe sepsis and septic shock have been associated with multiple time-sensitive factors. Those lacking in the study include timing of antibiotics, lactate level, mean arterial pressure less than 65, $ScvO_2$ less than 70%. These variables have important clinical implications on survival.

4. Another limitation is that the study looked only at mortality without examining other possible adverse effects of transfusion that could explain the longer hospital length of stay in the group of transfused patients.

Data concerning the negative effects of PRBC transfusion has been mounting over many years. The positive conclusion of this study, despite its limitations, highlights the need for the topic of transfusion in severe sepsis and septic shock to be revisited.

Z. Kobeissi, MD

Red blood cell transfusions are associated with lower mortality in patients with severe sepsis and septic shock: A propensity-matched analysis
Park DW, Chun B-C, Kwon S-S, et al (Korea Univ College of Medicine, Ansan; Korea Univ College of Medicine, Seoul; et al)
Crit Care Med 40:3140-3145, 2012

Objectives.—To evaluate the effects of transfusions in patients with severe sepsis and septic shock on mortality.

Design.—Propensity-matched analysis of a prospective observational database (April 2005 to February 2009).
Setting.—Twenty-two medical and surgical intensive care units in 12 teaching hospitals in Korea.
Patients.—One thousand fifty-four patients with community-acquired severe sepsis and septic shock.
Interventions.—None.
Measurements and Main Results.—Of the 1,054 patients, 407 (38.6%) received a blood transfusion. The mean pretransfusion hemoglobin level was 7.7 ± 1.2 g/dL. Transfused patients had higher 28-day and in-hospital mortality rates (32.7% vs. 17.3%; $p < .001$, 41.3% vs. 20.3%; $p < .001$, respectively) and a longer duration of hospital stay (21 [interquartile range, 10–35] vs. 13 [interquartile range, 8–24] days; $p < .001$), but were more severely ill at admission (lower systolic blood pressure, higher Acute Physiology and Chronic Health Evaluation II score, and Sequential Organ Failure Assessment score at admission). In 152 pairs matched according to the propensity score depending on patient transfusion status, transfused patients had a lower risk of 7-day (9.2% vs. 27.0%; $p < .001$), 28-day (24.3% vs. 38.8%; $p = .007$), and in-hospital mortality rates (31.6% vs. 42.8%; $p = .044$). After adjusting for blood transfusion as a time-dependent variable in multivariable analysis, blood transfusion was independently associated with lower risk of 7-day (hazard ratio 0.42, 95% confidence interval 0.19–0.50, $p = .026$), 28-day (hazard ratio 0.43, 95% confidence interval 0.29–0.62, $p < .001$), and in-hospital mortality (hazard ratio 0.51, 95% confidence interval 0.39–0.69, $p < .001$).
Conclusions.—In this observational study of patients with community-acquired severe sepsis and septic shock, red blood cell transfusions were associated with lower risk of mortality.

▶ Septic shock remains the single leading cause of death in intensive care units (ICUs). Investigators have been looking for targeted therapies to reduce mortality in this condition for decades, to little or no avail. As a broad statement, good supportive therapy, including appropriate and timely antibiotics, maintenance of stable hemodynamics and respiratory status, and adequate nutritional and metabolic support, are the mainstays of therapy, along with the avoidance of complications, such as gastrointestinal bleeding, deep vein thrombosis, and ventilator-associated pneumonia. Aggressive resuscitation such as with Early Goal Directed Therapy (EGDT) and the utilization of the sepsis bundles as advocated by the Surviving Sepsis Campaign employ essentially standard therapies in protocolized ways, although sometimes more vigorously than some practitioners are accustomed to. Most historical data that have evaluated the utility of packed red blood cell (PRBC) transfusion on outcomes in severe sepsis or septic shock have been disappointing, finding it to be of limited utility.

One possible exception was the original EGDT study by Rivers et al, in which PRBC transfusion was included as part of the algorithm to achieve an central venous oxygen saturation ≥70%. However, the individual impact of transfusion on outcome was not reported, although subjects in the treatment arm had overall better outcomes. In the study reviewed here, the investigators collected data on a prospective observational basis on more than 1000 patients with severe sepsis and septic shock admitted to a large number of medical and surgical ICUs to assess outcome differences based on the impact of PRBC transfusion.

Outcomes for transfused patients and nontransfused patients were compared in both crude and multivariate analyses, as is typical for studies of this design. In addition, 152 matched pairs from these 2 groups were compared using propensity-matching, a relatively recently developed statistical technique that attempts to account for the absence of randomization. In effect, it is an attempt to factor in the likelihood that a subject would have received the treatment being studied based on a variety of variables or characteristics, which are included in a logistic regression model used to predict the probability (or so-called "propensity") that the patient would have received the treatment under investigation. In both the crude and basic multivariate analyses, the patients receiving transfusions had worse outcomes as measured by a number of parameters. This is likely not unexpected because they were sicker as measured by a number of parameters and had lower hemoglobins. However, when the propensity matched pairs were evaluated, the transfused patients had lower 7- and 28-day and hospital mortality than did nontransfused patients. These findings are interesting, in that they are at odds with the significant preponderance of literature that has accumulated in the past 2 decades regarding the impact of PRBC transfusion on outcomes in a wide variety of critically ill patients. However, the authors point out that there have been other studies within the past few years also indicating that septic patients may benefit from PRBC transfusion.

Although several potential explanations are posited, no definitive ones are provided. Perhaps the most reasonable is that with the adoption of a restrictive transfusion strategy, relatively strict adherence may show benefit if practitioners limit transfusion to unstable patients with hemoglobins in the range of 7 g/dL, as appears to have been done in this study. Of course, as an observational study, it is limited by the nature of its design. In addition, although propensity matching is intended to improve the accuracy and validity of nonrandomized studies, this methodology has its detractors, who feel it has the potential to introduce its own confounding or biases into the analysis.[1]

Nevertheless, these findings add an interesting bit of food for thought to the critical care menu, and they may well open the door for a new prospective study on transfusion, this time targeting patients specifically with severe sepsis and septic shock.

D. R. Gerber, DO

Reference

1. Nuttall GA, Houle TT. Liars, damn liars, and propensity scores. *Anesthesiology.* 2008;108:3-4.

Initial resuscitation guided by the Surviving Sepsis Campaign recommendations and early echocardiographic assessment of hemodynamics in intensive care unit septic patients: A pilot study
Bouferrache K, Amiel J-B, Chimot L, et al (Univ Hosp Ambroise Paré, Boulogne, France; CHU de Limoges, France)
Crit Care Med 40:2821-2827, 2012

Objective.—To compare therapeutic interventions during initial resuscitation derived from echocardiographic assessment of hemodynamics and from the Surviving Sepsis Campaign guidelines in intensive care unit septic patients.

Design and Setting.—Prospective, descriptive study in two intensive care units of teaching hospitals.

Methods.—The number of ventilated patients with septic shock who were studied was 46. Transesophageal echocardiography was first performed (T1 < 3 hrs after intensive care unit admission) to adapt therapy according to the following predefined hemodynamic profiles: fluid loading (index of collapsibility of the superior vena cava ≥ 36%), inotropic support (left ventricular fractional area change < 45% without relevant index of collapsibility of the superior vena cava), or increased vasopressor support (right ventricular systolic dysfunction, unremarkable transesophageal echocardiography study consistent with sustained vasoplegia). Agreement for treatment decision between transesophageal echocardiography and Surviving Sepsis Campaign guidelines was evaluated. A second transesophageal echocardiography assessment (T2) was performed to validate therapeutic interventions.

Results.—Although transesophageal echocardiography and Surviving Sepsis Campaign approaches were concordant to manage fluid loading in 32 of 46 patients (70%), echocardiography led to the absence of blood volume expansion in the remaining 14 patients who all had a central venous pressure < 12 mm Hg. Accordingly, the agreement was weak between transesophageal echocardiography and Surviving Sepsis Campaign for the decision of fluid loading (κ: 0.37 [0.16;0.59]). With a cut-off value < 8 mm Hg for central venous pressure, κ was 0.33 [−0.03;0.69]. Inotropes were prescribed based on transesophageal echocardiography assessment in 14 patients but would have been decided in only four patients according to Surviving Sepsis Campaign guidelines. As a result, the agreement between the two approaches for the decision of inotropic support was weak (κ: 0.23 [−0.04;0.50]). No right ventricular dysfunction was observed. No patient had anemia and only three patients with transesophageal echocardiography documented left ventricular systolic dysfunction had a central venous oxygen saturation < 70%.

Conclusions.—A weak agreement was found in the prescription of fluid loading and inotropic support derived from early transesophageal echocardiography assessment of hemodynamics and Surviving Sepsis Campaign guidelines in patients presenting with septic shock.

▶ The optimal modality for hemodynamic assessment in early treatment of septic shock remains a much-debated issue. Research has evaluated static and dynamic parameters for assessing volume responsiveness. This article describes a prospective study in which the early use of transesophageal echocardiography (TEE) in mechanically ventilated septic shock patients was compared with the Surviving Sepsis Campaign (SSC) guidelines. In particular, the study evaluates early volume assessment with fluid loading and the implementation of inotropic support. In the 46 patients studied, a TEE was performed 2 separate times; early (< 3 hours) in their intensive care unit (ICU) stay and then again after intervention. The key results of the study were as follows: First, a large proportion of patients (30%) did not receive further volume expansion as would have been recommended by SSC guidelines for central venous pressure target because of their routine use of superior vena cava (SVC) collapsibility index to determine volume responsiveness. Second, an additional 10 patients were placed on inotropic therapy based on TEE evaluation of left ventricular (LV) function when compared with indications for starting inotropes if following the SSC guidelines. This led to an appropriate conclusion by the authors that their routine use of TEE may lead to less fluid administration and more frequent use of inotropes than if SSC guidelines were followed.

It is important to emphasize that the specific population studied was septic shock patients requiring mechanical ventilation. This is a key point in any discussion of volume responsiveness because all dynamic parameters for determining volume responsiveness have only been studied in appropriately sedated patients on mechanical ventilation with > 8 mL/kg tidal volume. In this article, the dynamic parameter used was an SVC collapsibility index of > 36%, which has a very well-reported sensitivity and specificity in predicting volume responsiveness. Additionally, the authors used transesophageal echocardiography for their hemodynamic assessment. Certainly, transthoracic echocardiography to aid in hemodynamic assessment in the ICU has become increasingly common, although it still would not be considered routine in clinical practice worldwide. However, TEE would be even less common as part of the ICU clinician's armamentarium for hemodynamic assessment. It is this issue that severely limits any major clinical impact from this study. An often-used argument in studies using echocardiography or other bedside ultrasound for critically ill patients is that the technique is very practitioner-dependent. This argument would be relevant here and possibly even more so with use of TEE as opposed to transthoracic echocardiogram.

Based on the design of the study, no conclusions can be made about clinical patient-oriented outcomes. However, this study makes some very important points. First, dynamic parameters for predicting volume responsiveness should be used when available in the appropriate patient as outlined previously. Second, targets for initiation of inotropic support, specifically a central venous oxygen saturation < 70%, often do not correlate with LV dysfunction based on echocardiographic visualization. Ultimately, whether use of echocardiography for hemodynamic assessment leads to improved patient-oriented outcomes is unclear.

B. Goodgame, MD

S. Zanotti, MD

Fever Control Using External Cooling in Septic Shock: A Randomized Controlled Trial

Schortgen F, Clabault K, Katsahian S, et al (Groupe Hospitalier Henri Mondor, Créteil, France; Centre Hospitalier Universitaire de Rouen, France; et al)

Am J Respir Crit Care Med 185:1088-1095, 2012

Rationale.—Fever control may improve vascular tone and decrease oxygen consumption, but fever may contribute to combat infection.

Objectives.—To determine whether fever control by external cooling diminishes vasopressor requirements in septic shock.

Methods.—In a multicenter randomized controlled trial, febrile patients with septic shock requiring vasopressors, mechanical ventilation, and sedation were allocated to external cooling (n = 101) to achieve normo-thermia (36.5−37°C) for 48 hours or no external cooling (n = 99). Vaso-pressors were tapered to maintain the same blood pressure target in the two groups. The primary endpoint was the number of patients with a 50% decrease in baseline vasopressor dose after 48 hours.

Measurements and Main Results.—Body temperature was significantly lower in the cooling group after 2 hours of treatment (36.8 ± 0.7 vs. 38.4 ± 1.1°C; $P < 0.01$). A 50% vasopressor dose decrease was significantly more common with external cooling from 12 hours of treatment (54 vs. 20%; absolute difference, 34%; 95% confidence interval [95% CI], −46 to −21; $P < 0.001$) but not at 48 hours (72 vs. 61%; absolute difference, 11%; 95% CI, −23 to 2). Shock reversal during the intensive care unit stay was significantly more common with cooling (86 vs. 73%; absolute difference,13%; 95% CI, 2 to 25; $P = 0.021$). Day-14 mortality was significantly lower in the cooling group (19 vs. 34%; absolute differ-ence, −16%; 95% CI, −28 to −4; $P = 0.013$).

Conclusions.—In this study, fever control using external cooling was safe and decreased vasopressor requirements and early mortality in septic shock.

▶ Fever in the intensive care unit (ICU) has been defined by the Society of Crit-ical Care Medicine as a temperature greater than 38.3°C. The incidence of fever in the ICU ranges from 23% to 70%, with approximately half of these cases being attributable to an infectious process. Fever is often considered a common finding in patients with sepsis. However, at presentation, 10% of septic patients are hypothermic and 35% are normothermic. Physician and staff response to fever varies institutionally. It is common for the patient to receive either pharmacologic or mechanical antipyretic therapy. Studies evaluating the effect of fever and its modulation on patient outcomes have yielded conflicting results. There are studies suggesting a beneficial effect of fever on patient outcomes in sepsis. In one study of 218 patients with gram-negative bacteremia, the presence of fever was found to have a positive correlation with survival.[1] In this study, failure to mount a febrile response within the first 24 hours was associated with increased mortality. Another study of prospectively collected data found that patients with a temperature greater than 101.3°F were 59% less likely to die when compared with patients with a normal temperature.[2] With regard to fever modulation, the Fever and Antipyretic in Critically ill patients Evaluation trial failed to show a mortality benefit in sepsis patients with external cooling.[3] Other studies have suggested that aggressive fever control is associated with higher mortality.

It is still unclear whether fever is globally beneficial or harmful in sepsis and perhaps more important whether modulation of fever improves patient outcomes. In this multicenter, randomized, controlled trial, the authors attempt to shine some light on this much-debated issue. Case study patients were allocated to external cooling with the objective of achieving normothermia (36.5°C to 37°C) during the study period of 48 hours versus no external cooling in the control group. The primary endpoint of the study was the number of patients with a 50% decrease in baseline vasopressor dose after 48 hours. Both groups had similar demographics with the exception of the cumulative dose of vasopressors (higher in the control group ($P = .03$)). The study found that the percentage of patients with a 50% vasopressor dose decrease versus baseline between 2 groups was not significantly different at 48 hours (primary endpoint). Shock reversal was significantly more common in the cooling group than in the control group (significance persisted after adjustment for severity of illness and vasopressor dose imbalance). The investigator proposed that beneficial effect of cooling was caused by decreased oxygen consumption along with early vasopressor sparing. Furthermore, the risk of death on Day 14 was significantly lower in the cooling group. However, this difference in mortality was not significant at ICU or hospital discharge. The incidence of acquired infections by Day 14 was 32.6 per 1000 ICU days in the cooling group and 23.8 per 1000 ICU days in the control group.

The use of targeted temperature management (TTM) has been found to be beneficial in other critically ill patient populations (hypothermia after cardiac arrest). This study is a preliminary evaluation of a TTM targeting normothermia in patients with severe sepsis and septic shock. Although the study results are of great interest, they by no means answer all our questions regarding this topic. Current clinical consensus recommends initiating treatment when fever is greater than 40°C with a goal to achieve a temperature range of 37.5°C to 38.4°C. Further research is needed to best define the value and the way to proceed with TTM in severe sepsis and septic shock.

M. Gajera, MD
S. Zanotti, MD

References

1. Bryant RE, Hood AF, Hood ED, et al. Factors affecting mortality of gram-negative rod bacteremia. *Arch Intern Med.* 1971;127:120-128.

2. Sanga R, Zanotti S, Schorr C, et al. Relation between temperature in the initial 24 hours in patients with severe sepsis or septic shock with mortality and length of stay in the ICU. *Crit Care.* 2012;16:P57.
3. Fever and Antipyretic in Critically ill patients Evaluation (FACE) Study Group; Lee BH, Inui D, Suh GY, et al. Association of body temperature and antipyretic treatments with mortality of critically ill patients with and without sepsis: multi-centered prospective observational study. *Crit Care.* 2012;16:R33.

Fever Control Using External Cooling in Septic Shock: A Randomized Controlled Trial

Schortgen F, Clabault K, Katsahian S, et al (Groupe Hospitalier Henri Mondor, Créteil, France; Centre Hospitalier Universitaire de Rouen, Rouen, France; et al)

Am J Respir Crit Care Med 185:1088-1095, 2012

Rationale.—Fever control may improve vascular tone and decrease oxygen consumption, but fever may contribute to combat infection.

Objectives.—To determine whether fever control by external cooling diminishes vasopressor requirements in septic shock.

Methods.—In a multicenter randomized controlled trial, febrile patients with septic shock requiring vasopressors, mechanical ventilation, and sedation were allocated to external cooling (n = 101) to achieve normo-thermia (36.5–37°C) for 48 hours or no external cooling (n = 99). Vaso-pressors were tapered to maintain the same blood pressure target in the two groups. The primary endpoint was the number of patients with a 50% decrease in baseline vasopressor dose after 48 hours.

Measurements and Main Results.—Body temperature was significantly lower in the cooling group after 2 hours of treatment (36.8 ± 0.7 vs. 38.4 ± 1.1°C; $P < 0.01$). A 50% vasopressor dose decrease was significantly more common with external cooling from 12 hours of treatment (54 vs. 20%; absolute difference, 34%; 95% confidence interval [95% CI], −46 to −21; $P < 0.001$) but not at 48 hours (72 vs. 61%; absolute difference, 11%; 95% CI, −23 to 2). Shock reversal during the intensive care unit stay was significantly more common with cooling (86 vs. 73%; absolute difference, 13%; 95% CI, 2 to 25; $P = 0.021$). Day-14 mortality was significantly lower in the cooling group (19 vs. 34%; absolute difference, −16%; 95% CI, −28 to −4; $P = 0.013$).

Conclusions.—In this study, fever control using external cooling was safe and decreased vasopressor requirements and early mortality in septic shock.

▶ Fever is one of the defining criteria for systemic inflammatory response and the varying degrees of sepsis.[1-3] Although fever control is intuitive, this study answers the question about whether it is efficacious. The authors demonstrate reduced use of vasoactive drugs, and remarkably, with a short 48-hour intervention, improved outcomes (Fig 5 in the original article).

These data are obtained from medical rather than surgical patients. In particular, neurosurgical patients are excluded. This is 1 patient group in which hyperthermia is clearly deleterious.

Why did outcome improve with external cooling? It is possible that demands on oxygen consumption were reduced.[4] Toxicity of vasopressor utilization was also decreased because these agents were required in smaller amounts. Although therapies combined with cooling are discussed, the etiology of septic shock is not revealed.

Quick examination of Fig 3 from the original article reveals that although the temperature difference was statistically significant, the "cooled" group did not have drastic temperature reduction. In summary, this work suggests that brief normalization of a temperature curve may improve outcome in patients with fever complicating severe infection.

D. J. Dries, MSE, MD

References

1. Su F, Nguyen ND, Wang Z, Cai Y, Rogiers P, Vincent JL. Fever control in septic shock: beneficial or harmful? *Shock.* 2005;23:516-520.
2. Ryan M, Levy MM. Clinical review: fever in intensive care unit patients. *Crit Care.* 2003;7:221-225.
3. Peres Bota D, Lopes Ferreira F, Mélot C, Vincent JL. Body temperature alterations in the critically ill. *Intensive Care Med.* 2004;30:811-816.
4. Manthous CA, Hall JB, Olson D, et al. Effect of cooling on oxygen consumption in febrile critically ill patients. *Am J Respir Crit Care Med.* 1995;151:10-14.

Physical and Mental Health in Patients and Spouses After Intensive Care of Severe Sepsis: A Dyadic Perspective on Long-Term Sequelae Testing the Actor–Partner Interdependence Model

Rosendahl J, Brunkhorst FM, Jaenichen D, et al (Friedrich-Schiller Univ, Jena, Germany)
Crit Care Med 41:69-75, 2013

Objective.—To examine the physical and mental long-term consequences of intensive care treatment for severe sepsis in patients and their spouses under consideration of a dyadic perspective using the Actor–Partner Interdependence Model.

Design.—Prospective study.

Setting.—Patients and spouses who had requested advice from the German Sepsis Aid's National Helpline were invited to participate.

Subjects.—We included 55 patients who survived severe sepsis and their spouses an average of 55 months after ICU discharge.

Measurements and Main Results.—The Hospital Anxiety and Depression Scale, the Short Form-12 Health Survey, the Posttraumatic Stress Scale-10, and the Giessen Subjective Complaints List-24 were used. The Actor–Partner Interdependence Model was tested using multilevel modeling with the actor effect representing the impact of a person's posttraumatic stress symptoms on his or her own mental health-related quality

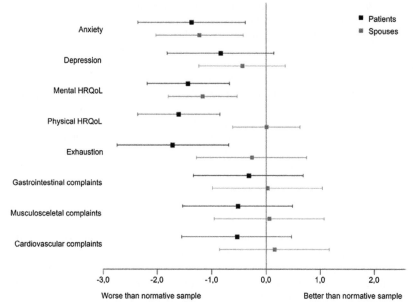

FIGURE 2.—Patients' and spouses' physical and mental health in comparison to normative samples. Differences expressed as standardized mean differences with 95% confidence interval. Mental health-related quality of life (HRQOL) = mental component summary of Short Form-12 Health Survey (SF-12); Physical HRQOL = physical component summary of SF-12. (Reprinted from Rosendahl J, Brunkhorst FM, Jaenichen D, et al. Physical and mental health in patients and spouses after intensive care of severe sepsis: a dyadic perspective on long-term sequelae testing the actor–partner interdependence model. *Crit Care Med.* 2013;41:69-75, with permission from the Society of Critical Care Medicine and Lippincott Williams & Wilkins.)

of life and the partner effect characterized by the impact of a person's post-traumatic stress symptoms on his or her partner's mental health-related quality of life. A significant proportion of patients and spouses (26%–42%) showed clinically relevant scores of anxiety and depression; approximately two thirds of both, patients and spouses, reported posttraumatic stress symptoms defined as clinically relevant. Compared with normative samples, patients reported greater anxiety, poorer mental and physical health-related quality of life, and greater exhaustion; spouses had an impaired mental health-related quality of life and increased anxiety. Testing the Actor–Partner Interdependence Model revealed that posttraumatic stress symptoms were related to patients' ($\beta = -0.71$, 95% confidence interval -0.88 to -0.54) and spouses' ($\beta = -0.62$, 95% confidence interval -0.79 to -0.46) own mental health-related quality of life. Posttraumatic stress symptoms further influenced the mental health-related quality of life of the respective other ($\beta = -0.18$, 95% confidence interval -0.35 to -0.003 for patients; $\beta = -0.15$, 95% confidence interval -0.32 to 0.02 for spouses).

Conclusions.—Interventions to treat posttraumatic stress symptoms after critical illness to improve mental health-related quality of life should not only include patients, but also consider spouses (Fig 2).

▶ There is a growing body of literature showing important long-term consequences in survivors of critical illness. Studies have shown increased impairment of physical and mental health associated with a large list of symptoms and problems such as weakness, cognitive impairment, disability, chronic pain, and mental disorders including depression, anxiety, and posttraumatic stress disorder. In this prospective study, the investigators evaluated 55 patients and their spouses for evidence of physical and mental health problems after surviving intensive care for severe sepsis. The novelty of this study was the evaluation of spouses and perhaps more interesting the evaluation of the patient-spouse dyad as 1 interdependent unit.

The results of this study showed that an average of 55 months after intensive care of severe sepsis, patients show significant impairment of physical and mental health—related quality of life. Furthermore, spouses reported significantly decreased mental health—related quality of life when compared with the normal population (Fig 2). The study found a significant dyadic association between patients and spouses regarding mental health. Anxiety and depression scores, posttraumatic stress symptoms, and mental health—related qualities of life were significantly related between patients and spouses.

Notwithstanding the limitations of this study, these results are an important addition to our evolving understanding of the long-term consequences of surviving severe sepsis-related critical illness. The results of this study strongly suggest that patients and their spouses act as emotionally interdependent entities with interrelated physical and mental health. Clinicians should think about the long-term effects on their patients as well as their families when counseling them in the intensive care unit.

S. Zanotti, MD

An evaluation of the diagnostic accuracy of the 1991 American College of Chest Physicians/Society of Critical Care Medicine and the 2001 Society of Critical Care Medicine/European Society of Intensive Care Medicine/ American College of Chest Physicians/American Thoracic Society/ Surgical Infection Society sepsis definition
Zhao H, Heard SO, Mullen MT, et al (Univ of Massachusetts Med School, Worcester; et al)
Crit Care Med 40:1700-1706, 2012

Objectives.—Limited research has been conducted to compare the test characteristics of the 1991 and 2001 sepsis consensus definitions. This study assessed the accuracy of the two sepsis consensus definitions among adult critically ill patients compared to sepsis case adjudication by three senior clinicians.

Design.—Observational study of patients admitted to intensive care units.
Setting.—Seven intensive care units of an academic medical center.
Patients.—A random sample of 960 patients from all adult intensive care unit patients between October 2007 and December 2008.
Intervention.—None.
Measurements and Main Results.—Sensitivity, specificity, and the area under the receiver operating characteristic curve for the two consensus definitions were calculated by comparing the number of patients who met or did not meet consensus definitions vs. the number of patients who were or were not diagnosed with sepsis by adjudication. The 1991 sepsis definition had a high sensitivity of 94.6%, but a low specificity of 61.0%. The 2001 sepsis definition had a slightly increased sensitivity but a decreased specificity, which were 96.9% and 58.3%, respectively. The areas under the receiver operating characteristic curve for the two definitions were not statistically different (0.778 and 0.776, respectively). The sensitivities and areas under the receiver operating characteristic curve of both definitions were lower at the 24-hr time window level than those of the intensive care unit stay level, though their specificities increased slightly. Fever, high white blood cell count or immature forms, low Glasgow coma score, edema, positive fluid balance, high cardiac index, low Pao_2/Fio_2 ratio, and high levels of creatinine and lactate were significantly associated with sepsis by both definitions and adjudication.
Conclusions.—Both the 1991 and the 2001 sepsis definition have a high sensitivity but low specificity; the 2001 definition has a slightly increased sensitivity but a decreased specificity compared to the 1991 definition. The diagnostic performances of both definitions were suboptimal. A parsimonious set of significant predictors for sepsis diagnosis is likely to improve current sepsis case definitions.

▶ Clinicians have recognized sepsis as an important disease for centuries. It is currently considered one of the leading causes of morbidity and mortality in critically ill patients. Sepsis is an important area of research in critical care, with millions of dollars invested in the search for new therapeutic interventions. Yet, despite all this, we are still trying to find clear, concise definitions that can help clinicians diagnose sepsis at the bedside. In 1991, the American College of Chest Physicians and the Society of Critical Care Medicine convened a conference in an attempt to provide a framework of standardized definitions for sepsis.[1] This consensus conference produced definitions for sepsis, severe sepsis, and septic shock and coined the term *systemic inflammatory response syndrome (SIRS)*. Although these definitions helped establish a common language for research, they often were criticized for their lack of specificity at the bedside. To this point, critics argued that SIRS was often found in critically ill patients and was not a good discriminator for sepsis/infection. In 2001, a new consensus conference was convened with the goal of revising and improving the 1991 definitions. The new definition expanded the SIRS criteria to include a list of general, inflammatory, hemodynamic, organ dysfunction, or tissue perfusion criteria.[2]

There has been a paucity of research evaluating the effect of the 1991 and 2001 definitions. In this study, the authors assessed the test characteristics (sensitivity, specificity, and area under the receiver operating characteristic [ROC] curve) of the 1991 and 2001 consensus definitions compared with sepsis case adjudication by 3 senior intensive care clinicians. The study found that the 1991 sepsis definition had a high sensitivity (94.6%) but a low specificity (61%). The 2001 sepsis definition had a slightly increased sensitivity (96.9%) but a decreased specificity (58.3%). The areas under the ROC curve were essentially the same for both definitions (0.778 and 0.776, respectively). The study utilized a logistic regression to identify specific criteria that were significantly associated with sepsis diagnosis both by the definitions and case adjudication. The criteria that were more likely to be associated with a final diagnosis of sepsis included fever, high white cell count or immature forms, low Glasgow coma score, edema, positive fluid balance, high cardiac index, low Pao_2/Fio_2 ratio, high level of creatinine, and high levels of lactate. Despite its limitations, this is an important study because it is the first to utilize a methodology to evaluate how the consensus definitions for sepsis perform. The bottom line is that both the 1991 and 2001 consensus definitions are suboptimal in the clinical arena. The results of this study may be important to consider in future attempts to refine our definitions of sepsis.

S. Zanotti, MD

References

1. Bone RC, Balk RA, Cerra FB, et al. Definitions for sepsis and organ failure and guidelines for the use of innovative therapies in sepsis. The ACCP/SCCM Consensus Conference Committee. American College of Chest Physicians/Society of Critical Care Medicine. *Chest.* 1992;101:1644-1655.
2. Levy MM, Fink MP, Marshall JC, et al. 2001 SCCM/ESICM/ACCP/ATS/SIS International Sepsis Definitions Conference. *Crit Care Med.* 2003;31:1250-1256.

Septic Shock Attributed to *Candida* Infection: Importance of Empiric Therapy and Source Control
Kollef M, Micek S, Hampton N, et al (Washington Univ School of Medicine, St Louis, MO; Barnes-Jewish Hosp, St Louis, MO; Hosp Informatics Group, St Louis, MO; et al)
Clin Infect Dis 54:1739-1746, 2012

Background.—Delayed treatment of candidemia has previously been shown to be an important determinant of patient outcome. However, septic shock attributed to *Candida* infection and its determinants of outcome have not been previously evaluated in a large patient population.

Methods.—A retrospective cohort study of hospitalized patients with septic shock and blood cultures positive for *Candida* species was conducted at Barnes-Jewish Hospital, a 1250-bed urban teaching hospital (January 2002—December 2010).

Results.—Two hundred twenty-four consecutive patients with septic shock and a positive blood culture for *Candida* species were identified. Death during hospitalization occurred among 155 (63.5%) patients. The hospital mortality rate for patients having adequate source control and antifungal therapy administered within 24 hours of the onset of shock was 52.8% (n = 142), compared to a mortality rate of 97.6% (n = 82) in patients who did not have these goals attained (*P* < .001). Multivariate logistic regression analysis demonstrated that delayed antifungal treatment (adjusted odds ratio [AOR], 33.75; 95% confidence interval [CI], 9.65−118.04; *P* = .005) and failure to achieve timely source control (AOR, 77.40; 95% CI, 21.52−278.38; *P* = .001) were independently associated with a greater risk of hospital mortality.

Conclusions.—The risk of death is exceptionally high among patients with septic shock attributed to *Candida* infection. Efforts aimed at timely source control and antifungal treatment are likely to be associated with improved clinical outcomes.

► Severe sepsis and septic shock are among the leading causes of morbidity and mortality in critically ill patients. The cornerstone of treatment for septic shock is based on rapid administration of appropriate antimicrobials, hemodynamic support, and source control when possible. There is a clear relationship between delays in the initiation of appropriate antimicrobials and increased mortality. The number of cases of septic shock with positive blood cultures for *Candida* is somewhere in the range of 15%. Over time, cases of septic shock resulting from *Candida* seem to be increasing. Septic shock due to *Candida* has traditionally been associated with very poor outcomes. Many clinicians attribute this to the fact that patients who develop septic shock from *Candida* are usually sicker patients with numerous comorbid conditions. Alternatively, others have pointed out that we usually recognize *Candida* as a potential cause of septic shock after a positive blood culture. By the nature of how long it takes for these blood cultures to be reported as positive, it is usually associated with significant delays in the initiation of appropriate antifungals. This delay in the initiation of appropriate antifungal therapy could also represent a significant factor in determining poor outcomes in fungal septic shock.

This study had 2 goals: (1) to evaluate the appropriateness of antimicrobial therapy prescribed for patients with septic shock attributed to *Candida* infection and (2) to examine the influence of appropriate antimicrobial therapy on patient outcomes. This single-center retrospective cohort study identified 224 consecutive patients with septic shock and a blood culture positive for *Candida* species. Overall hospital mortality was high at 63.5%. In patients with adequate source control and antifungal therapy administered within 24 hours of onset of septic shock, hospital mortality was 52.8%. In patients who did not meet these criteria, mortality was significantly higher (97.6%). Furthermore, multivariate logistic regression analysis demonstrated that delayed antifungal treatment and failure to achieve timely source control were independent factors associated with greater mortality.

This study shows the exceptionally high risk of death among patients with septic shock resulting from *Candida*. It also provides strong evidence of the importance of initiation of early appropriate antifungal therapy and timely source control. Considering how most arrive at a diagnosis of *Candida* as the cause of septic shock, it is evident that we need to start appropriate therapy much earlier than the results of blood cultures are finalized. Pending new methods to identify pathogens, clinicians should consider carefully the need to initiate early empiric antifungals in appropriate patients with septic shock.

S. Zanotti, MD

Effect of Bedside Ultrasonography on the Certainty of Physician Clinical Decisionmaking for Septic Patients in the Emergency Department
Haydar SA, Moore ET, Higgins GL III, et al (Maine Med Ctr, Portland)
Ann Emerg Med 60:346-358, 2012

Study Objective.—Sepsis protocols promote aggressive patient management, including invasive procedures. After the provision of point-of-care ultrasonographic markers of volume status and cardiac function, we seek to evaluate changes in emergency physician clinical decisionmaking and physician assessments about the clinical utility of the point-of-care ultrasonographic data when caring for adult sepsis patients.

Methods.—For this prospective before-and-after study, patients with suspected sepsis received point-of-care ultrasonography to determine cardiac contractility, inferior vena cava diameter, and inferior vena cava collapsibility. Physician reports of treatment plans, presumed causes of observed vital sign abnormalities, and degree of certainty were compared before and after knowledge of point-of-care ultrasonographic findings. The clinical utility of point-of-care ultrasonographic data was also evaluated.

Results.—Seventy-four adult sepsis patients were enrolled: 27 (37%) sepsis, 30 (40%) severe sepsis, 16 (22%) septic shock, and 1 (1%) systemic inflammatory response syndrome. After receipt of point-of-care ultrasonographic data, physicians altered the presumed primary cause of vital sign abnormalities in 12 cases (17% [95% confidence interval {CI} 8% to 25%]) and procedural intervention plans in 20 cases (27% [95% CI 17% to 37%]). Overall treatment plans were changed in 39 cases (53% [95% CI 41% to 64%]). Certainty increased in 47 (71%) cases and decreased in 19 (29%). Measured on a 100-mm visual analog scale, the mean clinical utility score was 65 mm (SD 29; 95% CI 58 to 72), with usefulness reported in all cases.

Conclusion.—Emergency physicians found point-of-care ultrasonographic data about cardiac contractility, inferior vena cava diameter, and inferior vena cava collapsibility to be clinically useful in treating adult patients with sepsis. Increased certainty followed acquisition of point-of-care ultrasonographic data in most instances. Point-of-care ultrasonography appears to be a useful modality in evaluating and treating adult sepsis patients.

▶ Following introduction of early goal-directed therapy and the publication of the Surviving Sepsis Campaign guidelines, many emergency departments initiated sepsis protocols to aid in early identification and treatment of severe sepsis and septic shock patients. As noted in this study and others, there has been a reluctance to adhere strictly to these guidelines partly due to assessment of central venous pressure and central venous oxygen saturation with the relatively invasive procedure of central venous catheter placement. Use of bedside ultrasound has been proposed as a potential noninvasive method to guide initial management in some of these patients. The objectives of this prospective questionnaire-based study were to determine if certain early bedside ultrasound interventions in septic patients affected physician decision-making or changed physician-perceived clinical utility of bedside ultrasound in septic patients. Clinical utility was defined as the degree to which the ultrasound data influenced their management decisions. Data were collected using a before-and-after questionnaire regarding treatment plans, degree of certainty, and clinical utility, as defined previously. The specific ultrasound interventions were assessment of inferior vena cava (IVC) diameter and collapsibility and a single measurement to estimate left ventricular (LV) ejection fraction. The main results are summarized as follows: First, change in treatment plan occurred more than 50% of the time. Second, 90% of treating clinicians perceived the ultrasound data to be of positive clinical utility.

The fundamental confounding issue with this study is whether the change in treatment plan was appropriate or not. The assumption by the authors in their discussion section is that the change in treatment plan was beneficial to the patient. This may have been the case but there is no way to know this based on the study design and the recorded outcomes. Simply more data, even when collected noninvasively, are not always a helpful or even ethical approach. It is quite unclear from the presented data that a 1-time evaluation of IVC diameter and collapsibility and LV function can lead to improved patient care regardless of whether it changes decision plans of treating physicians. Some examples of potential pitfalls would include the following: What treatment decisions can be reached after determining volume status by IVC diameter and/or collapsibility in a patient who is not in shock or having signs of systemic hypoperfusion (elevated serum lactate)? How does the clinician react to a relatively low ejection fraction in a severe sepsis patient who also appears to be underresuscitated based on IVC collapsibility? With IVC diameter and collapsibility, is the clinician making decisions about merely volume status or predicting fluid responsiveness?

In the authors' conclusion, they accurately state that clinicians caring for sepsis patients "considered point-of-care ultrasonographic data about cardiac contractility, inferior vena cava diameter and collapsibility to be clinically useful." This is simply perceived clinical utility and one should not infer that this provides evidence for actual clinical utility of bedside ultrasound in this specific setting. It is important to note 3 issues in regard to the assessment of clinical utility: First, the questionnaire was apparently immediately filled out after the ultrasound results were given to the treating clinician. Thus, clinical utility was assessed before seeing the results of any intervention. Second, the treating clinician did not perform the ultrasound. This means that the clinical utility was determined without taking into account the time needed to complete the procedure. This is often an issue in clinical practice, where decisions to use bedside ultrasound from patient to patient are at least partially based on the time needed to perform the procedure. Third, the time to perform the ultrasound was noted to be an average of 138 minutes after patient arrival. Considering these patients required informed consent and a large portion were critically ill, completing the ultrasound just over 2 hours after arrival seems to be quite an impressive feat. However, one could argue that in clinical practice, use of bedside ultrasound in the critically ill patient is done even sooner and may be even more clinically useful earlier on in the patient's stay.

B. Goodgame, MD
S. Zanotti, MD

C1-esterase inhibitor infusion increases survival rates for patients with sepsis
Igonin AA, Protsenko DN, Galstyan GM, et al (Sechenov Moscow Med Univ, Russia; Clinical City Hosp #7, Moscow, Russia; Hematology Res Centre, Moscow, Russia; et al)
Crit Care Med 40:770-777, 2012

Objectives.—Systemic inflammatory response variability displays differing degrees of organ damage and differing outcomes of sepsis. C1-esterase inhibitor, an endogenous acute-phase protein, regulates various inflammatory and anti-inflammatory pathways, including the kallikrein-kinin system and leukocyte activity. This study assesses the influence of high-dose C1-esterase inhibitor administration on systemic inflammatory response and survival in patients with sepsis.

Design.—Open-label randomized controlled study.

Setting.—Surgical and medical intensive care units of nine university and city hospitals.

Patients.—Sixty-one patients with sepsis.

Interventions.—Patients were randomized to receive either 12,000 U of C1-esterase inhibitor infusions in addition to conventional treatment or conventional treatment only (n = 41 C1-esterase inhibitor, 20 controls). Blood samples for measurement of C1-esterase inhibitor, complement components C3 and C4, and C-reactive protein concentrations were drawn on days 1, 3, 5, 7, 10, and 28.

Measurements and Main Results.—Quartile analysis of C1-esterase inhibitor activity in sepsis subjects revealed that the lowest quartile subgroup had similar activity levels (0.7–1.2 U/L), when compared to healthy volunteers ($p > .05$). These normal-level C1-esterase inhibitor sepsis patients nevertheless displayed increased C-reactive protein ($p = .04$) production and higher likelihoods of a more severe sepsis ($p = .001$). Overall, infusion

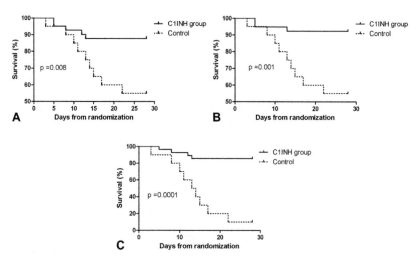

FIGURE 6.—*A*, All-cause mortality in the C1-esterase inhibitor (*C1INH*) (n = 41) and control (n = 20) groups; *p* = 0.008 (log rank Mantel-Cox). *B*, Sepsis-related mortality in the C1INH (n = 39) and control (n = 20) groups; *p* = 0.001 (log rank Mantel-Cox). *C*, Survival in the subgroup of Simplified Acute Physiology Score II >27. C1INH (n = 15) group vs. control group (n = 10); *p* = 0.0001 (log rank Mantel-Cox). Kaplan-Meier 28-day survival curves for the comparison of the treatment arm (C1-esterase inhibitor [*C1INH*] presented as *solid line*) and control arm (as *dashed line*) in subgroups stratified by the parameters of sepsis severity. (Reprinted from Igonin AA, Protsenko DN, Galstyan GM, et al. C1-esterase inhibitor infusion increases survival rates for patients with sepsis. *Crit Care Med.* 2012;40:770-777, with permission from the Society of Critical Care Medicine and Lippincott Williams & Wilkins.)

of C1-esterase inhibitor increased C1-esterase inhibitor ($p < .005$ vs. control on days 2, 3, and 5) functional activity, resulted in higher C3 levels ($p < .05$ vs. control on days 2 and 3), followed by decreased C-reactive protein ($p < .05$ vs. control on days 3 and 10). Simultaneously, C1-esterase inhibitor infusion in sepsis patients was associated with reduced all-cause mortality (12% vs. 45% in control, $p = .008$) as well as sepsis-related mortality (8% vs. 45% in control, $p = .001$) assessed over 28 days. The highest absolute reduction risk of 70% was achieved in sepsis patients with Simplified Acute Physiology Score II scores > 27.

Conclusion.—In the present study, patients in the lowest quartile of C1-esterase inhibitor activity in combination with high C-reactive protein demonstrated a higher risk of developing severe sepsis. In general, high-dose C1-esterase inhibitor infusion down-regulated the systemic inflammatory response and was associated with improved survival rates in sepsis patients, which could have important treatment and survival implications for individuals with C1-esterase inhibitor functional deficiency (Fig 6).

▶ With the recent withdrawal of recombinant human activated protein C from the market, the area of host response modulation in severe sepsis is once again orphan, with no approved treatments. After decades of failed clinical trials for novel host-modulating agents, it has become evident that patients with severe sepsis and septic shock have a variable inflammatory response. Therefore, it is unlikely that 1 agent blocking a specific aspect of the host response will work for all patients with sepsis. It seems that the future would hold treatments based on specific biomarkers or inflammatory patterns for individual patients. C1-esterase inhibitor (C1INH) is an endogenous acute-phase protein with regulatory actions of inflammatory and anti-inflammatory pathways. C1INH has important effects on the kallikrein-kinin system, the coagulation cascade, and leukocyte activity. These properties make C1INH an intriguing agent for treating severe sepsis. Furthermore, C1INH is already safely used to treat hereditary angioedema. In this open-label randomized study, the investigators evaluated the use of C1INH in the treatment of severe sepsis. The study also measured various inflammatory markers in each patient including levels of endogenous C1-esterase inhibitor activity. The most significant finding of this study was the association of C1INH administration at high doses with improved survival in sepsis patients (Fig 6). All-cause mortality and sepsis-related mortality were both improved significantly in the group of patients that received C1INH compared with the control group. Patients with increased severity as measured by a Simplified Acute Physiology Score II score of > 27 had the greatest benefit in mortality from treatment with C1INH. Finally, when patients were classified into quartiles based on C1-esterase inhibitor endogenous activity, the quartile with the lowest levels responded the best to the C1INH treatment. The results of this study should be considered preliminary. Many previous novel agents showed promise at this stage and later failed in larger confirmatory trials. However, the results of this study may offer a different approach to the evaluation of novel agents for the treatment of severe sepsis. This new approach would involve the use of biomarkers, specifically endogenous C1-esterase inhibitor activity, to identify a study group of patients with a higher likelihood of success.

S. Zanotti, MD

An evaluation of the diagnostic accuracy of the 1991 American College of Chest Physicians/Society of Critical Care Medicine and the 2001 Society of Critical Care Medicine/European Society of Intensive Care Medicine/ American College of Chest Physicians/American Thoracic Society/ Surgical Infection Society sepsis definition

Zhao H, Heard SO, Mullen MT, et al (Univ of Massachusetts Med School, Worcester; et al)

Crit Care Med 40:1700-1706, 2012

Objectives.—Limited research has been conducted to compare the test characteristics of the 1991 and 2001 sepsis consensus definitions. This study assessed the accuracy of the two sepsis consensus definitions among adult critically ill patients compared to sepsis case adjudication by three senior clinicians.

Design.—Observational study of patients admitted to intensive care units.

Setting.—Seven intensive care units of an academic medical center.

Patients.—A random sample of 960 patients from all adult intensive care unit patients between October 2007 and December 2008.

*Intervention.—*None.

*Measurements and Main Results.—*Sensitivity, specificity, and the area under the receiver operating characteristic curve for the two consensus definitions were calculated by comparing the number of patients who met or did not meet consensus definitions vs. the number of patients who were or were not diagnosed with sepsis by adjudication. The 1991 sepsis definition had a high sensitivity of 94.6%, but a low specificity of 61.0%. The 2001 sepsis definition had a slightly increased sensitivity but a decreased specificity, which were 96.9% and 58.3%, respectively. The areas under the receiver operating characteristic curve for the two definitions were not statistically different (0.778 and 0.776, respectively). The sensitivities and areas under the receiver operating characteristic curve of both definitions were lower at the 24-hr time window level than those of the intensive care unit stay level, though their specificities increased slightly. Fever, high white blood cell count or immature forms, low Glasgow coma score, edema, positive fluid balance, high cardiac index, low Pao_2/Fio_2 ratio, and high levels of creatinine and lactate were significantly associated with sepsis by both definitions and adjudication.

*Conclusions.—*Both the 1991 and the 2001 sepsis definition have a high sensitivity but low specificity; the 2001 definition has a slightly increased sensitivity but a decreased specificity compared to the 1991 definition. The diagnostic performances of both definitions were suboptimal. A parsimonious set of significant predictors for sepsis diagnosis is likely to improve current sepsis case definitions.

▶ This is a fascinating study using records from a computerized dataset of 1000 patients from 7 critical care units at a single hospital admitted between October 2007 and December 2008. Three senior intensivists used 2 definition systems to identify individuals having sepsis. Overall, a dramatic difference between the 2 definitions is not identified.[1,2]

Interestingly, these authors identify a number of biophysical parameters that support the diagnosis in the analysis conducted including fever, leukocytosis, Glasgow Coma Scale, edema, fluid balance, changes in cardiac index, partial pressure of arterial oxygen/fraction of inspired oxygen ratio, creatinine, and lactate level. Correlation between the clinicians reviewing cases was good but not outstanding. This reflects ambiguity that persists in identifying the patient with sepsis.

The authors are clear about limitations of this work. First, only adults admitted to this set of critical care units were employed. In many cases, data were incomplete. In some cases, conflicting information was recorded in the computerized medical record. Finally, the authors noted inconsistency in description and recording of organ failure within this patient group. All of these characteristics are consistent with utilization of data that were not gathered prospectively for the purpose of this trial.

Overall, it does not appear that we have gained significantly in diagnostic sophistication with a decade of evolution between the 2 scores.

D. J. Dries, MSE, MD

References

1. Bone RC, Balk RA, Cerra FB, et al. Definitions for sepsis and organ failure and guidelines for the use of innovative therapies in sepsis. The ACCP/SCCM Consensus Conference Committee. American College of Chest Physicians/Society of Critical Care Medicine. *Chest.* 1992;101:1644-1655.
2. Levy MM, Fink MP, Marshall JC, et al. 2001 SCCM/ESICM/ACCP/ATS/SIS International Sepsis Definitions Conference. *Crit Care Med.* 2003;31:1250-1256.

7 Metabolism/ Gastrointestinal/ Nutrition/ Hematology-Oncology

---

Fibrinogen function after severe burn injury
Schaden E, Hoerburger D, Hacker S, et al (Med Univ Of Vienna, Austria; et al)
Burns 38:77-82, 2012

Background.—Evidence regarding hypercoagulability in the first week after burn trauma is growing. This hypercoagulable state may partly be caused by increased fibrinogen levels. Rotational thrombelastometry offers a test which measures functional fibrinogen (FIBTEM®). To test the hypothesis that in patients with severe burn injury fibrinogen function changes over time, we simultaneously measured FIBTEM® and fibrinogen concentration early after burn trauma.

Methods.—After Ethics Committee approval consecutive patients with severe burn trauma admitted to the burn intensive care unit of the General Hospital of Vienna were included in the study. Blood examinations were done immediately and 12, 24 and 48 h after admission. At each time point fibrinogen level (Clauss) and 4 commercially available ROTEM® tests were performed.

Results.—20 consecutive patients were included in the study. Fibrinogen level and FIBTEM® MCF were within the reference range until 24 h after burn trauma but increased significantly 48 h after trauma. There was a significant correlation between FIBTEM® MCF and fibrinogen level ($R = 0.714$, $p < 0.001$).

Conclusion.—The results of this prospective observational clinical study show that fibrinogen function changes early after burn trauma and can be visualized by ROTEM® with the fibrinogen-sensitive FIBTEM® test.

▶ The systemic inflammatory response syndrome that develops following a significant thermal trauma or inhalation injury has been well described. The occurrence is considered part of the normal physiological response to burn injury and is not considered a separate diagnosis or a complication. Current definitions

177

for sepsis and infection have many criteria that are routinely found in burn patients, making these definitions less applicable to the burn patient population.[1] The authors' assertion that major blood loss is a routine part of surgery for burn wound excision and grafting is overstated, as more recent developments and use of multimodal intraoperative therapies have vastly decreased the need for transfusions. A more limited approach to packed red blood cell transfusions has been recommended as the negative effects of blood transfusions in burn patients have come to light.[2] With this background in mind, we must consider whether the knowledge of the fibrinogen levels at an earlier time point (40 minutes earlier with the FIBTEM®) has clinical application and relevance in the burn population. Even without clinical evidence of hypercoagulable states, many burn center physicians routinely administer deep vein thrombosis prophylaxis to burn patients starting at the time of admission. There are certain risk factors in burn patients that may place some patients at higher risk of clotting, but these are not universally accepted criteria. Data that extend beyond 48 hours showing changes in outcomes based on interventions regarding fibrinogen levels may provide more clinically relevant information in the future. Without data provided beyond the brief 48-hour time frame in this study, I am not changing my practice or ordering additional laboratory studies that just show up as another charge on a patient's hospital bill.

B. A. Latenser, MD, FACS

References

1. Greenhalgh DG, Saffle JR, Holmes JH IV, et al. American Burn Association consensus conference to define sepsis and infection in burns. *J Burn Care Res.* 2007;28:776-790.
2. Palmieri TL, Lee T, O'Mara MS, Greenhalgh DG. Effects of a restrictive blood transfusion policy on outcomes in children with burn injury. *J Burn Care Res.* 2007;28:65-70.

Five-Year Outcomes after Oxandrolone Administration in Severely Burned Children: A Randomized Clinical Trial of Safety and Efficacy
Porro LJ, Herndon DN, Rodriguez NA, et al (Shriners Hosps for Children-Galveston, Galveston, TX; et al)
J Am Coll Surg 214:489-504, 2012

Background.—Oxandrolone, an anabolic agent, has been administered for 1 year post burn with beneficial effects in pediatric patients. However, the long-lasting effects of this treatment have not been studied. This single-center prospective trial determined the long-term effects of 1 year of oxandrolone administration in severely burned children; assessments were continued for up to 4 years post therapy.

Study Design.—Patients 0 to 18 years old with burns covering >30% of the total body surface area were randomized to receive placebo (n = 152) or oxandrolone, 0.1 mg/kg twice daily for 12 months (n = 70). At hospital discharge, patients were randomized to a 12-week exercise program or to

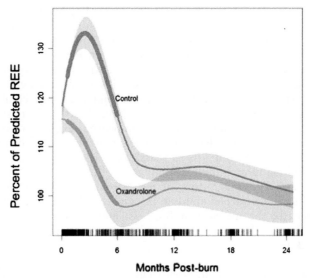

Months Post-burn

FIGURE 2.—Effect of oxandrolone on percent predicted resting energy expenditure (REE). Data are represented the loess-smoothed trend in REE with shading indicating ± standard error. Hatch marks across the bottom represent the density of sampled data at each time point (1,427 total observations). Time points at which differences are significant are indicated with wider lines ($p < 0.004$). (Reprinted from Porro LJ, Herndon DN, Rodriguez NA, et al. Five-year outcomes after oxandrolone administration in severely burned children: a randomized clinical trial of safety and efficacy. *J Am Coll Surg.* 2012;214:489-504, Copyright 2012, with permission from the American College of Surgeons.)

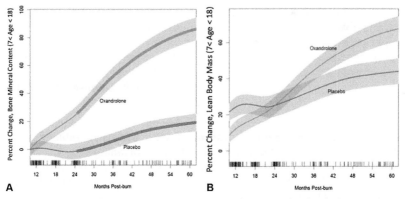

FIGURE 4.—Percent change in (A) total body bone mineral content and (B) lean body mass. Data are represented as the loess-smoothed trend in bone mineral content and in lean body mass with shading indicating ± standard error. Hatch marks across the bottom represent the density of the sampled data at each time point (572 total observations). Time points at which differences are significant are indicated with wider lines ($p < 0.001$). (Reprinted from Porro LJ, Herndon DN, Rodriguez NA, et al. Five-year outcomes after oxandrolone administration in severely burned children: a randomized clinical trial of safety and efficacy. *J Am Coll Surg.* 2012;214:489-504, Copyright 2012, with permission from the American College of Surgeons.)

standard of care. Resting energy expenditure, standing height, weight, lean body mass, muscle strength, bone mineral content (BMC), cardiac work, rate pressure product, sexual maturation, and concentrations of serum inflammatory cytokines, hormones, and liver enzymes were monitored.

Results.—Oxandrolone substantially decreased resting energy expenditure and rate pressure product, increased insulin-like growth factor-1 secretion during the first year after burn injury, and, in combination with exercise, increased lean body mass and muscle strength considerably. Oxandrolone-treated children exhibited improved height percentile and BMC content compared with controls. The maximal effect of oxandrolone was found in children aged 7 to 18 years. No deleterious side effects were attributed to long-term administration.

Conclusions.—Administration of oxandrolone improves long-term recovery of severely burned children in height, BMC, cardiac work, and muscle strength; the increase in BMC is likely to occur by means of insulin-like growth factor-1. These benefits persist for up to 5 years post burn (Figs 2 and 4).

▶ This is another elegant study from Herndon's laboratory at the Galveston Shriners' Hospital investigating oxandrolone use in severely burned children. The authors investigated many of the components of the improved (ie, decreased) resting energy expenditure, height percentiles, and bone mineral content with long-term oxandrolone therapy. Figs 2 and 4 demonstrate the most relevant findings in a very easy-to-read format. Certainly, the mechanisms by which oxandrolone has long-lasting effects are a little more clear and fascinating as they unfold. Only a lab with the robust resources such as those demonstrated here could adequately conduct a research project of this scope. It could be most illuminating to see what, if any, improved outcomes may be present in a comparably powered study of severely burned adults. Given the safety profile of long-term use, oxandrolone should be a routine part of the outpatient medication list for children who survive burns > 30% of their body surface area.

B. A. Latenser, MD, FACS

Red blood cell transfusion is associated with increased rebleeding in patients with nonvariceal upper gastrointestinal bleeding
Restellini S, Kherad O, Jairath V, et al (Geneva's Univ Hosps and Univ of Geneva, Switzerland; La Tour Hosp and Univ of Geneva, Switzerland; John Radcliffe Hosp, Oxford, UK; et al)
Aliment Pharmacol Ther 37:316-322, 2013

Background.—There exists considerable practice variation and little evidence to guide red blood cell (RBC) transfusion in patients with nonvariceal upper gastrointestinal bleeding (NVUGIB). Studies in other critically ill cohorts suggest associations between transfusions and adverse patient outcomes.

Aim.—To characterise any possible clinically-relevant association between RBC transfusion following NVUGIB with rebleeding and mortality.

Methods.—Observational study utilising the Canadian Registry of patients with Upper Gastrointestinal Bleeding and Endoscopy (RUGBE). Multivariable logistic regression models were used to examine and quantify independent associations between RBC transfusion and clinical outcomes.

Results.—Overall, 1677 patients were included (66.2 ± 16.8 years, 61.7% male, 2.5 ± 1.7 comorbid conditions, initial haemoglobin, 96.8 ± 27.2 g/L); 53.7% received RBC transfusions (2.9 ± 1.6 units of blood), 31.6% had haemodynamic instability, 5.1% fresh blood on rectal examination and 8.6% in the nasogastric tube aspirate. Endoscopic haemostasis was performed in 35.2%. Overall rebleeding (defined as continuous bleeding, rebleeding or surgery) and mortality rates were 17.9% and 5.4%, respectively. After adjusting for potential confounders, transfusion of RBC within 24 h of presentation was significantly and independently associated with an increased risk of rebleeding (OR: 1.8, 95% CI: 1.2−2.8), but not death (OR: 1.0, 95% CI: 0.6−1.8).

Conclusions.—This study suggests an association between RBC transfusion following NVUGIB and subsequent rebleeding, after appropriate and extensive adjustment for confounding. Prospective randomised trial evidence is needed to identify the most efficacious and cost-effective transfusional strategies in these patients.

▶ Transfusion is commonly used in patients with upper gastrointestinal bleeding (UGIB) both variceal and nonvariceal, often before either the source or extent of hemorrhage is fully defined, although practices vary widely between institutions and individuals. There are data that suggest that aggressive transfusion of packed red blood cells (PRBC) in variceal hemorrhage may exacerbate bleeding by elevating portal pressures, but specific parameters guiding the use of PRBC in nonvariceal bleeding are lacking. This observational study attempted to assess the impact of red cell transfusion on rebleeding and mortality in patients with nonvariceal UGIB. In this study, data on nearly 1700 patients admitted to 18 hospitals over a 4-year period were reviewed for a variety of historical, demographic, clinical, diagnostic, therapeutic, acuity, and outcome data. After adjustment for a variety of confounding factors in a multivariate analysis, PRBC transfusion was determined to be 1 of several independent predictors of rebleeding in the subjects evaluated, with an odds ratio of 1.8. Transfusion was not, however, a predictor of increased mortality. The mechanism for the increased rebleeding is not immediately obvious. Although the amount of platelets and fresh frozen plasma or other clotting factors transfused were not reported, dilutional and/or consumptive coagulopathy seem unlikely explanations, as the median number of units of PRBC transfused was 1 (interquartile ratio 1-2). Also, because these were nonvariceal bleeding patients, it is unlikely that any substantial number of rebleeding events can be attributed to an acute elevation in intravascular pressures after transfusion. Thus, as the authors point out, the relationship remains one of association at this time. Nevertheless, these are intriguing findings, and yet another area in which PRBC transfusion, traditionally felt to be not only safe but essential, may well be, in many instances, detrimental. Further prospective study is clearly warranted to validate and clarify these findings.

D. R. Gerber, DO

Outcome of Patients Who Refuse Transfusion After Cardiac Surgery: A Natural Experiment With Severe Blood Conservation

Pattakos G, Koch CG, Brizzio ME, et al (Cleveland Clinic, OH; et al)
Arch Intern Med 172:1154-1160, 2012

Background.—Jehovah's Witness patients (Witnesses) who undergo cardiac surgery provide a unique natural experiment in severe blood conservation because anemia, transfusion, erythropoietin, and antifibrinolytics have attendant risks. Our objective was to compare morbidity and long-term survival of Witnesses undergoing cardiac surgery with a similarly matched group of patients who received transfusions.

Methods.—A total of 322 Witnesses and 87 453 non-Witnesses underwent cardiac surgery at our center from January 1, 1983, to January 1, 2011. All Witnesses prospectively refused blood transfusions. Among non-Witnesses, 38 467 did not receive blood transfusions and 48 986 did. We used propensity methods to match patient groups and parametric multiphase hazard methods to assess long-term survival. Our main outcome measures were postoperative morbidity complications, in-hospital mortality, and long-term survival.

Results.—Witnesses had fewer acute complications and shorter length of stay than matched patients who received transfusions: myocardial infarction, 0.31% vs 2.8% ($P = .01$); additional operation for bleeding, 3.7% vs 7.1% ($P = .03$); prolonged ventilation, 6% vs 16% ($P \le .001$); intensive care unit length of stay (15th, 50th, and 85th percentiles), 24, 25, and 72 vs 24, 48, and 162 hours ($P < .001$); and hospital length of stay (15th, 50th, and 85th percentiles), 5, 7, and 11 vs 6, 8, and 16 days ($P < .001$). Witnesses had better 1-year survival (95%; 95% CI, 93%-96%; vs 89%; 95% CI, 87%-90%; $P = .007$) but similar 20-year survival (34%; 95% CI, 31%-38%; vs 32% 95% CI, 28%-35%; $P = .90$).

Conclusions.—Witnesses do not appear to be at increased risk for surgical complications or long-term mortality when comparisons are properly made by transfusion status. Thus, current extreme blood management strategies do not appear to place patients at heightened risk for reduced long-term survival.

▶ A substantial body of literature has accumulated in recent years that strongly indicates that patients undergoing cardiac surgery can not only tolerate lower hemoglobins than traditionally appreciated, but they may suffer both short- and long-term adverse effects from red cell transfusions. Such data have prompted some investigators to advocate increased diligence in blood conservation and blood management protocols in cardiac surgery. By reviewing outcomes in Jehovah's Witnesses, a population whose religious beliefs preclude the acceptance of red blood cells (and often other blood products as well) and comparing them with propensity-matched subjects undergoing cardiac surgery who were transfused, the authors attempted to perform what they deemed a natural observational study on the short- and long-term effects of red cell transfusion on outcomes in cardiac surgical patients. They found that Jehovah's Witnesses were significantly less likely to have several postoperative complications, including myocardial infarction, reoperation for bleeding, and prolonged mechanical ventilation. They also had shorter intensive care and overall postoperative lengths of stay. In addition, the Jehovah's Witnesses had lower short-term mortality compared with propensity-matched transfused patients, but this did not persist long term, measured at 20 years. While there are limitations inherent in this study, including its retrospective, observational design, certain inherent concerns with propensity matching, and the absence of some demographic comparison data (eg, while there are data on smoking history in the Jehovah's Witness and matched groups, there are no data on alcohol history), overall this study seems to provide yet more support for a cautious application of red cell transfusion, even in a population historically felt to be vulnerable to low hemoglobin values.

D. R. Gerber, DO

Impact of Blood Product Transfusion on Short and Long-Term Survival After Cardiac Surgery: More Evidence
Bhaskar B, Dulhunty J, Mullany DV, et al (The Prince Charles Hosp, Brisbane, Australia; Royal Brisbane and Women's Hosp, Australia)
Ann Thorac Surg 94:460-467, 2012

Background.—Despite the proven benefits in hemorrhagic shock, blood transfusions have been linked to increased morbidity and mortality. The short-term adverse effects of blood transfusion in cardiac surgical patients are well documented but there are very few studies that adequately assess the long-term survival. This study was undertaken to evaluate the effects of transfusion on both short-term and long-term survival after cardiac surgery.

Methods.—Data from 5,342 patients who underwent a cardiac surgical procedure from January 2002 to December 2005 at our institution were reviewed. The effect of transfusion of packed red blood cells (PRBC) and other blood products was tested in a 2-level approach of transfusion (any) versus no transfusion, and also a 4-level approach of transfusion (PRBC, other blood products, and both blood and blood products) versus no transfusion. Long-term survival data of these patients were obtained. Cox proportional hazard models, Kaplan-Meier survival plots, and hazard functions were used to compare the groups.

Results.—A total of 3,013 of the 5,342 study patients (56.4%) received transfusion during or within 72 hours of their cardiac surgery. Median time to death was significantly lower for patients who received transfusions; 1.15 years for PRC and 0.83 years for any transfusion, compared with

4.68 years in the non-transfused group. The overall 30-day mortality was 1.7%, but in patients who received transfusions (3.6%) was significantly higher than the non-transfused group (0.3%, $p < 0.001$). The 1-year mortality (overall 3.9%) in the transfused group (7.3%, $p < 0.001$) was also significantly higher than that in the non-transfused group (1.3%). The 5-year mortality rate in the transfused group was more than double that in the non-transfused group (16% vs 7%). After correction for comorbidities and other factors, transfusion was still associated with a 66% increase in mortality.

Conclusions.—This study suggests that blood or blood product transfusion during or after cardiac surgery is associated with increased short-term and long-term mortality. It reinforces the need for prospective randomized controlled studies for evaluation of restrictive transfusion triggers and objective clinical indicators for transfusion in the cardiac surgical patient population.

▶ Although formal guidelines for the use of packed red blood cells (PRBC) in the setting of cardiac surgery have been published by authoritative sources,[1] these products continue to be transfused far more liberally by many practitioners involved in the care of patients undergoing such surgery than current recommendations would suggest. In addition, an extensive volume of literature now exists that shows that cardiac surgical patients who receive PRBC, as a group, have a wide variety of worse outcomes than those who do not. What is particularly interesting is that the data indicate these adverse effects may continue for many years. To evaluate for this possibility, these investigators performed a retrospective analysis of data collected on more than 5000 patients undergoing cardiac surgery over a 4-year period. Just more than 56% received PRBC and other blood products, and approximately 69% of those (2077) received only PRBC. When assessed via a standard multivariate analysis, controlling for numerous risk factors and comorbidities as well as when subsequently evaluated using a propensity score, constructed attempting to estimate the probability of receiving a PRBC transfusion, red cell transfusion was identified as an independent risk factor for both early (30-day) and late (1- and 5-year) mortality. In addition, other short-term complications were found to be independently associated with transfusion and included a variety of infections (including severe sepsis) and renal dysfunction. As the authors note, there are plausible explanations for the increased short-term adverse effects seen with PRBC transfusion, including immunosuppression and proinflammatory effects. Higher short-term mortality could be at least partially ascribed to the higher acuity of the patients in this group (despite the adjustments made in the statistical analyses). However, this would no longer seem to be a factor at 5 years. These data, similar to those in some previous work, indicate that PRBC have acute detrimental effects in the cardiac surgical population. Because there is a significant body of literature indicating that these patients can tolerate hemoglobin levels significantly lower than those that had traditionally been considered safe, and with specific guidelines now available supporting this, practitioners should be increasingly wary when it comes to transfusing PRBC in this population, especially without a clear physiologic indication. These data, along with the other reported data indicating not only acute but prolonged adverse effects of transfusion in cardiac surgery patients, make it reasonable to wonder whether similar effects occur in other patient populations, including nonsurgical patients receiving PRBC. The answer could have significant implications for the treatment of many patients, especially those for whom transfusion may be an option but not a necessity. This would seem to be an area that is clearly ripe for investigation and potentially of great clinical utility.

D. R. Gerber, DO

Reference

1. Society of Thoracic Surgeons Blood Conservation Guideline Task Force; Ferraris VA, Brown JR, Despotis GJ. 2011 update to the society of Thoracic Surgeons and the Society of Cardiovascular Anesthesiologists blood conservation clinical practice guidelines. *Ann Thorac Surg.* 2011;91:944-982.

Red Blood Cell Transfusion: A Clinical Practice Guideline From the AABB
Carson JL, for the Clinical Transfusion Medicine Committee of the AABB
(UMDNJ—Robert Wood Johnson Med School, New Brunswick, NJ; et al)
Ann Intern Med 157:49-58, 2012

Description.—Although approximately 85 million units of red blood cells (RBCs) are transfused annually worldwide, transfusion practices vary widely. The AABB (formerly, the American Association of Blood Banks) developed this guideline to provide clinical recommendations about hemoglobin concentration thresholds and other clinical variables that trigger RBC transfusions in hemodynamically stable adults and children.

Methods.—These guidelines are based on a systematic review of randomized clinical trials evaluating transfusion thresholds. We performed a literature search from 1950 to February 2011 with no language restrictions. We examined the proportion of patients who received any RBC transfusion and the number of RBC units transfused to describe the effect of restrictive transfusion strategies on RBC use. To determine the clinical consequences of restrictive transfusion strategies, we examined overall mortality, nonfatal myocardial infarction, cardiac events, pulmonary edema, stroke, thromboembolism, renal failure, infection, hemorrhage, mental confusion, functional recovery, and length of hospital stay.

Recommendation 1.—The AABB recommends adhering to a restrictive transfusion strategy (7 to 8 g/dL) in hospitalized, stable patients (Grade: strong recommendation; high-quality evidence).

Recommendation 2.—The AABB suggests adhering to a restrictive strategy in hospitalized patients with preexisting cardiovascular disease and considering transfusion for patients with symptoms or a hemoglobin level of 8 g/dL or less (Grade: weak recommendation; moderate-quality evidence).

Recommendation 3.—The AABB cannot recommend for or against a liberal or restrictive transfusion threshold for hospitalized, hemodynamically stable patients with the acute coronary syndrome (Grade: uncertain recommendation; very low-quality evidence).
Recommendation 4.—The AABB suggests that transfusion decisions be influenced by symptoms as well as hemoglobin concentration (Grade: weak recommendation; low-quality evidence).

▶ As all clinicians involved in the care of the critically ill are acutely aware, anemia, whether present at the time of admission or developing over the course of hospitalization, is a problem ultimately affecting most intensive care unit patients. As data regarding the ability of patients to tolerate lower hemoglobin (Hgb) levels, as well as data concerning the adverse effects of transfused packed red blood cells (PRBC) and their often limited acute physiologic benefits in terms of ability to deliver oxygen to tissues increases, many practitioners have adopted a more restrictive approach to transfusion, using physiologic parameters and lower Hgb levels as the basis for clinical decisions for when to give PRBC. Even so, 15 million units of PRBC are transfused annually in the United States and 85 million worldwide. However, for most situations, specific guidelines have been lacking to assist in such decision making. This article, produced by a multidisciplinary group with expertise in a variety of relevant fields, evaluated the literature on the appropriate indications for PRBC transfusion in clinically stable patients under a variety of circumstances and subjected it to a well-defined and careful grading system to come up with recommendations. Most importantly, the group concludes overall that the general concept of a restrictive approach to transfusion in hemodynamically stable patients is well supported by the literature. This recommendation holds for medical and surgical patients and patients with a history of coronary artery disease, although the threshold for "restrictive" varied between 7 g/dL and 8 g/dL depending on the specific patient population. Only in patients with acute coronary syndrome (ACS) did the panel fail to make a recommendation. While acknowledging the extensive literature demonstrating a significant increase in adverse outcomes in patients with ACS who underwent transfusion when their Hgb levels were greater than approximately 8 g/dL, these data were essentially all retrospective or observational, so it didn't feel adequate enough to base any recommendations on.[1] It was noted that this was in contrast to the European Society of Cardiology, which recommends withholding transfusion in stable ACS patients with Hgb levels greater than 8 g/dL.[1] Overall, this set of guidelines fills an important gap for not only intensivists but surgeons and anyone involved in the care of the acutely ill, in-patient population. It provides relatively clear guidance on utilization of an important resource with a rational basis for these decisions. There is still room for individualization of therapy and allowances for clinical situations, and the authors address the issue of transfusion for relief of symptomatic anemia. Although questions remain to be answered about what, if any, the ultimate safe threshold is for transfusion in specific circumstances and in specific patient populations, these guidelines are a good resource now.

D. R. Gerber, DO

Reference

1. Task Force for Diagnosis and Treatment of Non-ST-Segment Elevation Acute Coronary Syndromes of European Society of Cardiology, Bassand JP, Hamm CW, Ardissino D, et al. Guidelines for the diagnosis and treatment of non-ST-segment elevation acute coronary syndromes. *Eur Heart J.* 2007;28: 1598-1660.

Is fresh-frozen plasma clinically effective? An update of a systematic review of randomized controlled trials

Yang L, Stanworth S, Hopewell S, et al (NHS Blood and Transplant, Oxford, UK; Addenbrooke's Hosp, Cambridge, UK; UK Cochrane Centre, Oxford)
Transfusion 52:1673-1686, 2012

Background.—The clinical use of frozen plasma (FP) continues to increase, both in prophylactic and in therapeutic settings. In 2004, a systematic review of all published randomized controlled trials (RCTs) revealed a lack of evidence that supported the efficacy of FP use. This is an update that includes all new RCTs published since the original review.

Study Design and Methods.—Trials involving transfusion of FP up to July 2011 were identified from searches of MEDLINE, EMBASE, CINAHL, *The Cochrane Library*, and the UKBTS/SRI Transfusion Evidence Library. Methodologic quality was assessed. The primary outcome measure was the effect of FP on survival.

Results.—Twenty-one new trials were eligible for inclusion. These covered prophylactic and therapeutic FP use in liver disease, in cardiac surgery, for warfarin anticoagulation reversal, for thrombotic thrombocytopenic purpura treatment, for plasmapheresis, and in other settings, including burns, shock, and head injury. The largest number of recent RCTs were conducted in cardiac surgery; meta-analysis showed no significant difference for FP use for the outcome of 24-hours postoperative blood loss (weighted mean difference, -35.24 mL; 95% confidence interval, -84.16 to 13.68 mL). Overall, there was no significant benefit for FP use across all the clinical conditions. Only two of the 21 trials fulfilled all the criteria for quality assessment.

Conclusion.—Combined with the 2004 review, 80 RCTs have investigated FP with no consistent evidence of significant benefit for prophylactic and therapeutic use across a range of indications evaluated. There has been little improvement in the overall methodologic quality of RCTs conducted in the past few years.

▶ Fresh frozen plasma (FFP) is one of the most commonly administered blood products, with nearly 6 million units having been produced for administration in the United States in 2009. It is given for a wide variety of purposes, but most often the indication is either to prevent or stop/control bleeding. Although as many as 30% of patients in intensive care units may have an elevated prothrombin times on testing, it is also estimated that as many as 50% may receive

FFP with no clinical evidence of bleeding. In this article, the authors reviewed the current state of the literature on the status of randomized clinical trials (RCT) evaluating the efficacy of FFP for a variety of common and some less common clinical uses. Although the total number of RCT was sizable (80), the number of subjects included in each study was often relatively small and numerous studies suffered from methodologic deficiencies. Meta-analyses were often employed to overcome these problems. In terms of clinically relevant situations, the most significant findings reported by the authors were as follows: International Normalized Ratio elevations resulting from warfarin corrected most rapidly in response to clotting factor concentrates, followed next by FFP, and most slowly in response to vitamin K administration. In patients with liver disease, 10 RCT looking at the use of FFP both therapeutically and prophylactically have failed to demonstrate clear benefit. In cardiac surgical patients, pooled data are available from 19 studies on a total of less than 1000 patients. No consistent benefit has been shown on the prevention or volume of postoperative bleeding with FFP. FFP has been demonstrated to be effective in the treatment of thrombotic thrombocytopenic purpura/hemolytic uremic syndrome, although some literature has questioned whether plasma exchange is truly superior to plasma infusion. FFP is used by some for a number of other indications, including disseminated intravascular coagulation, head injury, burns, and organophosphate poisoning, all with variable amounts and quality of literature to support such uses. As noted previously, even many of most common clinical uses of FFP have weak data supporting them. Better RCT are clearly needed to formally resolve some of these questions, but in the absence of active bleeding, the best data indicate that FFP is of limited if any utility. In the face of coagulopathy associated with the use of warfarin, coagulation factor replacement is a more rapid way to stop bleeding than FFP administration.

D. R. Gerber, DO

Bacterial Sepsis after Living Donor Liver Transplantation: The Impact of Early Enteral Nutrition
Ikegami T, Shirabe K, Yoshiya S, et al (Kyushu Univ, Fukuoka, Japan)
J Am Coll Surg 214:288-295, 2012

Background.—Bacterial sepsis is a significant problem that must be addressed after living donor liver transplantation (LDLT).

Study Design.—A retrospective analysis of 346 adult-to-adult LDLT patients was performed.

Results.—Forty-six patients (13.3%) experienced bacterial sepsis, with primary and secondary origins in 23.9% and 76.1%, respectively. Gram-negative bacteria accounted for 71.7% of the bacteria isolated. The 2-year cumulative graft survival rate in patients with bacterial sepsis was 45.7%. Patients with bacterial sepsis secondary to pneumonia (n = 12) had poorer 2-year graft survival rates (16.7%) than did those with primary or other types of secondary sepsis ($p = 0.004$). Multivariate analysis showed that intraoperative massive blood loss >10L ($p < 0.001$) and no

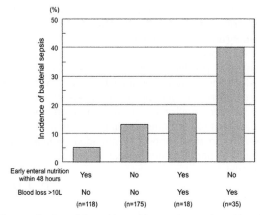

FIGURE 3.—The rate of early graft loss with or without early enteral nutrition within 48 hours after operation and/or intraoperative blood loss >10L. (Reprinted from Ikegami T, Shirabe K, Yoshiya S, et al. Bacterial sepsis after living donor liver transplantation: the impact of early enteral nutrition. *J Am Coll Surg.* 2012;214:288-295, Copyright 2012, with permission from the American College of Surgeons.)

TABLE 3.—Multivariate Analysis for Bacterial Sepsis

Variables	Odds ratio	95% Confidence Interval		*p* Value
		Lower	Upper	
Intraoperative blood loss >10L, yes	4.32	1.82	9.38	<0.001
Early enteral nutrition within 48 h, no	3.26	1.41	7.57	0.005
Hospitalized status, yes	2.43	0.98	5.96	0.053
MELD score >20, yes	2.03	0.89	4.65	0.093
PVP >20 mmHg at closure, yes	1.12	0.49	1.81	0.781

MELD, Model for End-Stage Liver Disease; PVP, portal venous pressure.

enteral feeding started within 48 hours after transplantation ($p = 0.005$) were significant risk factors for bacterial sepsis. Among patients who received enteral nutrition, the incidences of bacterial sepsis in patients who received enteral nutrition within 48 hours (n = 135) or later than 48 hours (n = 57) were 5.9% and 21.0%, respectively ($p = 0.002$). The incidence of early graft loss was 8-fold higher in recipients with massive intraoperative blood loss without early enteral nutrition ($p < 0.001$).

Conclusions.—Early enteral nutrition was associated with significantly reduced risk of developing bacterial sepsis after LDLT (Fig 3, Table 3).

▶ This large Japanese experience identifies 2 factors that were strongly related to bacterial sepsis, and in turn, graft loss. These factors were massive blood loss (> 10 L) and failure to initiate enteral nutrition within 48 hours of transplantation. Remarkably, in multivariate analysis, the Model for End-Stage Liver Disease (MELD) score did not fall out as an independent predictor of bacterial sepsis despite the fact that patients with bacterial sepsis had higher MELD scores (Table 3).

The impact of enteral nutrition, or nutrition support in general, on outcome is difficult to tease out of most studies (Fig 3). I found it hard to overlook the impact of massive blood loss (and the requirement, therefore, for massive transfusion) on the results obtained. However, many of the pathogens identified were either multidrug-resistant gram-positives, or in most cases, gram-negatives with potential abdominal and intestinal origin. Certainly, there is a rationale for enteral nutrition as supportive of biliary tree function and as a preventive measure for intestinal mucosal atrophy with preservation of intestinal structure and function.[1,2] When they indicate initiation of enteral nutrition, the authors do not indicate whether full caloric support or partial support is provided. However, another recent study suggests that even partial caloric support with enteral nutrition may provide good clinical outcome.[3]

D. J. Dries, MSE, MD

References

1. Moore FA, Moore EE. The evolving rationale for early enteral nutrition based on paradigms of multiple organ failure: a personal journey. *Nutr Clin Pract.* 2009;24: 297-304.
2. Heyland DK, Drover JW, Dhaliwal R, Greenwood J. Optimizing the benefits and minimizing the risks of enteral nutrition in the critically ill: role of small bowel feeding. *JPEN J Parenter Enteral Nutr.* 2002;26:S51-S57.
3. National Heart, Lung, and Blood Institute Acute Respiratory Distress Syndrome (ARDS) Clinical Trials Network, Rice TW, Wheeler AP, Thompson BT, et al. Initial trophic vs full enteral feeding in patients with acute lung injury: the EDEN randomized trial. *JAMA.* 2012;307:795-803.

8 Neurologic: Traumatic and Non-traumatic

Continuous electroencephalography monitoring for early prediction of neurological outcome in postanoxic patients after cardiac arrest: a prospective cohort study
Cloostermans MC, van Meulen FB, Eertman CJ, et al (Univ of Twente, Enschede, The Netherlands; Medisch Spectrum Twente, Enschede, The Netherlands)
Crit Care Med 40:2867-2875, 2012

Objective.—To evaluate the value of continuous electroencephalography in early prognostication in patients treated with hypothermia after cardiac arrest.
Design.—Prospective cohort study.
Setting.—Medical intensive care unit.
Patients.—Sixty patients admitted to the intensive care unit for therapeutic hypothermia after cardiac arrest.
Intervention.—None.
Measurements and Main Results.—In all patients, continuous electroencephalogram and daily somatosensory evoked potentials were recorded during the first 5 days of admission or until intensive care unit discharge. Neurological outcomes were based on each patient's best achieved Cerebral Performance Category score within 6 months. Twenty-seven of 56 patients (48%) achieved good neurological outcome (Cerebral Performance Category score 1–2).
At 12 hrs after resuscitation, 43% of the patients with *good neurological* outcome showed continuous, diffuse slow electroencephalogram rhythms, whereas this was never observed in patients with poor outcome. The sensitivity for predicting *poor neurological outcome* of low-voltage and isoelectric electroencephalogram patterns 24 hrs after resuscitation was 40% (95% confidence interval 19%–64%) with a 100% specificity (confidence interval 86%–100%), whereas the sensitivity and specificity of absent somatosensory evoked potential responses during the first 24 hrs were 24% (confidence interval 10%–44%) and 100% (confidence interval: 87%–100%), respectively. The negative predictive value for poor outcome of low-voltage and isoelectric electroencephalogram patterns was 68% (confidence interval 50%–81%) compared to 55% (confidence interval 40%–60%) for bilateral somatosensory evoked potential absence, both

with a positive predictive value of 100% (confidence interval 63%−100% and 59%−100% respectively). Burst-suppression patterns after 24 hrs were also associated with poor neurological outcome, but not inevitably so. *Conclusions.*—In patients treated with hypothermia, electroencephalogram monitoring during the first 24 hrs after resuscitation can contribute to the prediction of both good and poor neurological outcome. Continuous patterns within 12 hrs predicted good outcome. Isoelectric or low-voltage electroencephalograms after 24 hrs predicted poor outcome with a sensitivity almost two times larger than bilateral absent somatosensory evoked potential responses.

▶ Accurate neurologic prognosis of patients undergoing therapeutic hypothermia after cardiac arrest not only is useful to physicians to identify when continuation of treatment is futile, but is also important to patients' families. Currently there is no known algorithm that is both sensitive and specific regarding predicting prognosis. Bilateral absent short-latency somatosensory evoked potential (SSEP) testing is the most predictive of poor outcome with specificity of 100% but poor sensitivity of only about 25%. In this single-center prospective cohort study, continuous electroencephalogram (EEG) was performed on 56 consecutive patients in order to determine if continuous EEG may have a role in predicting neurologic outcome in patients undergoing therapeutic hypothermia after cardiac arrest. Patients were followed for 6 months and the best cerebral performance category score during that time was used to classify patients as having a good or poor neurologic outcome. Low-voltage and isoelectric EEG patterns observed during the first 24 hours after resuscitation correlated to a 40% sensitivity for predicting poor neurologic outcome while being 100% specific. Given the small sample size, the confidence interval was 86% to 100%. This study illustrates the encouraging potential for continuous EEG to predict neurologic outcome in patients undergoing therapeutic hypothermia after cardiac arrest. However, further study is needed to confirm the results.

R. T. Bourdon, MD

Implementation of Adapted PECARN Decision Rule for Children With Minor Head Injury in the Pediatric Emergency Department
Bressan S, Romanato S, Mion T, et al (Univ of Padova, Italy; et al)
Acad Emerg Med 19:801-807, 2012

Objectives.—Of the currently published clinical decision rules for the management of minor head injury (MHI) in children, the Pediatric Emergency Care Applied Research Network (PECARN) rule, derived and validated in a large multicenter prospective study cohort, with high methodologic standards, appears to be the best clinical decision rule to accurately identify children at very low risk of clinically important traumatic brain injuries (ciTBI) in the pediatric emergency department (PED). This study describes the implementation of an adapted version of the PECARN rule in a tertiary care academic PED in Italy and evaluates implementation success, in terms of medical staff adherence and satisfaction, as well as its effects on clinical practice.

Methods.—The adapted PECARN decision rule algorithms for children (one for those younger than 2 years and one for those older than 2 years) were actively implemented in the PED of Padova, Italy, for a 6-month testing period. Adherence and satisfaction of medical staff to the new rule were calculated. Data from 356 visits for MHI during PECARN rule implementation and those of 288 patients attending the PED for MHI in the previous 6 months were compared for changes in computed tomography (CT) scan rate, ciTBI rate (defined as death, neurosurgery, intubation for longer than 24 hours, or hospital admission at least for two nights associated with TBI) and return visits for symptoms or signs potentially related to MHI. The safety and efficacy of the adapted PECARN rule in clinical practice were also calculated.

Results.—Adherence to the adapted PECARN rule was 93.5%. The percentage of medical staff satisfied with the new rule, in terms of usefulness and ease of use for rapid decision-making, was significantly higher (96% vs. 51%, $p < 0.0001$) compared to the previous, more complex, internal guideline. CT scan was performed in 30 patients (8.4%, 95% confidence interval [CI] = 6% to 11.8%) in the implementation period versus 21 patients (7.3%, 95% CI = 4.8% to 10.9%) before implementation. A ciTBI occurred in three children (0.8%, 95% CI = 0.3 to 2.5) during the implementation period and in two children (0.7%, 95% CI = 0.2 to 2.5) in the prior 6 months. There were five return visits (1.4%) postimplementation and seven (2.4%) before implementation ($p = 0.506$). The safety of use of the adapted PECARN rule in clinical practice was 100% (95% CI = 36.8 to 100; three of three patients with ciTBI who received CT scan at first evaluation), while efficacy was 92.3% (95% CI = 89 to 95; 326 of 353 patients without ciTBI who did not receive a CT scan).

Conclusions.—The adapted PECARN rule was successfully implemented in an Italian tertiary care academic PED, achieving high adherence and satisfaction of medical staff. Its use determined a low CT scan rate that was unchanged compared to previous clinical practice and showed an optimal safety and high efficacy profile. Strict monitoring is mandatory to evaluate the long-lasting benefit in patient care and/or resource utilization.

▶ Minor head injury is common in the pediatric population. There is a strong movement to reduce computed tomography (CT) scan use in this population. A study published 3 years ago by the Pediatric Emergency Care Applied Research Network (PECARN) devised and validated a decision rule for patients younger than 18 years of age with minor head trauma. A decision rule is only effective if it is used. The current study examined how well this decision rule could be implemented in an Italian pediatric emergency department. The study used a before and after design with a primary aim of determining staff adherence to the rule and satisfaction with the rule. Staff members were educated with a dedicated teaching session, email, posters, and pocket cards. As previously, the decision rule performed perfectly, not missing any significant intracranial injuries. Adherence to the adapted PECARN rule was 93.5%. A total of 96% of the medical staff were satisfied with the rule, and 8.4% of patients underwent CT after the rule was implemented versus 7.3% before. This difference was not statistically significant. Interestingly, the CT scan rate was much lower than typical in the United States. The authors did note a concern that their CT rate would increase significantly after implementation because the CT rate in the PECARN study was just over 35%. This study shows that the PECARN head CT rule can be adopted with good adherence and great satisfaction. Now, if only we could figure out how to safely achieve such low CT rates in the United States.

M. D. Zwank, MD

Cognitive and Neurologic Outcomes after Coronary-Artery Bypass Surgery
Selnes OA, Gottesman RF, Grega MA, et al (Johns Hopkins Univ School of Medicine, Baltimore, MD; et al)
N Engl J Med 366:250-257, 2012

Background.—Even though patients who are undergoing coronary revascularization procedures are older and sicker than previously, the mortality for coronary-artery bypass grafting (CABG) is declining. However, adverse neurologic outcomes such as stroke and cognitive decline are still a primary concern. Attempts to reduce these problems are beginning to focus on patient-related risk factors rather than procedure-related factors.

Stroke Analysis and Prevention.—Recent data indicate that neurologic injury may be related to hypoperfusion and the systemic inflammatory response as much as to macroembolization or microembolization. A combination of factors has also been suggested. Patient factors that may contribute include older age, history of stroke, history of hypertension, and diabetes, which have shown the ability to predict postoperative neurologic complications. These share a focus on the health of the blood vessels. Anemia may also contribute to stroke and other adverse outcomes. Preoperative subclinical vascular disease of the brain may be able to predict postoperative neurologic complications as well. In fact, patient-related factors such as arteriosclerotic burden are more important predictors of stroke risk than type of surgery done. Preventive efforts now are being individualized for high-risk patients. Statin medications are being used for nearly all CABG patients and duplex ultrasonography of the carotid artery is routine before CABG. However, preventive efforts for high-risk patients are being individualized to achieve better results. Intraoperative epiaortic ultrasonography helps determine the location and severity of aortic plaque. Intraoperatively, near-infrared spectroscopy is used to monitor patients and assess cerebral-tissue oxygenation and adequacy of perfusion. Transcranial Doppler studies may prove useful as well.

Cognitive Decline Analysis and Prevention.—From 20% to 46% of candidates for CABG have impaired cognitive performance before surgery.

Predictors of baseline cognitive performance include age, presence or absence of hypertension, educational level, and preexisting imaging abnormalities. Preoperative cognitive testing may detect high-risk patients. Although short-term cognitive deficits are common postoperatively and not peculiar to CABG patients, these symptoms generally resolve within 3 months. However, long-term cognitive decline, lasting several years after surgery, can occur even in nonsurgical patients with diagnosed coronary artery disease. The risk of cognitive decline after coronary revascularization procedures has shown closer links to the degree of preoperative cerebrovascular disease than to the surgical procedure performed. More consistent control postoperatively of modifiable risk factors for cardiovascular and cerebrovascular disease, along with the use of lipid-lowering drugs and beta-blocking agents, may reduce the risk of long-term cognitive impairment.

Conclusions.—Patient-related risk factors have a more profound effect on short- and long-term neurologic deficits than procedure-related risk factors, such as on-pump versus off-pump surgery. Thus risk of postoperative stroke or cognitive decline should not dictate the choice of surgical therapy for patients with coronary artery disease.

▶ coronary-artery bypass grafting (CABG) is performed in patients who are already at high risk for a cerebrovascular event. Despite the attempt to move to off-pump surgical techniques, the rates of adverse neurologic outcomes have not changed. The preoperative cognitive state is a big risk factor for postoperative cognitive decline. Postoperative cognitive decline may be seen in the short and long term. Some centers have moved to screening for cerebrovascular events in these high-risk patients with magnetic resonance imaging and neuropsychological testing to medically optimize their treatments and, hopefully, outcomes. The effect of statin use in known high-risk patients has not been studied; however, preoperative aspirin does not reduce the risk of postoperative stroke, but it does lower in-hospital mortality.

Previously, the mechanism of stroke was thought to be intraoperative embolism, but relative hypoperfusion or a systemic inflammatory response may also be potential etiologies. Evaluation of the aorta with ultrasound scan may guide decisions about the safety of cross-clamping in the presence of plaque. Carotid ultrasound scan is now part of the routine preoperative workup as well. Whether outcomes are improved with carotid surgery before CABG is unknown at this time. Transcranial Doppler can detect cerebral microemboli but is of limited usefulness clinically. A thorough assessment of patient-related risk factors and focus on minimizing the impact of these is probably the best approach to maximize the neurologic outcome of these patients after coronary revascularization. It is also very important to know each patient's baseline cognitive function preoperatively. Most of these patient-centered preventative strategies still need to be tested in randomized, controlled trials, and there is no standard of care regarding them at this time.

M. Gardecki, MD

Timing of neuroprognostication in postcardiac arrest therapeutic hypothermia
Perman SM, Kirkpatrick JN, Reitsma AM, et al (Univ of Pennsylvania School of Medicine, Philadelphia)
Crit Care Med 40:719-724, 2012

Objective.—Early assessment of neurologic recovery is often challenging in survivors of cardiac arrest. Further, little is known about when to assess neurologic status in comatose, postarrest patients receiving therapeutic hypothermia. We sought to evaluate timing of prognostication in cardiac arrest survivors who received therapeutic hypothermia.

Design.—A retrospective chart review of consecutive postarrest patients receiving therapeutic hypothermia (protocol: 24-hr maintenance at target temperature followed by rewarming over 8 hrs). Data were abstracted from the medical chart, including documentation during the first 96 hrs post arrest of "poor" prognosis, diagnostic tests for neuroprognostication, consultations used for determination of prognosis, and outcome at discharge.

Setting.—Two academic urban emergency departments.

Patients.—A total of 55 consecutive patients who underwent therapeutic hypothermia were reviewed between September 2005 and April 2009.

Intervention.—None.

Results.—Of our cohort of comatose postarrest patients, 59% (29 of 49) were male, and the mean age was 56 ± 16 yrs. Chart documentation of "poor" or "grave" prognosis occurred "early": during induction, maintenance of cooling, rewarming, or within 15 hrs after normothermia in 57% (28 of 49) of cases. Of patients with early documentation of poor prognosis, 25% (seven of 28) had care withdrawn within 72 hrs post arrest, and 21% (six of 28) survived to discharge with favorable neurologic recovery. In the first 96 hrs post arrest: 88% (43 of 49) of patients received a head computed tomography, 90% (44 of 49) received electroencephalography, 2% (one of 49) received somatosensory evoked potential testing, and 71% (35 of 49) received neurology consultation.

Conclusions.—Documentation of "poor prognosis" occurred during therapeutic hypothermia in more than half of patients in our cohort. Premature documentation of poor prognosis may contribute to early decisions to withdraw care. Future guidelines should address when to best prognosticate in postarrest patients receiving therapeutic hypothermia.

▶ In this interesting retrospective study, Perman et al attempt to evaluate the rate of neurologic prognostication after cardiac arrest. They reviewed the charts of 55 consecutive cardiac arrest patients admitted to 2 different medical settings. The authors observed that prognostication as "poor," "grave," or "grim" occurred early (within 15 hours of hypothermia protocol) in 57% of patients. Of these, 25% had care withdrawn and 21% were discharged with favorable outcome. The importance of this study is that despite the robust effects of hypothermia on outcomes after cardiac arrest, physicians still attempt to provide prognosis on the basis of early clinical and paraclinical information. The study calls for an over-all reappraisal of how we approach neurologic prognostication in an attempt to provide the best care for these patients.

F. Rincon, MD

Acute lung injury in critical neurological illness
Hoesch RE, Lin E, Young M, et al (Johns Hopkins Univ School of Medicine, Baltimore, MD)
Crit Care Med 40:587-593, 2012

Objective.—Acute lung injury and acute respiratory distress syndrome have been reported in a significant proportion of patients with critical neurologic illness. Our aim was to identify risk factors for acute lung injury/acute respiratory distress syndrome in this population.

Design.—Prospective, observational study.

Setting.—A 22-bed, adult neurosciences critical care unit at a tertiary care hospital.

Patients.—Primary neurologic disorder, mechanical ventilation > 48 hrs.

Interventions.—None.

Measurements and Main Results.—A total of 192 patients were enrolled with a range of neurologic disorders. Among these, 68 (35%) were diagnosed with acute lung injury/acute respiratory distress syndrome. In a multivariate logistic regression analysis, independent risk factors for acute lung injury/acute respiratory distress syndrome were pneumonia (odds ratio [95% confidence interval] 3.12 [1.5−6.0], $p = .002$), circulatory shock (2.2 [1.07−4.57], $p = .03$), and absence of a gag or cough reflex (3.41 [1.34−8.68], $p = .01$). Neither neurologic diagnosis nor neurologic severity, assessed with the Glasgow Coma Scale, was significantly associated with the development of acute lung injury/acute respiratory distress syndrome.

Conclusion.—Acute lung injury/acute respiratory distress syndrome occurred in more than one third of mechanically ventilated neurosciences critical care unit patients. Loss of the cough or gag reflex is strongly predictive of acute lung injury/acute respiratory distress syndrome, while neurologic diagnosis and Glasgow Coma Scale are not. Lower brainstem dysfunction, a clinical marker of neurologic injury not captured by the Glasgow Coma Scale, is a risk factor for acute lung injury/acute respiratory distress syndrome and could inform decisions regarding airway protection and mechanical ventilation.

▶ In this interesting article, Hoesch et al evaluate the prevalence and risk factors of acute respiratory distress syndrome and acute lung injury (ARDS/ALI) in a cohort of neurological patients. The authors used strict methods to ascertain ARDS/ALI based on the American/European Consensus Conference on ARDS/ALI. ARDS/ALI was confirmed with exclusion of high left atrial pressures in 68/108 patients initially diagnosed with "possible ARDS/ALI," and interestingly, only 5 patients underwent measurements of pulmonary occlusion pressures reflecting current trends in use of pulmonary artery catheters. The incidence of ARDS/ALI increases with age and exposure to several important risk factors such as sepsis, transfusions, and trauma. In this small cohort, the authors found no significant risk from age or neurological disease type or severity, but the main suspects were confirmed (pneumonia and shock). The authors found that the neurological patients with absent gag/cough reflex were at higher risk of ARDS/ALI, which may have explained the high risk of pneumonia seen in the cohort. Though outcomes except for duration of mechanical ventilation were not statistically significant, the lack of differences may have been related to the sample size. The study is important for critical care specialists dealing with these patients in the intensive care unit; however, it does not provide enough information on the heterogeneity of the ARDS/ALI syndrome within different types of brain injury.

F. Rincon, MD

Magnesium for aneurysmal subarachnoid haemorrhage (MASH-2): a randomised placebo-controlled trial
Mees SMD, Algra A, Vandertop WP, et al (Univ Med Ctr, Utrecht, The Netherlands; Academic Med Ctr Amsterdam and VU Univ Med Ctr, The Netherlands; et al)
Lancet 380:44-49, 2012

Background.—Magnesium sulphate is a neuroprotective agent that might improve outcome after aneurysmal subarachnoid haemorrhage by reducing the occurrence or improving the outcome of delayed cerebral ischaemia. We did a trial to test whether magnesium therapy improves outcome after aneurysmal subarachnoid haemorrhage.

Methods.—We did this phase 3 randomised, placebo-controlled trial in eight centres in Europe and South America. We randomly assigned (with computer-generated random numbers, with permuted blocks of four, stratified by centre) patients aged 18 years or older with an aneurysmal pattern of subarachnoid haemorrhage on brain imaging who were admitted to hospital within 4 days of haemorrhage, to receive intravenous magnesium sulphate, 64 mmol/day, or placebo. We excluded patients with renal failure or bodyweight lower than 50 kg. Patients, treating physicians, and investigators assessing outcomes and analysing data were masked to the allocation. The primary outcome was poor outcome—defined as a score of 4–5 on the modified Rankin Scale—3 months after subarachnoid haemorrhage, or death. We analysed results by intention to treat. We also updated a previous meta-analysis of trials of magnesium treatment for aneurysmal subarachnoid haemorrhage. This study is registered with controlled-trials.com (ISRCTN 68742385) and the EU Clinical Trials Register (EudraCT 2006-003523-36).

Findings.—1204 patients were enrolled, one of whom had his treatment allocation lost. 606 patients were assigned to the magnesium group (two lost to follow-up), 597 to the placebo (one lost to follow-up). 158 patients (26·2%) had poor outcome in the magnesium group compared with 151 (25·3%) in the placebo group (risk ratio [RR] 1·03, 95% CI 0·85—1·25). Our updated meta-analysis of seven randomised trials involving 2047 patients shows that magnesium is not superior to placebo for reduction of poor outcome after aneurysmal subarachnoid haemorrhage (RR 0.96, 95% CI 0·84—1·10).

Interpretation.—Intravenous magnesium sulphate does not improve clinical outcome after aneurysmal subarachnoid haemorrhage, therefore routine administration of magnesium cannot be recommended.

▶ Magnesium, a mineral with calcium channel blocking activity and neuroprotective properties, has been studied for several applications in medicine, including stroke and subarachnoid hemorrhage (SAH).[1] In this clinical trial (Magnesium for Aneurysmal Subarachnoid Haemorrhage-2), the investigators attempted to test the hypothesis that magnesium infusions would be associated with less delayed cerebral ischemia (DCI) after SAH. However, intravenous magnesium was not associated with improved outcome after SAH. Subgroup analyses failed to identify groups that may have benefited from this therapy. The explanation of these findings may be related to the complexity of the physiopathology of SAH, vasospasm, and the onset of DCI. The effect of other variables, such as cardiac dysfunction, fever, inflammation, hydrocephalus, among others, may not be therapeutic targets of magnesium infusions. Perhaps clinical trials testing a combination of therapies for the prevention of DCI are the way of the future.

F. Rincon, MD

Reference

1. Diringer MN, Bleck TP, Claude Hemphill J, et al. Critical care management of patients following aneurysmal subarachnoid hemorrhage: recommendations from the Neurocritical Care Society's Multidisciplinary Consensus Conference. *Neurocrit Care.* 2011;15:211-240.

Anemia and brain oxygen after severe traumatic brain injury
Oddo M, Levine JM, Kumar M, et al (Univ of Pennsylvania, Philadelphia)
Intensive Care Med 38:1497-1504, 2012

Purpose.—To investigate the relationship between hemoglobin (Hgb) and brain tissue oxygen tension ($PbtO_2$) after severe traumatic brain injury (TBI) and to examine its impact on outcome.

Methods.—This was a retrospective analysis of a prospective cohort of severe TBI patients whose $PbtO_2$ was monitored. The relationship between Hgb—categorized into four quartiles (≤ 9; 9—10; 10.1—11; >11 g/dl)—and $PbtO_2$ was analyzed using mixed-effects models. Anemia with compromised $PbtO_2$ was defined as episodes of Hgb ≤ 9 g/dl with simultaneous

$PbtO_2 < 20$ mmHg. Outcome was assessed at 30 days using the Glasgow outcome score (GOS), dichotomized as favorable (GOS 4—5) vs. unfavorable (GOS 1—3).

Results.—We analyzed 474 simultaneous Hgb and $PbtO_2$ samples from 80 patients (mean age 44 ± 20 years, median GCS 4 (3—7)). Using Hgb >11 g/dl as the reference level, and controlling for important physiologic covariates (CPP, PaO_2, $PaCO_2$), Hgb ≤ 9 g/dl was the only Hgb level that was associated with lower $PbtO_2$ (coefficient −6.53 (95 % CI −9.13; −3.94), $p < 0.001$). Anemia with simultaneous $PbtO_2 < 20$ mmHg, but not anemia alone, increased the risk of unfavorable outcome (odds ratio 6.24 (95% CI 1.61; 24.22), $p = 0.008$), controlling for age, GCS, Marshall CT grade, and APACHE II score.

Conclusions.—In this cohort of severe TBI patients whose $PbtO_2$ was monitored, a Hgb level no greater than 9 g/dl was associated with compromised $PbtO_2$. Anemia with simultaneous compromised $PbtO_2$, but not anemia alone, was a risk factor for unfavorable outcome, irrespective of injury severity.

► Regimens and thresholds for transfusion in critically ill neurologic patients vary substantially for medical/surgical patients. Although not substantiated by clinical evidence, the thresholds for transfusion in critically ill neurologic patients may be higher than those recommended for medical/surgical patients. Recent experiments, like this one by Oddo et al, suggest that anemia in the setting of brain hypoxia, as determined by partial brain tissue oxygenation ($PbtO_2$), are detrimental for survival after severe traumatic brain injury. The study shows that $PbtO_2$ may be an important tool for monitoring of these patients, and that transfusions based solely on guidelines or recommendations may not be enough to improve patient outcomes.

F. Rincon, MD

Will Delays in Treatment Jeopardize the Population Benefit From Extending the Time Window for Stroke Thrombolysis?
Pitt M, Monks T, Agarwal P, et al (Univ of Exeter Med School, UK; JDA Software, Hyderabad, India; et al)
Stroke 43:2992-2997, 2012

Background and Purpose.—Pooled analyses show benefits of intravenous alteplase (recombinant tissue-type plasminogen activator) treatment for acute ischemic stroke up to 4.5 hours after onset despite marketing approval for up to 3 hours. However, the benefit from thrombolysis is critically time-dependent and if extending the time window reduces treatment urgency, this could reduce the population benefit from any extension.

Methods.—Based on 3830 UK patients registered between 2005 to 2010 in the Safe Implementation of Treatments in Stroke—International Stroke Thrombolysis Registry (SITS-ISTR), a Monte Carlo simulation was used to model recombinant tissue-type plasminogen activator treatment up to 4·5 hours from onset and assess the impact (numbers surviving with little or no disability) from changes in hospital treatment times associated with this extended time window.

Results.—We observed a significant relation between time remaining to treat and time taken to treat in the UK SITS-ISTR data set after adjustment for censoring. Simulation showed that as this "deadline effect" increases, an extended treatment time window entails that an increasing number of patients are treated at a progressively lower absolute benefit to a point where the population benefit from extending the time window is entirely negated.

Conclusions.—Despite the benefit for individual patients treated up to 4.5 hours after onset, the population benefit may be reduced or lost altogether if extending the time window results in more patients being treated but at a lower absolute benefit. A universally applied reduction in hospital arrival to treatment times of 8 minutes would confer a population benefit as large as the time window extension.

▶ In this excellent study, the coined phrase *time is brain* is perfectly substantiated. The authors reviewed data on more than 3000 patients registered in stroke trials. Although the window for intravenous tissue plasminogen activator (tPA) as part of the emergency management of ischemic stroke has been extended to 4.5 hours, based on the results of the ECASS-III study, the benefit of thrombolysis is still time dependent. Regardless of the time window, increasing this time frame may result in an overall reduction in the sense of urgency by practitioners. This could negate the overall effect of tPA in the population. In this computer simulation, a reduction in hospital arrival to treatment time of only 8 minutes would be associated with an overall outcome benefit. The bottom line is not to rely on the extended time window to administer tPA but to do it as fast as possible when indicated.

F. Rincon, MD

Decompressive Hemicraniectomy in Patients With Supratentorial Intracerebral Hemorrhage
Fung C, Murek M, Z'Graggen WJ, et al (Univ Hosp, Bern, Switzerland; et al)
Stroke 43:3207-3211, 2012

Background and Purpose.—Decompressive craniectomy (DC) lowers intracranial pressure and improves outcome in patients with malignant middle cerebral artery stroke. Its usefulness in intracerebral hemorrhage (ICH) is unclear. The aim of this study was to analyze feasibility and safety of DC without clot evacuation in ICH.

Methods.—We compared consecutive patients (November 2010–January 2012) with supratentorial ICH treated with DC without hematoma evacuation and matched controls treated by best medical treatment. DC measured at least 150 mm and included opening of the dura. We analyzed clinical (age, sex, pathogenesis, Glasgow Coma Scale, National Institutes of Health Stroke Scale), radiological (signs of herniation, side and size of hematoma, midline shift, hematoma expansion, distance to surface), and surgical (time to and indication for surgery) characteristics. Outcome at 6 months was dichotomized into good (modified Rankin Scale 0–4) and poor (modified Rankin Scale 5–6).

Results.—Twelve patients (median age 48 years; interquartile range 35–58) with ICH were treated by DC. Median hematoma volume was 61.3 mL (interquartile range 37–83.5 mL) and median preoperative Glasgow Coma Scale was 8 (interquartile range 4.3–10). Four patients showed signs of herniation. Nine patients had good and 3 had poor outcomes. Three patients (25%) of the treatment group died versus 8 of 15 (53%) of the control group. There were 3 manageable complications related to DC.

Conclusions.—DC is feasible in patients with ICH. Based on this small cohort, DC may reduce mortality. Larger prospective cohorts are warranted to assess safety and efficacy.

▶ Decompressive hemicraniectomy (DHC) is a life-saving intervention currently indicated for the management of malignant middle cerebral artery infarction. The role of DHC in other types of brain injury has been studied, particularly after traumatic brain injury, with no substantial effect on outcome. The role of DHC after intracerebral hemorrhage (ICH) was studied by Fung et al in an elegant matched case-control study. The limitations of the study are related to its retrospective nature, the mixed characteristic of the cohort (both spontaneous and coagulopathic ICHs were included), and the sample size. However, this study is important because it supports the role of DHC after ICH as a life-saving procedure. The effect on outcomes remains to be answered. Importantly, whether the combination of other neuroprotective therapies such as hypothermia in combination with surgery could be a potential therapy for ICH remains to be answered by future clinical trials.

F. Rincon, MD

Tight glycemic control increases metabolic distress in traumatic brain injury: A randomized controlled within-subjects trial
Vespa P, McArthur DL, Stein N, et al (UCLA School of Medicine)
Crit Care Med 40:1923-1929, 2012

Objective.—To determine the effects of tight glycemic control on brain metabolism after traumatic brain injury using brain positron emission tomography and microdialysis.

Design.—Single-center, randomized controlled within-subject crossover observational trial.

Setting.—Academic intensive care unit.

Methods.—We performed a prospective, unblinded randomized controlled within-subject crossover trial of tight (80–110 mg/dL) vs. loose

(120–150 mg/dL) glycemic control in patients with severe traumatic brain injury to determine the effects of glycemic control on brain glucose metabolism, as measured by [^{18}F] deoxy-D-glucose brain positron emission tomography. Brain microdialysis was done simultaneously.

Measurements and Main Results.—Thirteen severely injured traumatic brain injury patients underwent the study between 3 and 8 days (mean 4.8 days) after traumatic brain injury. In ten of these subjects, global brain and gray matter tissues demonstrated higher glucose metabolic rates while glucose was under tight control as compared with loose control (3.2 ± 0.6 vs. 2.4 + 0.4, $p = .02$ [whole brain] and 3.8 ± 1.4 vs. 2.9 ± 0.8, $p = .05$ [gray matter]). However, the responses were heterogeneous with pericontusional tissue demonstrating the least state-dependent change. Cerebral microdialysis demonstrated more frequent critical reductions in glucose ($p = .02$) and elevations of lactate/pyruvate ratio ($p = .03$) during tight glycemic control.

Conclusion.—Tight glycemic control results in increased global glucose uptake and an increased cerebral metabolic crisis after traumatic brain injury. The mechanisms leading to the enhancement of metabolic crisis are unclear, but delivery of more glucose through mild hyperglycemia may be necessary after traumatic brain injury.

▶ Traumatic brain injury (TBI) is common, occurring in 1.7 million people per year. There is an immediate injury and a delayed secondary injury that occurs that may be due to unmet metabolic demands. This study done by Vespa et al included 13 severe TBI patients in a randomized controlled within subject crossover trial using cerebral microdialysis and F-18-fluorodeoxyglucose-positron emission tomography (PET) to monitor the effects of different blood glucose treatment strategies. Patients were kept in a glucose range of 80 to 110 mg/dL or 120 to 150 mg/dL for 24 hours, and then a PET scan obtained and the patients crossed over to the other glucose range for 24 hours, after which a PET scan was repeated. The measured arterial oxygenation and intracranial pressure values were not statistically different. Hypoglycemia (< 50 mg/ dL) was not seen in any subjects. However, critically low values of cerebral glucose and high lactate/pyruvate ratios seen on microdialysis results were statistically more likely to occur in the tight glucose control group. The PET scans tended to show an increase in glucose metabolism mostly localized to cortical gray matter; however, the exact patterns varied among the 13 patients. This was also affected by the presence of seizures, which increased metabolic demand, or use of high doses of sedating drugs, which decreased it. Ultimately the injured brain seems to go through a period where it is potentially detrimental to deprive it of glucose through a tight glycemic control strategy. Another important point from this article is that during this study no patient had hypoglycemic events measured from serum values, although frequent critically low glucose values were obtained from the microdialysis catheter readings. This may imply a much more liberal glucose strategy is appropriate for TBI patients.

M. Gardecki, MD

Placebo-Controlled Trial of Amantadine for Severe Traumatic Brain Injury

Giacino JT, Whyte J, Bagiella E, et al (JFK Johnson Rehabilitation Inst, Edison, NJ; Albert Einstein Healthcare Network, Elkins Park, PA; Columbia Univ, NY; et al)

N Engl J Med 366:819-826, 2012

Background.—Amantadine hydrochloride is one of the most commonly prescribed medications for patients with prolonged disorders of consciousness after traumatic brain injury. Preliminary studies have suggested that amantadine may promote functional recovery.

Methods.—We enrolled 184 patients who were in a vegetative or minimally conscious state 4 to 16 weeks after traumatic brain injury and who were receiving inpatient rehabilitation. Patients were randomly assigned to receive amantadine or placebo for 4 weeks and were followed for 2 weeks after the treatment was discontinued. The rate of functional recovery on the Disability Rating Scale (DRS; range, 0 to 29, with higher scores indicating greater disability) was compared over the 4 weeks of treatment (primary outcome) and during the 2-week washout period with the use of mixed-effects regression models.

Results.—During the 4-week treatment period, recovery was significantly faster in the amantadine group than in the placebo group, as measured by the DRS score (difference in slope, 0.24 points per week; $P = 0.007$), indicating a benefit with respect to the primary outcome measure. In a pre-specified subgroup analysis, the treatment effect was similar for patients in a vegetative state and those in a minimally conscious state. The rate of improvement in the amantadine group slowed during the 2 weeks after treatment (weeks 5 and 6) and was significantly slower than the rate in the placebo group (difference in slope, 0.30 points per week; $P = 0.02$). The overall improvement in DRS scores between baseline and week 6 (2 weeks after treatment was discontinued) was similar in the two groups. There were no significant differences in the incidence of serious adverse events.

Conclusions.—Amantadine accelerated the pace of functional recovery during active treatment in patients with post-traumatic disorders of consciousness. (Funded by the National Institute on Disability and Rehabilitation Research; ClinicalTrials.gov number, NCT00970944.)

▶ Most patients with severe traumatic brain injury (TBI) are discharged from acute care in either a vegetative or minimally conscious state. No intervention previously has been shown to improve the outcome or rate of recovery. This is a prospective, randomized, double-blind, placebo-controlled study examining the use of amantadine in promoting recovery in patients with severe TBI in either a vegetative or minimally conscious state. Although both groups had improvement in the Disability Rating Score, the amantadine group had a faster rate of recovery in the 4-week treatment period, but the effect diminished during the 2-week washout period. Limitations of this study include the use of other potentially confounding psychoactive medications and the inability to control for standard rehabilitation treatments. In addition, as the authors pointed out, the study was not able to measure the long-term effects of prolonged treatment. Despite the limitations, amantadine appears to be effective in promoting rapid recovery in the acute rehabilitation period in patients in a vegetative or minimally conscious state after TBI. However, this effect is not sustained.

L. Ng, MD, MPH

Factors influencing intracranial pressure monitoring guideline compliance and outcome after severe traumatic brain injury
Biersteker HAR, Andriessen TMJC, Horn J, et al (Radboud Univ Nijmegen Med Ctr, The Netherlands; Univ of Amsterdam, The Netherlands; et al)
Crit Care Med 40:1914-1922, 2012

Objective.—To determine adherence to Brain Trauma Foundation guidelines for intracranial pressure monitoring after severe traumatic brain injury, to investigate if characteristics of patients treated according to guidelines (ICP+) differ from those who were not (ICP-), and whether guideline compliance is related to 6-month outcome.
Design.—Observational multicenter study.
Patients.—Consecutive severe traumatic brain injury patients (≥ 16 yrs, n = 265) meeting criteria for intracranial pressure monitoring.
Measurements and Main Results.—Data on demographics, injury severity, computed tomography findings, and patient management were registered. The Glasgow Outcome Scale Extended was dichotomized into death (Glasgow Outcome Scale Extended = 1) and unfavorable outcome (Glasgow Outcome Scale Extended 1—4). Guideline compliance was 46%. Differences between the monitored and nonmonitored patients included a younger age (median 44 vs. 53 yrs), more abnormal pupillary reactions (52% vs. 32%), and more intracranial pathology (subarachnoid hemorrhage 62% vs. 44%; intraparenchymal lesions 65% vs. 46%) in the ICP+ group. Patients with a total intracranial lesion volume of ~ 150 mL and a midline shift of ~ 12 mm were most likely to receive an intracranial pressure monitor and probabilities decreased with smaller and larger lesions and shifts. Furthermore, compliance was low in patients with no (Traumatic Coma Databank score I -10%) visible intracranial pathology. Differences in case-mix resulted in higher a *priori* probabilities of dying (median 0.51 vs. 0.35, $p < .001$) and unfavorable outcome (median 0.79 vs. 0.63, $p < .001$) in the ICP+ group. After correction for baseline and clinical characteristics with a propensity score, intracranial pressure monitoring guideline compliance was not associated with mortality (odds ratio 0.93, 95% confidence interval 0.47—1.85, $p = .83$) nor with unfavorable outcome (odds ratio 1.81, 95% confidence interval 0.88—3.73, $p = .11$).
Conclusions.—Guideline noncompliance was most prominent in patients with minor or very large computed tomography abnormalities. Intracranial pressure monitoring was not associated with 6-month outcome, but multiple baseline differences between monitored and nonmonitored patients

underline the complex nature of examining the effect of intracranial pressure monitoring in observational studies.

▶ Currently, the Brain Trauma Foundation (BTF) guidelines recommend intracranial pressure (ICP) monitoring in severe traumatic brain injury (TBI) based on data suggesting that this results in a reduction in mortality. However, efficacy as well as compliance have varied among studies. This study examines demographic and injury characteristics associated with BTF guideline compliance and whether compliance is a predictor for long-term outcome after severe TBI. This study confirmed poor compliance with BTF guidelines, with less than 50% of eligible patients having an ICP monitor inserted, mainly in the population with a 40% to 60% chance of death. In addition, there was no difference in 6-month mortality between the 2 groups. This study raises the question of whether ICP monitor insertion is necessary in patients with severe TBI or perhaps only necessary in certain populations of patients with TBI.

L. Ng, MD, MPH

A Randomized Trial of Tenecteplase versus Alteplase for Acute Ischemic Stroke

Parsons M, Spratt N, Bivard A, et al (Univ of Newcastle, New South Wales, Australia; et al)
N Engl J Med 366:1099-1107, 2012

Background.—Intravenous alteplase is the only approved treatment for acute ischemic stroke. Tenecteplase, a genetically engineered mutant tissue plasminogen activator, is an alternative thrombolytic agent.

Methods.—In this phase 2B trial, we randomly assigned 75 patients to receive alteplase (0.9 mg per kilogram of body weight) or tenecteplase (0.1 mg per kilogram or 0.25 mg per kilogram) less than 6 hours after the onset of ischemic stroke. To favor the selection of patients most likely to benefit from thrombolytic therapy, the eligibility criteria were a perfusion lesion at least 20% greater than the infarct core on computed tomographic (CT) perfusion imaging at baseline and an associated vessel occlusion on CT angiography. The coprimary end points were the proportion of the perfusion lesion that was reperfused at 24 hours on perfusion-weighted magnetic resonance imaging and the extent of clinical improvement at 24 hours as assessed on the National Institutes of Health Stroke Scale (NIHSS, a 42-point scale on which higher scores indicate more severe neurologic deficits).

Results.—The three treatment groups each comprised 25 patients. The mean ($\pm$ SD) NIHSS score at baseline for all patients was 14.4 $\pm$ 2.6, and the time to treatment was 2.9 $\pm$ 0.8 hours. Together, the two tenecteplase groups had greater reperfusion ($P = 0.004$) and clinical improvement ($P < 0.001$) at 24 hours than the alteplase group. There were no significant between-group differences in intracranial bleeding or other serious adverse events. The higher dose of tenecteplase (0.25 mg per kilogram) was superior to the lower dose and to alteplase for all efficacy outcomes, including absence of serious disability at 90 days (in 72% of patients, vs. 40% with alteplase; $P = 0.02$).

Conclusions.—Tenecteplase was associated with significantly better reperfusion and clinical outcomes than alteplase in patients with stroke who were selected on the basis of CT perfusion imaging. (Funded by the Australian National Health and Medical Research Council; Australia New Zealand Clinical Trials Registry number, ACTRN12608000466347.)

▶ Acute ischemic stroke (AIS) remains the third leading cause of death among Americans, the majority of which are ischemic in nature. Alteplase (t-PA) is the only thrombolytic agent approved for the management of AIS within a 4.5-hour window. The genetically engineered t-PA, tenecteplase, has demonstrated pharmacokinetic properties, which suggest an advantage over alteplase in recanalization via improved clot penetration. This phase 2B trial compared tenecteplase and alteplase through imaging and clinical outcomes in the acute and long-term period. The investigators randomized 75 patients with AIS evaluated by computed tomography perfusion and angiography who met specific inclusion criteria to 3 groups: alteplase, tenecteplase 0.1 mg/kg, and tenecteplase 0.25 mg/kg. Participants started thrombolytic therapy within 6 hours of symptom onset. Magnetic resonance imaging and National Institutes of Health Stroke Scale scoring was done at 24 hours and 90 days. The pooled tenecteplase group was significantly superior to alteplase for reperfusion and clinical improvement at 24 hours. There was no significant difference in the safety outcomes between the groups. The higher dose of tenecteplase demonstrated improved imaging and clinical outcomes in comparison to alteplase, whereas the lower dose only showed significant benefit in clinical measures at 24 hours in comparison to alteplase. These results suggest that tenecteplase offers improved reperfusion and clinical success without a loss in safety through a possible dose-response relationship. The study's major drawback was the strict inclusion criteria targeting the patients most likely to benefit from thrombolytic therapy, thus limiting generalizability. Patients were selected from 3 Australian stroke centers, which begs the question if a comparable trial could be attempted in the United States. The authors are currently pursuing a phase III trial, which is justified by their results. This study offers the exciting possibility of a thrombolytic alternative with improved outcomes, but not at the expense of safety.

J. Baker, MS

Poststroke delirium incidence and outcomes: Validation of the Confusion Assessment Method for the Intensive Care Unit (CAM-ICU)
Mitasova A, Kostalova M, Bednarik J, et al (Univ Hosp and Masaryk Univ, Brno, Czech Republic; et al)
Crit Care Med 40:484-490, 2012

Objective.—To describe the epidemiology and time spectrum of delirium using Diagnostic and Statistical Manual of Mental Disorders,

Fourth Edition criteria and to validate a tool for delirium assessment in patients in the acute poststroke period.

Design.—A prospective observational cohort study.

Setting.—The stroke unit of a university hospital.

Patients.—A consecutive series of 129 patients with stroke (with infarction or intracerebral hemorrhage, 57 women and 72 men; mean age, 72.5 yrs; age range, 35–93 yrs) admitted to the stroke unit of a university hospital were evaluated for delirium incidence.

Interventions.—None.

Measurements and Main Results.—Criterion validity and overall accuracy of the Czech version of the Confusion Assessment Method for the Intensive Care Unit (CAM-ICU) were determined using serial daily delirium assessments with CAM-ICU by a junior physician compared with delirium diagnosis by delirium experts using the Diagnostic and Statistical Manual of Mental Disorders, Fourth Edition criteria that began the first day after stroke onset and continued for at least 7 days. Cox regression models using time-dependent covariate analysis adjusting for age, gender, prestroke dementia, National Institutes of Stroke Health Care at admission, first-day Sequential Organ Failure Assessment, and asphasia were used to understand the relationships between delirium and clinical outcomes. An episode of delirium based on reference Diagnostic and Statistical Manual assessment was detected in 55 patients with stroke (42.6%). In 37 of these (67.3%), delirium began within the first day and in all of them within 5 days of stroke onset. A total of 1003 paired CAM-ICU/Diagnostic and Statistical Manual of Mental Disorders daily assessments were completed. Compared with the reference standard for diagnosing delirium, the CAM-ICU demonstrated a sensitivity of 76% (95% confidence interval [CI] 55% to 91%), a specificity of 98% (95% CI 93% to 100%), an overall accuracy of 94% (95% CI 88% to 97%), and high interrater reliability ($\kappa = 0.94$; 95% CI 0.83–1.0). The likelihood ratio of the CAM-ICU in the diagnosis of delirium was 47 (95% CI 27–83). Delirium was an independent predictor of increased length of hospital stay (hazard ratio 1.63; 95% CI 1.11–2.38; $p = .013$).

Conclusions.—Poststroke delirium may frequently be detected provided that the testing algorithm is appropriate to the time profile of poststroke delirium. Early (first day after stroke onset) and serial screening for delirium is recommended. CAM-ICU is a valid instrument for the diagnosis of delirium and should be considered an aid in delirium screening and assessment in future epidemiologic and interventional studies in patients with stroke.

▶ Mitasova et al report on the incidence of delirium in a cohort of stroke patients admitted to the intensive care unit (ICU) by comparing 2 methods of diagnosis: the commonly used ICU-Confusion Assessment Method (CAM) bedside assessment method compared with a standard of Diagnostic and Statistical Manual of Mental Disorders, 4th ed. (DSM-IV) criteria performed by experts (neuropsychologists). In this interesting prospective observational study, the incidence of delirium was as high as 43% using DSM-IV criteria and the accuracy of ICU-CAM was 93% (sensitivity 76%, specificity 98%, positive predictive value 94%). The study used strong statistical analysis to account for potential confounders such as National Institutes of Health Stroke Scale and symptoms of focal brain injury such as aphasia. Although the study did not demonstrate a significant effect on mortality, the presence of delirium after stroke was associated with prolonged length of stay. The results of this study support the use of the ICU-CAM for recognition of delirium in stroke patients.

F. Rincon, MD

Delirium in Acute Stroke: A Systematic Review and Meta-Analysis
Shi Q, Presutti R, Selchen D, et al (The Univ of Western Ontario, Ontario, Canada; Univ of Toronto, Canada)
Stroke 43:645-649, 2012

Background and Purpose.—Delirium is common in the early stage after hospitalization for an acute stroke. We conducted a systematic review and meta-analysis to evaluate the outcomes of acute stroke patients with delirium.

Methods.—We searched MEDLINE, EMBASE, CINAHL, Cochrane Library databases, and PsychInfo for relevant articles published in English up to September 2011. We included observational studies for review. Two reviewers independently assessed studies to determine eligibility, validity, and quality. The primary outcome was inpatient mortality and secondary outcomes were mortality at 12 months, institutionalization, and length of hospital stay.

Results.—Among 78 eligible studies, 10 studies (n=2004 patients) met the inclusion criteria. Stroke patients with delirium had higher inpatient mortality (OR, 4.71; 95% CI, 1.85—11.96) and mortality at 12 months (OR, 4.91; 95% CI, 3.18—7.6) compared to nondelirious patients. Patients with delirium also tended to stay longer in hospital compared to those who did not have delirium (mean difference, 9.39 days; 95% CI, 6.67—12.11) and were more likely to be discharged to a nursing homes or other institutions (OR, 3.39; 95% CI, 2.21—5.21).

Conclusions.—Stroke patients with development of delirium have unfavorable outcomes, particularly higher mortality, longer hospitalizations, and a greater degree of dependence after discharge. Early recognition and prevention of delirium may improve outcomes in stroke patients.

▶ In this interesting systematic review and meta-analysis, Shi et al study the impact of acute delirium in a population of stroke patients. Delirium has been associated with higher morbidity and mortality in hospitalized patients, and stroke patients are not an exemption. The study used statistical analysis to account for heterogeneity among point estimates. The reported incidence of delirium was as high as 48%. In all analyses, in-hospital and 12-month mortality was significantly higher in delirious patients. Unfortunately, the study does not elaborate on risk factors, but I suspect that age, medical co-morbidities, and medications could be the usual suspects. Nevertheless, this study is important because it identifies another potentially treatable derangement in stroke patients beyond temperature, glucose, and hemoglobin levels. Early identification of delirium with conventional bedside tools may improve stroke patient outcomes.

F. Rincon, MD

A Randomized and Blinded Single-Center Trial Comparing the Effect of Intracranial Pressure and Intracranial Pressure Wave Amplitude-Guided Intensive Care Management on Early Clinical State and 12-Month Outcome in Patients With Aneurysmal Subarachnoid Hemorrhage

Eide PK, Bentsen G, Sorteberg AG, et al (Oslo Univ Hosp—Rikshospitalet, Norway)
Neurosurgery 69:1105-1115, 2011

Background.—In patients with aneurysmal subarachnoid hemorrhage (SAH), preliminary results indicate that the amplitude of the single intracranial pressure (ICP) wave is a better predictor of the early clinical state and 6-month outcome than the mean ICP.

Objective.—To perform a randomized and blinded single-center trial comparing the effect of mean ICP vs mean ICP wave amplitude (MWA)-guided intensive care management on early clinical state and outcome in patients with aneurysmal SAH.

Methods.—Patients were randomized to 2 different types of ICP management: maintenance of mean ICP less than 20 mm Hg and MWA less than 5 mm Hg. Early clinical state was assessed daily using the Glasgow Coma Scale. The primary efficacy variable was 12-month outcome in terms of the Rankin Stroke Score.

Results.—Ninety-seven patients were included in the study. There were no significant differences in treatment between the 2 groups apart from a larger volume of cerebrospinal fluid drained during week 1 in the MWA group. There was a tendency toward higher Glasgow Coma Scale scores in the MWA group during weeks 1 ($P = .08$) and 2 ($P = .07$). Outcome in terms of Rankin Stroke Score at 12 months was significantly better in the MWA group ($P < .05$).

Conclusion.—This randomized and blinded trial disclosed a significant better primary efficacy variable (Rankin Stroke Score after 12 months) in the MWA patient group. We suggest that proactive intensive care management with MWA-tailored cerebrospinal fluid drainage during the first week improves aneurysmal SAH outcome.

▶ Subarachnoid hemorrhage is often a devastating diagnosis, carrying a 50% mortality rate, with 33% of survivors requiring lifelong care. Preventing secondary brain damage by maximizing cerebral perfusion pressure is a mainstay of intensive care unit management of these patients. In order to do this, strict attention must be paid to patients' intracranial pressures (ICP). In this randomized and blinded single-center trial, 2 methods of monitoring ICP were used, comparing patient outcomes at 12 months using the modified Rankin stroke scale. The first method involved traditional ICP monitoring using a pressure transducer. The goal was to keep the ICP less than 20 mm Hg. The second method involved measuring the mean ICP wave amplitude (MWA) less than 5 mm Hg. MWA reflects intracranial compliance, and while some patients may have a normal ICP, they may still have an elevated MWA, reflecting decreased intracranial compliance. Results of the study showed that a higher volume of cerebrospinal fluid was drained from patients in the MWA group, which was expected. During the first 2 weeks of treatment, the Glasgow coma scale numbers of those in the MWA group were higher than those in the traditional ICP monitoring group. At 12 months, patients in the MWA group had significantly better Rankin stroke scores, reflected especially in those with minimal to no residual disability. This study was small (N = 97) and performed at a single center. Although the patients and those who reevaluated the patients 12 months after their ictus were blinded to the patient's study group, the doctors and nurses involved in their daily care obviously were not. This introduces the possibility of examiner bias. However, despite these shortcomings, this study indicates a clear need for further examination of this advanced monitoring modality.

T. Clark, MD

An evaluation of three measures of intracranial compliance in traumatic brain injury patients
Howells T, Lewén A, Sköld MK, et al (Uppsala Univ, Sweden)
Intensive Care Med 38:1061-1068, 2012

Purpose.—To compare intracranial pressure (ICP) amplitude, ICP slope, and the correlation of ICP amplitude and ICP mean (RAP index) as measures of compliance in a cohort of traumatic brain injury (TBI) patients.

Methods.—Mean values of the three measures were calculated in the 2-h periods before and after surgery (craniectomies and evacuations), and in the 12-h periods preceding and following thiopental treatment, and during periods of thiopental coma. The changes in the metrics were evaluated using the Wilcoxon test. The correlations of 10-day mean values for the three metrics with age, admission Glasgow Motor Score (GMS), and Extended Glasgow Outcome Score (GOSe) were evaluated. Patients under and over 60 years old were also compared using the Student t test. The correlation of ICP amplitude with systemic pulse amplitude was analyzed.

Results.—ICP amplitude was significantly correlated with GMS, and also with age for patients 35 years old and older. The correlations of ICP slope and the RAP index with GMS and with age were not significant. All three metrics indicated significant improvements in compliance following surgery and during thiopental coma. None of the metrics were significantly correlated with outcome, possibly due to confounding effects

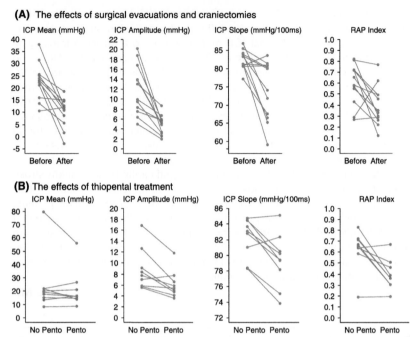

(A) The effects of surgical evacuations and craniectomies

ICP Mean (mmHg)   ICP Amplitude (mmHg)   ICP Slope (mmHg/100ms)   RAP Index

(B) The effects of thiopental treatment

ICP Mean (mmHg)   ICP Amplitude (mmHg)   ICP Slope (mmHg/100ms)   RAP Index

FIGURE 2.—Effects of surgery (craniectomies and evacuations) (a) and thiopental treatment (b) on mean ICP and the three compliance metrics. (With kind permission from Springer Science+Business Media. Reprinted from Howells T, Lewén A, Sköld MK, et al. An evaluation of three measures of intracranial compliance in traumatic brain injury patients. *Intensive Care Med.* 2012;38:1061-1068.)

of treatment factors. The correlation of systemic pulse amplitude with ICP amplitude was low ($R = 0.18$), only explaining 3% of the variance.

Conclusions.—This study provides further validation for all three of these features of the ICP waveform as measures of compliance. ICP amplitude had the best performance in these tests (Fig 2).

▶ The measurement of intracranial pressure in the setting of brain injury is valuable, particularly in the setting of severe traumatic brain injury (TBI). Similarly, the estimation of brain compliance is useful for predicting higher risk of intracranial pressure (ICP) elevation or crisis. However, the determination of intracranial compliance is difficult at the bedside. In this elegant experiment, Howells et al compare 3 different methods to determine brain compliance: ICP amplitude, ICP slope, and the correlation of ICP amplitude and ICP mean (RAP index) in a prospective cohort of TBI patients, and correlate these methods with a 6-month clinical outcome. Among the 3 measurements, the ICP amplitude correlated very well with the severity of the injury, the effect of surgery, and medical therapy (thiopental, Fig 2). Other measurements had significant but less prominent correlations. None of the measurements correlated with a 6-month outcome. The effects of surgery and other treatments were not accounted for in the analysis. This study is important, as it provides further validation about different measurements of the compliance of the brain not normally determined from ICP measurements alone.

F. Rincon, MD

Cardiac and central vascular functional alterations in the acute phase of aneurysmal subarachnoid hemorrhage
Papanikolaou J, Makris D, Karakitsos D, et al (Univ of Thessaly, Greece; General State Hosp of Athens, Greece; et al)
Crit Care Med 40:223-232, 2012

Objectives.—To investigate aortic functional alterations in the acute phase of aneurysmal subarachnoid hemorrhage and to evaluate the relationship between potential cardiovascular alterations and delayed cerebral infarctions or poor Glasgow Outcome Scale score at discharge from critical care unit.

Design.—Prospective observational study.

Setting.—Critical Care Departments of two tertiary centers.

Patients.—Thirty-seven Patients with aneurysmal subarachnoid hemorrhage.

Interventions.—Patients were evaluated at two time points: on admission (acute aneurysmal subarachnoid hemorrhage phase) and at least 21 days later (stable aneurysmal subarachnoid hemorrhage state). At baseline, the severity of aneurysmal subarachnoid hemorrhage was assessed clinically (Hunt and Hess scale) and radiologically (brain computed tomography Fisher grading). Aortic elasticity was evaluated by Doppler-derived pulse-wave velocity and left ventricular function by echocardiography. Serum B-type natriuretic peptide and troponin I were also assessed at the same time points.

Measurements and Main Results.—At the acute phase, 23 Patients (62%) were found to present supranormal pulse-wave velocity and 14 Patients (38%) presented left ventricular systolic dysfunction; there were significant associations between pulse-wave velocity values and left ventricular ejection fraction ($p < .001$). Left ventricular ejection fraction and pulse-wave velocity were both associated with Hunt and Hess ($p \leq .004$) and Fisher grading ($p \leq .03$). Left ventricular ejection fraction and pulse-wave velocity were improved between acute aneurysmal subarachnoid hemorrhage and stable state ($p \leq .005$); changes ($\Delta\%$) were greater in Patients who initially had regional wall motion abnormalities compared to Patients who had not ($28.7\% \pm 10.2\%$ vs. $2.4\% \pm 1.8\%$ [$p = .002$] and $-17.9\% \pm 3.7\%$ vs. $-3.5\% \pm 4.7\%$ [$p = .045$], respectively). Pulse-wave velocity/left ventricular ejection fraction ratio was the only independent predictor for delayed cerebral infarctions. Left ventricular ejection fraction, B-type natriuretic peptide, pulse-wave velocity, and pulse-wave velocity/left ventricular ejection fraction showed significant diagnostic performance for predicting delayed cerebral infarctions or poor Glasgow Outcome Scale score (1–3).

Conclusions.—Our findings suggest that significant cardiovascular alterations in left ventricular function and in aortic stiffness occur during the early phase of aneurysmal subarachnoid hemorrhage. These phenomena were associated with adverse outcomes in this study and their role in the pathogenesis of delayed neurologic complications warrants further investigation.

▶ In this prospective observational study of 37 patients admitted with an acute aneurysmal subarachnoid hemorrhage (SAH), the authors sought to evaluate aortic functional alterations in the setting of SAH as well as to determine if cardiovascular alterations had a prognostic significance in predicting delayed cerebral infarctions (DCI; defined as a new hypodense lesion on a follow-up cerebral computed tomography [CT] scan that was not found on a CT scan 48 hours after aneurysm occlusion and not attributable to other causes) and poor neurologic outcomes (PNO; defined as Glasgow Outcomes Scale scores between 1 and 3). The study found that patients with acute SAH presented with left ventricular systolic dysfunction (left ventricular ejection fraction; LVEF) parameters, aortic stiffness (pulse wave velocity; PWV), and elevated brain natriuretic peptide (BNP) and troponin I levels as compared with when they were at a stable SAH state. Patients with PNO and DCI also had significantly worse LVEF and higher BNP levels during acute SAH. Patients with DCI were also found to have stiffer aortas/higher PWV values. Intractable intracranial hypertension and PWF/LVEF ratio (a combined sonographic index that the researchers introduced to incorporate both aortic stiffness and LV systolic dysfunction) were found to be independent predictors of PNO ($P < 0.04$) and DCI ($P < 0.04$), respectively. Limitations to the study included the small sample size and diminished precision and interobserver reproducibility in regard to assessment of LV segmental wall motion. There was also a lack of stratification of poor outcomes when grading SAH, which may be able to provide more clinically significant insight. Therefore, further studies should be undertaken with stronger sample sizes and an analysis of patients with differing levels of severity of SAH to further solidify these preliminary findings.

S. Siow, MD

Closure or Medical Therapy for Cryptogenic Stroke with Patent Foramen Ovale
Furlan AJ, for the CLOSURE I Investigators (Univ Hosps Case Med Ctr, Cleveland, OH; et al)
N Engl J Med 366:991-999, 2012

Background.—The prevalence of patent foramen ovale among patients with cryptogenic stroke is higher than that in the general population. Closure with a percutaneous device is often recommended in such patients, but it is not known whether this intervention reduces the risk of recurrent stroke.

Methods.—We conducted a multicenter, randomized, open-label trial of closure with a percutaneous device, as compared with medical therapy alone, in patients between 18 and 60 years of age who presented with a cryptogenic stroke or transient ischemic attack (TIA) and had a patent foramen ovale. The primary end point was a composite of stroke or transient ischemic attack during 2 years of follow-up, death from any cause during the first 30 days, or death from neurologic causes between 31 days and 2 years.

Results.—A total of 909 patients were enrolled in the trial. The cumulative incidence (Kaplan—Meier estimate) of the primary end point was 5.5% in the closure group (447 patients) as compared with 6.8% in the medical-therapy group (462 patients) (adjusted hazard ratio, 0.78; 95% confidence interval, 0.45 to 1.35; $P = 0.37$). The respective rates were 2.9% and 3.1% for stroke ($P = 0.79$) and 3.1% and 4.1% for TIA ($P = 0.44$). No deaths occurred by 30 days in either group, and there were no deaths from neurologic causes during the 2-year follow-up period. A cause other than paradoxical embolism was usually apparent in patients with recurrent neurologic events.

Conclusions.—In patients with cryptogenic stroke or TIA who had a patent foramen ovale, closure with a device did not offer a greater benefit than medical therapy alone for the prevention of recurrent stroke or TIA. (Funded by NMT Medical; ClinicalTrials.gov number, NCT00201461.)

▶ The prevalence of patent foramen ovale (PFO) in the general population is roughly 20% to 25%, and it has been shown in autopsy studies that patients < 55 years of age with cryptogenic stroke had a nearly 56% incidence of PFO. It is often recommended that patients opt for percutaneous closure of a PFO based on data from the CLOSURE I trial. This well-designed prospective, multi-center, randomized, open-label trial aimed to compare the efficacy of STARflex septal closure system with medical management in reducing the recurrence of stroke and transient ischemic attack (TIA) in patients with cryptogenic stroke who were found to have a PFO and no other reason for their stroke. A total of 909 patients, aged 18 to 60, were randomized between the 2 groups and the end composite of stroke or TIA in 2 years was found to be 5.5% for the percutaneous closure group and 6.8% for the medical management group ($P = .37$). This study produced a relatively balanced set of baseline characteristics for the 2 study groups. It was found that there was a slightly higher prevalence of hypertension ($P = .08$), hypercholesterolemia ($P = .05$), and moderate/substantial PFO shunting ($P = .07$) in the closure group. Also, in the intention-to-treat analysis, the composite end point of TIA or stroke for the 2 groups actually showed that 20/23 in the closure group and 22/29 in the medical group demonstrated a possible alternative later in the trial, suggesting that not all participants suffered cryptogenic stroke. Finally, with only 909 patients, the study had power only to detect a 2/3 difference between the 2 groups, suggesting that a much larger sample size or longer follow-up period was needed. The importance of this study is that patients with PFO and cryptogenic stroke will not have better outcomes with a closure device rather than medical management. This study as well as CLOSURE I show that closure device placement does cause a significant increase in atrial fibrillation in patients. Further research needs to be done looking at patients with repeated TIA or stroke after medical management who may benefit from closure device placement as well as a younger population who may benefit more long-term.

K. Vakharia, MD

Midlevel practitioners can safely place intracranial pressure monitors
Young PJ, Bowling WM (Hurley Med Ctr, Flint, MI)
J Trauma Acute Care Surg 73:431-434, 2012

Background.—Neurosurgical coverage is a challenge for many trauma centers. Midlevel practitioners (MLPs) can extend coverage by sharing the workload. Our objective was to determine whether the complication rates for intracranial pressure (ICP) monitor placement were similar between neurosurgeons and MLPs.

Methods.—After obtaining institutional review board approval, the trauma registry at a Level I trauma center was searched for all ICP monitors placed between June 2005 and March 2010. Complications were classified as major or minor. The study was designed as a noninferiority trial with a 5% absolute difference in major complications defined as acceptable, a priori. Time to monitor placement was a secondary outcome and was analyzed by Wilcoxon rank sum and multiple linear regression.

Results.—One hundred seven patients were identified. Fifteen patients were excluded (inserted by trauma surgeon or MLP under direct supervision, ventricular drain, or inserted at an outside facility). Of the remaining 92, 22 were inserted by neurosurgeons and 70 by MLPs. There was one major complication (cerebrospinal fluid leak) in a monitor placed by an MLP. The difference in complication rates was significantly less than 5% (1.4% vs. 0%, $p = 0.0128$). The minor complication rate was higher for MLPs (5.7% vs. 0%, $p = 0.80$). Craniotomy and placement on third shift were associated with shorter times to monitor placement. Nine monitors were inserted at the time of craniotomy, eight of them by the neurosurgeon.

Conclusion.—ICP monitors can be safely placed by midlevel practitioners with major complication rates not different from those of neurosurgeons.

▶ This retrospective trial at an urban level I trauma center in Michigan examined complications associated with intracranial pressure monitor placement. Major complications were defined as hemorrhage, infection, or cerebrospinal fluid leak. Minor complications include malfunction or malposition. The primary outcome studied was major complication rate.

Similar to a report from the 1990s by Kaups and coworkers, midlevel practitioners in this trauma center were safely able to place intracranial pressure monitors.[1] This is important because this program lacks postgraduate surgical trainees to perform this common procedure. Thus, midlevel practitioners can extend the effectiveness of the neurosurgeons.

Midlevel practitioners learn to do this procedure by first assisting in the operating room and learning ward management. The next step in training for these midlevel practitioners is emergency response to trauma patients followed by training specific to the neurosurgery service. Finally, qualified midlevel practitioners undergo a series of intracranial pressure monitor insertions under direct supervision of neurosurgical staff. It is valuable to note that the hospital, its neurosurgeons, and its midlevel practitioners have agreed to this program as essential for trauma program maintenance.

D. J. Dries, MSE, MD

Reference

1. Kaups KL, Parks SN, Morris CL. Intracranial pressure monitor placement by midlevel practitioners. *J Trauma.* 1998;45:884-886.

A Trial of Intracranial-Pressure Monitoring in Traumatic Brain Injury

Chesnut RM, Temkin N, Carney N, et al (Univ of Washington, Seattle; Oregon Health and Science Univ, Portland; et al)
N Engl J Med 367:2471-2481, 2012

Background.—Intracranial-pressure monitoring is considered the standard of care for severe traumatic brain injury and is used frequently, but the efficacy of treatment based on monitoring in improving the outcome has not been rigorously assessed.

Methods.—We conducted a multicenter, controlled trial in which 324 patients 13 years of age or older who had severe traumatic brain injury and were being treated in intensive care units (ICUs) in Bolivia or Ecuador were randomly assigned to one of two specific protocols: guidelines-based management in which a protocol for monitoring intraparenchymal intracranial pressure was used (pressure-monitoring group) or a protocol in which treatment was based on imaging and clinical examination (imaging—clinical examination group). The primary outcome was a composite of survival time, impaired consciousness, and functional status at 3 months and 6 months and neuropsychological status at 6 months; neuropsychological status was assessed by an examiner who was unaware of protocol assignment. This composite measure was based on performance across 21 measures of functional and cognitive status and calculated as a percentile (with 0 indicating the worst performance, and 100 the best performance).

Results.—There was no significant between-group difference in the primary outcome, a composite measure based on percentile performance across 21 measures of functional and cognitive status (score, 56 in the pressure-monitoring group vs. 53 in the imaging—clinical examination group; $P = 0.49$). Six-month mortality was 39% in the pressure-monitoring group and 41% in the imaging—clinical examination group $(P = 0.60)$. The median length of stay in the ICU was similar in the two groups (12 days in the pressure-monitoring group and 9 days in the imaging—clinical examination group; $P = 0.25$), although the number of days of brain-specific treatments (e.g., administration of hyperosmolar fluids and the use of hyperventilation) in the ICU was higher in the imaging—clinical examination group than in the pressure-monitoring group (4.8 vs. 3.4, $P = 0.002$). The distribution of serious adverse events was similar in the two groups.

Conclusions.—For patients with severe traumatic brain injury, care focused on maintaining monitored intracranial pressure at 20 mm Hg or less was not shown to be superior to care based on imaging and clinical examination. (Funded by the National Institutes of Health and others; ClinicalTrials.gov number, NCT01068522.)

▶ At first glance, the reader could be surprised at the outcome of this study. Intracranial pressure monitoring and management has been held as a gold standard for care of the brain-injured patient. This study calls the role of a long-accepted monitoring strategy into question.[1] On further examination, however, these results are not so surprising. Clinical assessment is compared with intracranial pressure monitoring. The ultimate determination of outcome is physical examination (Fig 1 in the original article). Changes in physical examination should lead to intervention. In general, these changes will parallel changes in intracranial pressure. However, intracranial pressure is a global measure of what is truly a regional phenomenon. Blunt or penetrating head trauma affects regions of the brain in different ways dependent on location relative to injury.

In an excellent editorial, Ropper points out that it is not the total intracranial pressure but rather the specific area of the brain sustaining compression or other injury that has the greatest effect on outcome. Thus, clinical findings reflecting damage at zones such as the midbrain, thalamus, and reticular-activating system may be more sensitive than simple measurement of intracranial pressure.[2]

If neurologic examination is obscured by medication administration, particularly administration of muscle relaxants and heavy sedation, intracranial pressure monitoring is a reasonable choice.

In time, I hope to see trials with a longer monitoring horizon than the 6-month interval employed here.

D. J. Dries, MSE, MD

References

1. Brain Trauma Foundation; American Association of Neurological Surgeons; Congress of Neurological Surgeons; Joint Section on Neurotrauma and Critical Care AANS/CNS; Bratton SL, Chestnut RM, Ghajar J, et al. Guidelines for the management of severe traumatic brain injury. VIII. Intracranial pressure thresholds. *J Neurotrauma*. 2007;24:S55-S58.
2. Ropper AH. Brain in a box [editorial]. *N Engl J Med*. 2012;367:2539-2541.

Blast-related mild traumatic brain injury is associated with a decline in self-rated health amongst US military personnel
Heltemes KJ, Holbrook TL, MacGregor AJ, et al (Naval Health Res Ctr, San Diego, CA)
Injury 43:1990-1995, 2012

Introduction.—Mild traumatic brain injury (MTBI) has emerged as the preeminent injury of combat from the recent conflicts in Iraq and Afghanistan. Very little is known about short- and long-term outcomes after combat-related MTBI. As a measure of outcome after injury, self-rated health is a reliable, widely used measure that assesses perceived health. The primary aim of this study was to determine the effect of combat-related MTBI on self-reported health status after return from deployment. The secondary objective was to examine predictors of a decline in self-reported health status amongst US service members with MTBI, as compared to those service members with other minor non-TBI injuries.

Patients and Methods.—MTBI cases and an injured comparison group were identified from the Expeditionary Medical Encounter Database records of 1129 male, US service members who experienced blast-related injuries in Iraq from March 2004 to March 2008. Self-rated health was assessed from the routinely administered pre- and post-deployment health assessment questionnaires by the following question, "Overall, how would you rate your health during the past month?" Possible responses were "poor", "fair", "good", "very good", or "excellent." A distinction was made between minor and major negative changes in health (i.e., very good to fair) based on these self-rated health outcomes captured post-injury.

Results.—For all personnel, post-injury levels of self-rated health were statistically significantly worse than pre-injury health rating. At 6 months post-injury, service members with MTBI were 5 times more likely to report a major negative change in health as compared to members with other mild injuries. This association was independent of age, rank, branch

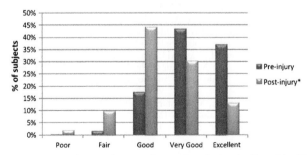

FIGURE.—Frequency distribution of pre- and post-injury levels of self-rated health ($N = 1129$). *Statistically significant difference Wilcoxon matched pairs signed-ranks test, $Z = 19.21$, $P < .001$. (Reprinted from Heltemes KJ, Holbrook TL, MacGregor AJ, et al. Blast-related mild traumatic brain injury is associated with a decline in self-rated health amongst US military personnel. *Injury.* 2012;43:1990-1995, with permission from Elsevier.)

of service, Injury Severity Score, mental health diagnosis prior to injury, and having been referred to a health care professional.

Discussion.—Blast-related injuries, specifically MTBI, during deployment have negative consequences on service members' perception of health. Future research is needed to improve our understanding of the overall effects of MTBI on health and quality of life (Fig).

▶ Self-rated health status is a valuable predictor of outcome among patients sustaining injury. Patients with traumatic brain injury (TBI) report more post-concussive symptoms even when evaluated months after injury. In fact, many of our evaluation tools should extend to 1 year or more in the head injury population.[1-5]

This study uses a military "before and after" scale to assess the outcome of minor TBI secondary to combat-related blast injury. As the data indicate, individuals sustaining minor TBI clearly have poorer health-related assessment after deployment in which these injuries occur.

These early outcomes contradict studies of civilian populations suggesting improvement in outcomes in the first months after minor TBI. Data were obtained 6 months after injury. It would be interesting to see outcome-related data at a later timeframe. A great strength of this work is the availability of "before and after" data (Fig). An obvious limitation is the lack of a validated medical tool in making this assessment. The assessment employed here has not been previously validated. Nonetheless, these data support a growing concern that TBI among military personnel may be the greatest adverse outcome and one with a lengthy, ill-defined horizon.[5,6]

D. J. Dries, MSE, MD

References

1. Emanuelson I, Andersson Holmkvist E, Björklund R, Stålhammar D. Quality of life and post-concussion symptoms in adults after mild traumatic brain injury: a population-based study in western Sweden. *Acta Neurol Scand.* 2003;108: 332-338.
2. Findler M, Cantor J, Haddad L, Gordon W, Ashman T. The reliability and validity of the SF-36 health survey questionnaire for use with individuals with traumatic brain injury. *Brain Inj.* 2001;15:715-723.
3. Steadman-Pare D, Colantonio A, Ratcliff G, Chase S, Vernich L. Factors associated with perceived quality of life many years after traumatic brain injury. *J Head Trauma Rehabil.* 2001;16:330-342.
4. Hawthorne G, Gruen RL, Kaye AH. Traumatic brain injury and long-term quality of life: findings from an Australian study. *J Neurotrauma.* 2009;26:1623-1633.
5. Okie S. Traumatic brain injury in the war zone. *N Engl J Med.* 2005;352: 2043-2047.
6. McCrea M, Iverson GL, McAllister TW, et al. An integrated review of recovery after mild traumatic brain injury (MTBI): implications for clinical management. *Clin Neuropsychol.* 2009;23:1368-1390.

Performance of the Canadian CT Head Rule and the New Orleans Criteria for Predicting Any Traumatic Intracranial Injury on Computed Tomography in a United States Level I Trauma Center
Papa L, Stiell IG, Clement CM, et al (Orlando Regional Med Ctr, FL; Univ of Ottawa, Ontario, Canada; Ottawa Health Res Inst, Ontario, Canada; et al)
Acad Emerg Med 19:2-10, 2012

Objectives.—This study compared the clinical performance of the Canadian CT Head Rule (CCHR) and the New Orleans Criteria (NOC) for detecting any traumatic intracranial lesion on computed tomography (CT) in patients with a Glasgow Coma Scale (GCS) score of 15. Also assessed were ability to detect patients with "clinically important" brain injury and patients requiring neurosurgical intervention. Additionally, the performance of the CCHR was assessed in a larger cohort of those presenting with GCS of 13 to 15.
Methods.—This prospective cohort study was conducted in a U.S. Level I trauma center and enrolled a consecutive sample of mildly head-injured adults who presented to the emergency department (ED) with witnessed loss of consciousness, disorientation or amnesia, and GCS 13 to 15. The rules were compared in the group of patients with GCS 15. The primary outcome was prediction of "any traumatic intracranial injury" on CT. Secondary outcomes included "clinically important brain injury" on CT and need for neurosurgical intervention.
Results.—Among the 431 enrolled patients, 314 patients (73%) had a GCS of 15, and 22 of the 314 (7%) had evidence of a traumatic intracranial lesion on CT. There were 11 of 314 (3.5%) who had "clinically important" brain injury, and 3 of 314 (1.0%) required neurosurgical intervention. The NOC and CCHR both had 100% sensitivity (95% confidence interval [CI] = 82% to 100%), but the CCHR was more specific for detecting any traumatic intracranial lesion on CT, with a specificity of 36.3% (95% CI = 31% to 42%) versus 10.2% (95% CI = 7% to 14%) for NOC. For "clinically important" brain lesions, the CCHR and the NOC had similar sensitivity (both 100%; 95% CI = 68% to 100%), but the specificity was 35% (95% CI = 30% to 41%) for CCHR and 9.9% (95% CI = 7% to 14%) for NOC. When the rules were compared for predicting need for neurosurgical intervention, the sensitivity was equivalent at 100% (95% CI = 31% to 100%) but the CCHR had a higher specificity at 80.7% (95% CI = 76% to 85%) versus 9.6% (95% CI = 7% to 14%) for NOC. Among all 431 patients with a GCS score 13 to 15, the CCHR had sensitivities of 100% (95% CI = 84% to 100%) for 27 patients with clinically important brain injury and 100% (95% CI = 46% to 100%) for five patients requiring neurosurgical intervention.
Conclusions.—In a U.S. sample of mildly head-injured patients, the CCHR and the NOC had equivalently high sensitivities for detecting any traumatic intracranial lesion on CT, clinically important brain injury,

and neurosurgical intervention, but the CCHR was more specific. A larger cohort will be needed to validate these findings.

▶ The Canadian CT Head Rule (CCHR) and the New Orleans Criteria (NOC) are 2 validated clinical decision rules aimed at guiding the decision to obtain head computed tomography (CT) in patients with head trauma. Both rules have been studied extensively in various countries. This is the first study to prospectively apply both rules to patients at a trauma center in the United States. While the CCHR was originally developed to detect clinically important brain injury, in this study, it was tested to detect any traumatic intracranial injury. Four hundred thirty-one patients were enrolled, 314 with a Glascow Coma Score (GCS) of 15 and 22 with traumatic injury on CT. Among patients with GCS of 15, both rules performed perfectly (sensitivity 100%) across the spectrum of injuries, including any injury (n = 22), clinically important injury (n = 11), and those requiring neurosurgical intervention (n = 3). Because of the relatively small number of enrolled patients, the confidence intervals for these sensitivities ranged from 68% to 100%. The CCHR was more specific in all categories. This study adds to the body of evidence supporting the use of these 2 rules. In an effort to provide quality care and to reduce the radiation burden associated with CT use, clinicians should be applying one of these rules in their daily practice. Which rule depends on a clinician's relative concern for radiation exposure versus detecting injury. The NOC has a lower specificity and leads to higher rates of CT scanning but detects any intracranial injury. The CCHR is more specific and, therefore, results in less CT scanning but is only validated to detect clinically significant injuries (as defined by a large group of neurosurgeons). The current study shows both rules are great at detecting intracranial injury, so decide which one best matches your practice style and use it.

M. D. Zwank, MD

9 Renal

Predicting Acute Kidney Injury Among Burn Patients in the 21st Century:
A Classification and Regression Tree Analysis
Schneider DF, Dobrowolsky A, Shakir IA, et al (Loyola Univ Med Ctr, Maywood, IL)
J Burn Care Res 33:242-251, 2012

Historically, acute kidney injury (AKI) carried a deadly prognosis in the burn population. The aim of this study is to provide a modern description of AKI in the burn population and to develop a prediction tool for identifying patients at risk for late AKI. A large multi-institutional database, the Glue Grant's Trauma-Related Database, was used to characterize AKI in a cohort of critically ill burn patients. The authors defined AKI according to the RIFLE criteria and categorized AKI as early, late, or progressive. They then used Classification and Regression Tree (CART) analysis to create a decision tree with data obtained from the first 48 hours of admission to predict which subset of patients would develop late AKI. The accuracy of this decision tree was tested in a separate, single-institution cohort of burn patients who met the same criteria for entry into the Glue Grant study. Of the 220 total patients analyzed from the Glue Grant cohort, 49 (22.2%) developed early AKI, 39 (17.7%) developed late AKI, and 16 (7.2%) developed progressive AKI. The group with progressive AKI was statistically older, with more comorbidities and with the worst survival when compared with those with early or late AKI. Using CART analysis, a decision tree was developed with an overall accuracy of 80% for the development of late AKI for the Glue Grant dataset. The authors then tested this decision tree on a smaller dataset from our own institution to validate this tool and found it to be 73% accurate. AKI is common in severe burns with notable differences between early, late, and progressive AKI. In addition, CART analysis provided a predictive model for early identification of patients at highest risk for developing late AKI with proven clinical accuracy.

▶ These authors have taken the well-known RIFLE (risk, injury, failure, loss, and end-stage kidney) classification for kidney injury and focused on defining a prediction model early in the hospitalization course of burn patients that translates into a useful prediction model for developing acute kidney injury at a later point in time. The rationale for developing this tool is that the pathophysiology for patients developing multiple organ dysfunction syndrome is multifactorial and the associated mortality rate in burn patients is high. Using an analysis model unfamiliar to surgery and burn trauma care specifically requires a bit of explaining, but the authors do so in the introduction and methods section on Classification and Regression Tree (CART). I refer those brief and easily understandable sections to you for further details.

What we discover from this study is that the timing of acute kidney injury (AKI) affects outcomes significantly. Those with progressive AKI fared the worst, which is not surprising as they were the oldest group with the most comorbidities. Defining this group of patients early in their hospital course may lead to different resuscitation or renal protocol strategies to keep them alive and off dialysis. In the grander scheme, perhaps CART methodology will be useful in other critical areas of burn care and defining prevention strategies for morbidities such as ventilator associated pneumonia.

B. A. Latenser, MD, FACS

Body mass index and acute kidney injury in the acute respiratory distress syndrome
Soto GJ, Frank AJ, Christiani DC, et al (Montefiore Med Ctr, Bronx, NY; Massachusetts General Hosp, Boston; Harvard School of Public Health, Boston, MA)
Crit Care Med 40:2601-2608, 2012

Objectives.—Obesity is increasingly encountered in intensive care units but the relationship between obesity and acute kidney injury is unclear. We aimed to evaluate whether body mass index was associated with acute kidney injury in the acute respiratory distress syndrome and to examine the association between acute kidney injury and mortality in patients with and without obesity.

Design.—Retrospective study.

Setting.—Massachusetts General Hospital and Beth Israel Deaconess Medical Center.

Patients.—Seven hundred fifty-one patients with acute respiratory distress syndrome.

Interventions.—None.

Measurements and Main Results.—Acute kidney injury was defined as meeting the "Risk" category according to modified Risk, Injury, Failure, Loss, End-stage criteria based on creatinine and glomerular filtration rate because urine output was only available on the day of intensive care unit admission. Body mass index was calculated from height and weight at intensive care unit admission. The prevalence of acute kidney injury increased significantly with increasing weight ($p = .01$). The odds of acute kidney injury were twice in obese and severely obese patients compared to patients with normal body mass index, after adjusting for predictors of acute kidney injury (age, diabetes, Acute Physiology and Chronic Health Evaluation III, aspiration, vasopressor use, and thrombocytopenia [platelets $\leq 80,000/mm^3$]). After adjusting for the same predictors, body mass index was significantly associated with acute kidney injury (odds ratio$_{adj}$ 1.20 per 5 kg/m^2

increase in body mass index, 95% confidence interval 1.07—1.33). On multivariate analysis, acute kidney injury was associated with increased acute respiratory distress syndrome mortality (odds ratio$_{adj}$ 2.76, 95% confidence interval 1.72—4.42) whereas body mass index was associated with decreased mortality (odds ratio$_{adj}$ 0.81 per 5 kg/m^2 increase in body mass index, 95% confidence interval 0.71—0.93) after adjusting for mortality predictors.

Conclusions.—In acute respiratory distress syndrome patients, obesity is associated with increased development of acute kidney injury, which is not completely explained by severity of illness or shock. Although increased body mass index is associated with decreased mortality, acute kidney injury remained associated with higher mortality even after adjusting for body mass index.

▶ This study is taken from a large dataset gathered over 10 years at 2 hospitals in the Harvard University system. Patients with acute respiratory distress syndrome (ARDS) were followed, with outcomes and molecular markers studied. This data analysis is directed at the controversy in the literature regarding the impact of obesity on outcomes in patients with acute kidney injury, a common complication in critical care, and ARDS using standard international definitions.[1-4]

A remarkable association between body mass index (BMI), ARDS, and adverse outcomes was identified, with a highly reliable 60-day follow-up. Although increased BMI was not tied to mortality, renal insufficiency was associated with this parameter. The authors indicate that comorbidities did not contribute to this outcome but admit in the discussion that data on resuscitation, cardiovascular comorbidities, which could contribute to renal insufficiency, and the rigor of obesity scoring other than BMI calculation were limited. All of these concerns reflect the problem with using a dataset directed at one question to obtain information on a related problem. It is inevitable that relevant data will be excluded.

This article can be recommended for its extensive dataset, consistent pattern of care, and the rigor employed by these investigators. Given the prevalence of acute kidney injury of greater than 60% in this cohort, the bedside clinician must watch for this complication in the intensive care unit population who have respiratory failure. Finally, the rapid onset of acute kidney injury in this population suggests that resuscitation in these patients requires further investigation.[3]

D. J. Dries, MSE, MD

References

1. Uchino S, Kellum JA, Bellomo R, et al. Beginning and Ending Supportive Therapy for the Kidney (BEST Kidney) Investigators. Acute renal failure in critically ill patients: a multinational, multicenter study. *JAMA.* 2005;294:813-818.
2. Mehta RL, Pascual MT, Soroko S, et al. Program to Improve Care in Acute Renal Disease. Spectrum of acute renal failure in the intensive care unit: the PICARD experience. *Kidney Int.* 2004;66:1613-1621.
3. Wiedemann HP, Wheeler AP, Bernard GR, et al. National Heart, Lung, and Blood Institute Acute Respiratory Distress Syndrome (ARDS) Clinical Trials Network. Comparison of two fluid-management strategies in acute lung injury. *N Engl J Med.* 2006;354:2564-2575.
4. Rubenfeld GD, Caldwell E, Peabody E, et al. Incidence and outcomes of acute lung injury. *N Engl J Med.* 2005;353:1685-1693.

Association Between a Chloride-Liberal vs Chloride-Restrictive Intravenous Fluid Administration Strategy and Kidney Injury in Critically Ill Adults

Yunos NM, Bellomo R, Hegarty C, et al (Monash Univ Sunway Campus, Malaysia; Austin Hosp, Melbourne, Australia; et al)
JAMA 308:1566-1572, 2012

Context.—Administration of traditional chloride-liberal intravenous fluids may precipitate acute kidney injury (AKI).

Objective.—To assess the association of a chloride-restrictive (vs chloride-liberal) intravenous fluid strategy with AKI in critically ill patients.

Design, Setting, and Patients.—Prospective, open-label, sequential period pilot study of 760 patients admitted consecutively to the intensive care unit (ICU) during the control period (February 18 to August 17, 2008) compared with 773 patients admitted consecutively during the intervention period (February 18 to August 17, 2009) at a university-affiliated hospital in Melbourne, Australia.

Interventions.—During the control period, patients received standard intravenous fluids. After a 6-month phase-out period (August 18, 2008, to February 17, 2009), any use of chloride-rich intravenous fluids (0.9% saline, 4% succinylated gelatin solution, or 4% albumin solution) was restricted to attending specialist approval only during the intervention period; patients instead received a lactated solution (Hartmann solution), a balanced solution (Plasma-Lyte 148), and chloride-poor 20% albumin.

Main Outcome Measures.—The primary outcomes included increase from baseline to peak creatinine level in the ICU and incidence of AKI according to the risk, injury, failure, loss, end-stage (RIFLE) classification. Secondary post hoc analysis outcomes included the need for renal replacement therapy (RRT), length of stay in ICU and hospital, and survival.

Results.—Chloride administration decreased by 144 504 mmol (from 694 to 496 mmol/patient) from the control period to the intervention period. Comparing the control period with the intervention period, the mean serum creatinine level increase while in the ICU was 22.6 μmol/L (95% CI, 17.5-27.7 μmol/L) vs 14.8 μmol/L (95% CI, 9.8-19.9 μmol/L) ($P = .03$), the incidence of injury and failure class of RIFLE-defined AKI was 14% (95% CI, 11%-16%; n = 105) vs 8.4% (95% CI, 6.4%-10%; n = 65) ($P < .001$), and the use of RRT was 10% (95% CI, 8.1%-12%; n = 78) vs 6.3% (95% CI, 4.6%-8.1%; n = 49) ($P = .005$). After adjustment for covariates, this association remained for incidence of injury and failure class of RIFLE-defined AKI (odds ratio, 0.52 [95% CI, 0.37-0.75]; $P < .001$) and use of RRT (odds ratio, 0.52 [95% CI, 0.33-0.81]; $P = .004$). There were no differences in hospital mortality, hospital or ICU length of stay, or need for RRT after hospital discharge.

Conclusion.—The implementation of a chloride-restrictive strategy in a tertiary ICU was associated with a significant decrease in the incidence of AKI and use of RRT.

TABLE 2.—Composition of Trial Fluids[a]

	0.9% Saline	Hartmann	4% Gelatin	Plasma-Lyte 148	Albumin 4%	Albumin 20%
Sodium	150	129	154	140	140	48-100
Potassium	0	5	0	5	0	0
Chloride	150	109	120	98	128	19
Calcium	0	2	0	0	0	0
Magnesium	0	0	0	1.5	0	0
Lactate	0	29	0	0	0	0
Acetate	0	0	0	27	0	0
Gluconate	0	0	0	23	0	0
Octanoate	0	0	0	0	6.4	32

[a]All concentrations in mmol/L.

Trial Registration.—clinicaltrials.gov Identifier: NCT00885404 (Table 2).

▶ This fascinating study follows up the observation that hyperchloremia causes renal vasoconstriction, decreases glomerular filtration rate, and compromises renal function in selected patient groups.[1-3]

This is a "before and after" study that did not use informed consent because treatment was considered unit protocol and data collection did not require patient contact. Control patients received normal saline, a 4% gelatin solution, and 4% albumin in sodium chloride whereas study patients, during the second trial interval, received a lactated crystalloid solution containing a smaller amount of chloride, a balanced buffered solution and a 20% albumin solution (Table 2). The authors achieved remarkable success in changing the amount of chloride exposure in patients in study intervals during 2008 and 2009. Biochemical parameters and the use of renal replacement therapy appear to support reduction in chloride exposure for critical care patients (Fig 1 in the original article).

The mechanism behind the results observed remains unclear. Afferent arteriolar vasoconstriction has been implicated in renal injury with chloride exposure along with increased thromboxane release. With exposure to chloride, the kidney is more responsive to vasoconstrictors including angiotensin II receptor blockers.

Perhaps the most important intervention between the control and study groups is elimination of the gelatin solution from control patients. The synthetic colloids have independently been associated with renal injury. In this case, control patients received gelatin combined with a significant amount of chloride.[4]

Clearly this is hypothesis-generating work. Nonetheless, with multiple fluid choices available, the intensivist may reconsider the amount of chloride given to the critically ill patient.

D. J. Dries, MSE, MD

References

1. Yunos NM, Kim IB, Bellomo R, et al. The biochemical effects of restricting chloride-rich fluids in intensive care. *Crit Care Med.* 2011;39:2419-2424.

2. Yunos NM, Bellomo R, Story D, Kellum J. Bench-to-bedside review: chloride in critical illness. *Crit Care.* 2010;14:226.
3. Chowdhury AH, Cox EF, Francis ST, Lobo DN. A randomized, controlled, double-blind crossover study on the effects of 2-L infusions of 0.9% saline and plasma-lyte® 148 on renal blood flow velocity and renal cortical tissue perfusion in healthy volunteers. *Ann Surg.* 2012;256:18-24.
4. Bayer O, Reinhart K, Kohl M, et al. Effects of fluid resuscitation with synthetic colloids or crystalloids alone on shock reversal, fluid balance, and patient outcomes in patients with severe sepsis: a prospective sequential analysis. *Crit Care Med.* 2012;40:2543-2551.

10 Trauma and Overdose

Embolization for Multicompartmental Bleeding in Patients in Hemodynamically Unstable Condition: Prognostic Factors and Outcome
Bize PE, Duran R, Madoff DC, et al (Univ Hosp of Lausanne, Vaud, Switzerland; New York Presbyterian Hosp; et al)
J Vasc Interv Radiol 23:751-760.e4, 2012

Purpose.—To determine prognostic factors and evaluate outcomes of transcatheter arterial embolization in severely injured patients in hemodynamically unstable condition with multicompartmental bleeding.

Materials and Methods.—Between June 2000 and May 2008, 36 consecutive patients treated with transcatheter arterial embolization for major retroperitoneal bleeding associated with at least one additional source of bleeding were retrospectively reviewed. Mean Injury Severity Score (ISS) was 49.4 ± 15.8. Univariate and multivariate analyses were performed to identify parameters associated with failure of embolization, need for additional surgery to control bleeding, and fatal outcome at 30 d.

Results.—Embolization was technically successful in 35 of 36 patients (97.2%) and resulted in immediate and sustained (>24 h) hemodynamic improvement in 29 (80.5%). Additional hemostatic surgery was necessary after embolization in six patients (16.6%). Fifteen patients (41.6%) died within 30 d. Failure to restore hemodynamic stability was correlated with the rate of administration of packed red blood cells ($P = .014$), rate of administration of fresh frozen plasma (FFP; $P = .031$), and systolic blood pressure (SBP) immediately before embolization ($P = .002$). The need for additional surgery was correlated with FFP administration rate before embolization ($P = .0002$) and hemodynamic success ($P = .003$). Death was correlated with Glasgow Coma Scale score at admission ($P = .001$), ISS ($P = .014$), New Injury Severity Score ($P = .016$), number of injured sites ($P = .012$), SBP before embolization ($P = .042$), need for vasopressive drugs before embolization ($P = .037$), and hemodynamic success ($P = .0004$).

Conclusions.—In patients in hemodynamically unstable condition, transcatheter arterial embolization effectively controls bleeding and improves hemodynamic stability. Immediate survival is related to hemodynamic condition before embolization, and 30-d mortality is mainly related to associated brain trauma.

▶ This was a retrospective study from 2000 to 2008 to evaluate the efficacy of transcatheter arterial embolization (TAE) in a group of 36 trauma patients with a mean Injury Severity Score of 49.4 presenting with major retroperitoneal bleeding, an additional source of bleeding in another anatomic compartment, and hemodynamic instability. In 94% of patients, whole-body computed tomography (CT) scanning found the source of bleeding. TAE was performed as the first intervention for hemodynamic control in 30 patients. Clinical success was achieved in 80.5%, which was defined as a ≥ 20% improvement in systolic blood pressure for 24 hours and a decrease in vasoactive drug use. In 30 of 36 patients who presented after the initial whole-body CT and before surgical intervention for hemodynamic control, 29 cases resulted in technical success. Only 2 patients required subsequent surgery for hemodynamic control. One patient in this group died of a bleeding complication, whereas other deaths were secondary to craniocerebral injury. In all patients, 7 of 36 required surgery to control retroperitoneal venous bleeding. In the 36 patients undergoing TAE, no intra-abdominal sepsis was observed.

This approach to hemodynamic control in the hemodynamically unstable trauma patient is appealing compared with damage control surgery in that it is less invasive, has high rates of technical and clinical success, and no observed intra-abdominal sepsis. The major drawback to the transcatheter approach is the inferiority of controlling mesenteric and retroperitoneal venous bleeding for which surgical intervention is superior. The current paradigm for the role of TAE in the treatment of active arterial bleeding in acute trauma is currently limited to hemodynamically stable patients with intraperitoneal bleeding or unstable patients with bleeding limited to the pelvis. The design of this study limits widespread adoption of this approach; however, it provides promising preliminary data indicating that a paradigm shift of the role of TAE may be on the horizon.

A. F. Miller, MD

S. Zanotti, MD

Debunking the survival bias myth: Characterization of mortality during the initial 24 hours for patients requiring massive transfusion
Brown JB, The Inflammation and the Host Response to Injury Investigators (Univ of Pittsburgh Med Ctr, PA; et al)
J Trauma Acute Care Surg 73:358-364, 2012

Background.—Controversy surrounds the optimal ratios of blood (packed red blood cell [PRBC]), plasma (fresh frozen plasma [FFP]) and platelet (PLT) use for patients requiring massive transfusion (MT) owing to possible survival bias in previous studies. We sought to characterize mortality during the first 24 hours while controlling for time varying effects of transfusion to minimize survival bias.

Methods.—Data were obtained from a multicenter prospective cohort study of adults with blunt injury and hemorrhagic shock. MT was defined as 10 U of PRBC or more over 24 hours. High FFP/PRBC (≥ 1:1.5) and PLT/PRBC (≥ 1:9) ratios at 6, 12, and 24 hours were compared with low ratio groups. Cox proportional hazards regression was used to determine the independent association of high versus low ratios with mortality at 6,

12, and 24 hours while controlling for important confounders. Cox proportional hazards regression was repeated with FFP/PRBC and PLT/PRBC ratios analyzed as time-dependent covariates to account for fluctuation over time. Mortality for more than 24 hours was treated as survival.

Results.—In the MT cohort (n = 604), initial base deficit, lactate, and international normalized ratio were similar across high and low ratio groups. High 6-hour FFP/PRBC and PLT/PRBC ratios were independently associated with a reduction in mortality risk at 6, 12, and 24 hours (hazard ratio [HR] range, 0.20–0.41, $p < 0.05$). These findings were consistent for 12-hour and 24-hour ratios. When analyzed as time-dependent covariates, a high FFP/PRBC ratio was associated with a 68% (HR, 0.32; 95% confidence interval [CI], 0.12–0.87, $p = 003$) reduction in 24-hour mortality, and a high PLT/PRBC ratio was associated with a 96% (HR, 0.04; 95% CI, 0.01–0.94, $p = 004$) reduction in 24-hour mortality. Subgroup analysis revealed that a high 1:1 ratio ($\geq 1:1.5$) had a significant 24-hour survival benefit relative to a high 1:2 (1:1.51−1:2.50) ratio group at both 6 hours (HR, 0.19; 95% CI, 0.03–0.86, $p = 003$) and 24 hours (HR, 0.25; 95% CI, 0.06–0.95, $p = 004$), suggesting a dose-response relationship. A high FFP/PRBC or PLT/PRBC ratio was not associated with development of multiple-organ failure, nosocomial infection, or adult respiratory distress syndrome in a 28-day Cox proportional hazards regression.

Conclusion.—Despite similar degrees of early shock and coagulopathy, high FFP/PRBC and PLT/PRBC ratios are associated with a survival benefit as early as 6 hours and throughout the first 24 hours, even when time-dependent fluctuations of component transfusion are accounted for. This suggests that the observed mortality benefit associated with high component transfusion ratios is unlikely owing to survivor bias and that early attainment of high transfusion ratios may significantly lower the risk of mortality in MT patients.

▶ Hemorrhage is a leading cause of death among trauma patients. In recent years, massive transfusion (MT) protocols have become widely adopted in the treatment of trauma patients, in which higher ratios of fresh frozen plasma (FFP) and platelets (PLT) to packed red blood cells (PRBC) are administered during the resuscitation of patients with life-threatening bleeding. While it has been postulated a high ratio of FFP and PLT to red cells is associated with improved survival, there remains debate as to the optimal ratios of these supplementary products to PRBC. Some observers are of the opinion that any benefit seen is the result of a survival bias because the patients receiving high ratios live long enough to achieve these additional products and, thus, ratios. In this study, the investigators evaluated data collected prospectively from a multicenter cohort study of nearly 2000 trauma patients. Massive transfusion was defined as 10 or more units of PRBC in the first 24 hours. The thresholds separating high and low FFP/PRBC and PLT/PRBC were ≥1:1.5 and ≥1:1.9, respectively. Data for mortality were assessed at 6, 12, and 24 hours for the high and low ratio groups. Groups were also compared for several other outcome variables. Approximately 600 patients received MT overall. Both high FFP/PRBC and high PLT/PRBC ratios were associated with decreased mortality at various time points in the initial 24 hours. Despite the higher volume of additional blood products, the subjects in the high ratio group did not have an increased incidence of multiple organ failure, nosocomial infection, or acute respiratory distress syndrome. Subjects in the low FFP/PRBC group had higher 24-hour transfusion requirements, however, as did patients in the low PLT/PRBC group at 6 hours. By removing the confounder of survival bias and evaluating the results on a time-dependent basis, these findings lend strong support to the notion of high ratios of products to PRBC as part of a massive transfusion protocol. Coagulopathy and ongoing bleeding is often as much of a concern as the initial injury. Consumption of platelets and clotting factors, in association with inadequate replacement, cannot be compensated for by replacement of red cells and attempts at surgical hemostasis alone. Presumably, the same principles can be extrapolated to massively bleeding medical patients, but that population is harder to study. Many have underlying coagulopathy to begin with, and the numbers of such patients, while perhaps large in the aggregate, are relatively small at any individual institution compared with the number of patients with severe hemorrhage seen at major trauma centers, making formal study difficult. For those caring for medical patients, it will probably be necessary to simply apply what is learned from the trauma literature and evaluate its utility in the medical population on a case-by-case basis.

D. R. Gerber, DO

Debunking the survival bias myth: Characterization of mortality during the initial 24 hours for patients requiring massive transfusion
Brown JB, The Inflammation and the Host Response to Injury Investigators (Univ of Pittsburgh Med Ctr, PA; et al)
J Trauma Acute Care Surg 73:358-364, 2012

Background.—Controversy surrounds the optimal ratios of blood (packed red blood cell [PRBC]), plasma (fresh frozen plasma [FFP]) and platelet (PLT) use for patients requiring massive transfusion (MT) owing to possible survival bias in previous studies. We sought to characterize mortality during the first 24 hours while controlling for time varying effects of transfusion to minimize survival bias.

Methods.—Data were obtained from a multicenter prospective cohort study of adults with blunt injury and hemorrhagic shock. MT was defined as 10 U of PRBC or more over 24 hours. High FFP/PRBC ($\geq$1:1.5) and PLT/PRBC ($\geq$1:9) ratios at 6, 12, and 24 hours were compared with low ratio groups. Cox proportional hazards regression was used to determine the independent association of high versus low ratios with mortality at 6, 12, and 24 hours while controlling for important confounders. Cox proportional hazards regression was repeated with FFP/PRBC and PLT/PRBC ratios analyzed as time-dependent covariates to account for fluctuation over time. Mortality for more than 24 hours was treated as survival.

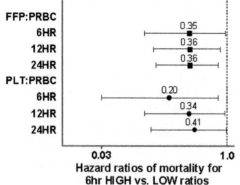

FIGURE 1.—Hazard ratios from Cox proportional hazards regression for mortality at 6, 12, and 24 hours in the 6-hour FFP/PRBC and PLT/PRBC ratio groups. HR indicates high compared with low ratio groups. *Bars* indicate 95% CIs. (Reprinted from Brown JB, The Inflammation and the Host Response to Injury Investigators. Debunking the survival bias myth: characterization of mortality during the initial 24 hours for patients requiring massive transfusion. *J Trauma Acute Care Surg.* 2012;73:358-364, with permission from Lippincott Williams & Wilkins.)

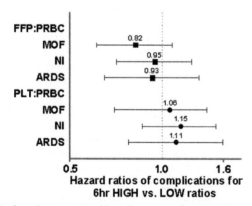

FIGURE 2.—HRs from Cox proportional hazards regression for MOF, NI, and ARDS in the 6-hour FFP/PRBC and PLT/PRBC ratio groups. HR indicates high compared with low ratio groups. *Bars* indicate 95% CIs. (Reprinted from Brown JB, The Inflammation and the Host Response to Injury Investigators. Debunking the survival bias myth: characterization of mortality during the initial 24 hours for patients requiring massive transfusion. *J Trauma Acute Care Surg.* 2012;73:358-364, with permission from Lippincott Williams & Wilkins.)

Results.—In the MT cohort (n = 604), initial base deficit, lactate, and international normalized ratio were similar across high and low ratio groups. High 6-hour FFP/PRBC and PLT/PRBC ratios were independently associated with a reduction in mortality risk at 6, 12, and 24 hours (hazard ratio [HR] range, 0.20–0.41, $p < 0.05$). These findings were consistent for 12-hour and 24-hour ratios. When analyzed as time-dependent covariates, a high FFP/PRBC ratio was associated with a 68% (HR, 0.32; 95% confidence interval [CI], 0.12–0.87, $p = 0.03$) reduction in 24-hour mortality, and a high PLT/PRBC ratio was associated with a 96% (HR, 0.04; 95% CI, 0.01−0.94, $p = 0.04$) reduction in 24-hour mortality. Subgroup analysis revealed that a high 1:1 ratio ($\geq$1:1.5) had a significant 24-hour survival benefit relative to a high 1:2 (1:1.51−1:2.50) ratio group at both 6 hours (HR, 0.19; 95% CI, 0.03−0.86, $p = 0.03$) and 24 hours (HR, 0.25; 95% CI, 0.06−0.95, $p = 0.04$), suggesting a dose-response relationship. A high FFP/PRBC or PLT/PRBC ratio was not associated with development of multiple-organ failure, nosocomial infection, or adult respiratory distress syndrome in a 28-day Cox proportional hazards regression.

Conclusion.—Despite similar degrees of early shock and coagulopathy, high FFP/PRBC and PLT/PRBC ratios are associated with a survival benefit as early as 6 hours and throughout the first 24 hours, even when time-dependent fluctuations of component transfusion are accounted for. This suggests that the observed mortality benefit associated with high component transfusion ratios is unlikely owing to survivor bias and that early attainment of high transfusion ratios may significantly lower the risk of mortality in MT patients (Figs 1 and 2).

▶ Data for this trial were obtained from the massive database of The Inflammation and the Host Response to Injury Collaborative Program, also known as the Glue Grant. This multicenter trial was conducted over an 8-year period in 7 selected trauma centers. Enrolled patients showed signs of shock as reflected in vital signs and metabolic parameters.[1]

This dataset was queried for patients receiving massive transfusion to address the question of survival bias in early trials. Writers describing the literature for massive transfusion practice suggest that a survival bias clouds the results of many studies.[2] These writers argue that survival benefit seen in patients receiving a high fresh-frozen plasma to packed red blood cell or platelet to packed red blood cell ratio is present because these individuals lived long enough to achieve high ratios. Many studies evaluate ratios achieved at the 24-hour point after injury.[3,4] Data obtained from the Glue Grant sites are ideal for review of questions regarding massive transfusion practice because patients in this study received care based on fixed protocols. Notably, however, massive transfusion practice was not rigorously standardized.

In these patients, identified by similar degrees of early shock and coagulopathy, high fresh-frozen plasma to packed red blood cell and platelet to packed red blood cell ratios were associated with survival benefit as early as 6 hours after injury and throughout the first 24 hours following the traumatic incident. This finding was consistent at all time points at which the patient groups with differing transfusion ratios were determined (Fig 1).

A second important observation was the lack of independent association with the development of multiple organ failure, acute respiratory failure, or other organ dysfunction related to massive transfusion in these patients (Fig 2).

The most important limitation of this work comes from the nature of the secondary data analysis. The Glue Grant was not designed to address the specific issues addressed here. Thus, potential confounders were not prospectively identified and controlled. However, this is a large patient group obtained from multiple trauma centers with rigorous attempts at practice standardization. In this respect, data provided from these trauma centers are unique.

D. J. Dries, MSE, MD

References

1. Moore FA, McKinley BA, Moore EE, et al. Inflammation and the Host Response to Injury, a large-scale collaborative project: patient-oriented research core— standard operating procedures for clinical care. III. Guidelines for shock resuscitation. *J Trauma.* 2006;61:82-89.
2. Dries DJ. The contemporary role of blood products and components used in trauma resuscitation. *Scand J Trauma Resusc Emerg Med.* 2010;18:63.
3. Snyder CW, Weinberg JA, McGwin G Jr, et al. The relationship of blood product ratio to mortality: survival benefit or survival bias? *J Trauma.* 2009;66:358-364.
4. Brohi K, Singh J, Heron M, Coats T. Acute traumatic coagulopathy. *J Trauma.* 2003;54:1127-1130.

Stress-Induced Hyperglycemia, Not Diabetic Hyperglycemia, Is Associated With Higher Mortality in Trauma

Kerby JD, Griffin RL, MacLennan P, et al (Univ of Alabama at Birmingham)
Ann Surg 256:446-452, 2012

Objectives.—To identify all trauma patients with diabetes and compare diabetic hyperglycemia (DH) patients with those with stress-induced hyperglycemia (SIH).

Background.—SIH has been shown to result in worse outcomes after trauma. The presence of diabetes mellitus (DM) or occult DM within the cohort confounded previous studies. We identified 2 distinct populations of trauma patients with SIH or DH to determine the impact of hyperglycemia on these 2 groups.

Methods.—Admission glycosylated hemoglobin (HbA1c), glucose levels, and comorbidity data were collected over a 2-year period. DM was determined by patient history or admission HbA1c 6.5% or more. SIH was determined by absence of DM and admission glucose 200 mg/dL or more. Cox proportional hazards models [adjusted for age, sex, injury mechanism, and injury severity score] were used to calculate risk ratios (RRs) and associated 95% confidence intervals (CIs) for outcomes of interest.

Results.—During the study period, 6852 trauma patients were evaluated, and 5117 had available glucose, HbA1c, and comorbidity data. Patients with SIH had an over twofold increase in mortality risk (RR 2.41, 95% CI 1.81—3.23), and patients with DH had a nonsignificant, near-50% increase in mortality risk (RR 1.47, 95% CI 0.92—2.36). Risk of pneumonia was similarly higher for both the DH (RR 1.49, 95% CI 1.03—2.17) and the SIH (RR 1.44, 95% CI 1.08—1.93).

Conclusions.—DM is common in patients with hyperglycemia after trauma. As opposed to DH, SIH is associated with higher mortality after

TABLE 1.—Criteria for Diagnosis of Diabetes[13]

HbA1c ≥ 6.5%. The test should be performed in a laboratory using a method that is NGSP certified and standardized to the DCCT assay*
OR
Fasting plasma glucose ≥ 126 mg/dL (7.0 mmol/L). Fasting os defined as no caloric intake for at least 8 h*
OR
2-h plasma glucose ≥ 200 mg/dL (11.1) mmol/L during an Oral Glucose Tolerance Test. The test should be performed as described by the World Health Organization, using a glucose load containing the equivalent of 75 g anhydrous glucose dissolved in water*
OR
In a patient with classic symptoms of hyperglycemia or hyperglycemic crisis, a random plasma glucose ≥ 200 mg/dL (11.1 mmol/L)

Editor's Note: Please refer to original journal article for full references.
NGSP indicates National glycohemoglobin standardization program; DCCT, iabetes control and complications trial.
*In the absence of unequivocal hyperglycemia, criteria 1—3 should be confirmed by repeat testing.

trauma. Further research is warranted to identify mechanisms causing hyperglycemia and subsequent worse outcomes after trauma (Table 1).

▶ A number of well-publicized studies highlight the potential risk associated with hyperglycemia in both the setting of critical illness and in the setting of trauma.[1,2] These investigators segregate patients with preexisting diabetes, as identified by HbA1c levels from patients having hyperglycemia without evidence of diabetes. The excellent trauma database at the University of Alabama is used for this trial.

In Table 1, the authors' criteria for diabetes are given. Although I do not argue with these parameters, I doubt that glucose tolerance testing was done in the trauma unit. I suspect that the key to diagnosis was the HbA1c level.

Using their extensive database, the authors demonstrate that hyperglycemia, associated with stress rather than underlying diabetes, contributes to mortality despite adjustment for age, gender, mechanism of injury, and Injury Severity Score. Stress-induced hyperglycemia, however, is a marker for the physiologic impact of injury and probably should not be managed as 1 more comorbidity. This may explain why multicenter trials such as Normoglycaemia in Intensive Care Evaluation and Survival Using Glucose Algorithm Regulation fail to demonstrate a reduction in mortality for patients with tight glycemic control.[2,3]

D. J. Dries, MSE, MD

References

1. Scalea TM, Bochicchio GV, Bochicchio KM, Johnson SB, Joshi M, Pyle A. Tight glycemic control in critically injured trauma patients. *Ann Surg.* 2007;246: 605-610.
2. van den Berghe G, Wouters P, Weekers F, et al. Intensive insulin therapy in critically ill patients. *N Engl J Med.* 2001;345:1359-1367.
3. Finfer S, Chittock DR, Su SY, et al; NICE-SUGAR Investigators. Intensive versus conventional glucose control in critically ill patients. *N Engl J Med.* 2009;360: 1283-1297.

Long-Term Propranolol Use in Severely Burned Pediatric Patients: A Randomized Controlled Study

Herndon DN, Rodriguez NA, Diaz EC, et al (Shriners Hosps for Children—Galveston, TX; et al)
Ann Surg 256:402-411, 2012

Objective.—To determine the safety and efficacy of propranolol given for 1 year on cardiac function, resting energy expenditure, and body composition in a prospective, randomized, single-center, controlled study in pediatric patients with large burns.

Background.—Severe burns trigger a hypermetabolic response that persists for up to 2 years postburn. Propranolol given for 1 month postburn

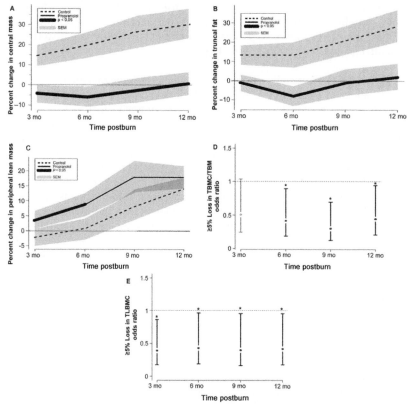

FIGURE 3.—Effect of propranolol on body composition. Percentage of change in central mass (A), truncal fat (B), and peripheral lean mass (C). In all panels, data are expressed as the percentage of change from patient baseline and are shown as the Loess smoothed trend, with shading indicating standard error of the mean. (D, E) Comparison of the likelihood of losing 5% or more of (D) total bone mineral content/total body mass and (E) total lumbar bone mineral content in control and propranolol-treated patients. Data are expressed as the odds ratios. *Significant difference at $P < 0.05$. (Reprinted from Herndon DN, Rodriguez NA, Diaz EC, et al. Long-term propranolol use in severely burned pediatric patients: a randomized controlled study. *Ann Surg.* 2012;256:402-411, with permission from Lippincott Williams & Wilkins.)

blunts this response. Whether propranolol administration for 1 year after injury provides a continued benefit is currently unclear.

Methods.—One-hundred seventy-nine pediatric patients with more than 30% total body surface area burns were randomized to control (n = 89) or 4 mg/kg/d propranolol (n = 90) for 12 months postburn. Changes in resting energy expenditure, cardiac function, and body composition were measured acutely at 3, 6, 9, and 12 months postburn. Statistical analyses included techniques that adjusted for non-normality, repeated-measures, and regression analyses. $P < 0.05$ was considered significant.

Results.—Long-term propranolol treatment significantly reduced the percentage of the predicted heart rate and percentage of the predicted resting energy expenditure, decreased accumulation of central mass and central fat, prevented bone loss, and improved lean body mass accretion. There were very few adverse effects from the dose of propranolol used.

Conclusions.—Propranolol treatment for 12 months after thermal injury, ameliorates the hyperdynamic, hypermetabolic, hypercatabolic, and osteopenic responses in pediatric patients. This study is registered at clinicaltrials.gov: NCT00675714 (Fig 3).

▶ This is the latest in a series of studies examining the hypermetabolic response to burn injury in a pediatric population. Propranolol, as a nonselective beta-antagonist, was administered in a randomized controlled trial to 90 patients for up to 12 months after burn injury. No difference in mortality is seen. The impact on vital signs at a dose of 4 mg/kg/day of propranolol is surprisingly small. This is the first long-term outcome data from these investigators.[1]

Specific data demonstrated a reduction in burn-related elevation in heart rate in patients receiving propranolol. Body mass and favorable changes in body composition after severe burn injury were more prominent in patients receiving propranolol (Fig 3). A more modest effect on metabolic response as seen with metabolic cart data was identified. Adverse events including hypotension, bradycardia, hypoglycemia, cardiac arrhythmias, respiratory arrest, and death were no different between the 2 groups. Sepsis was the cause of death in all cases.

These authors continue studies with propranolol administration to blunt the hyperdynamic response after burns. Quality of outcome, if not mortality, seems to be improved in patients treated with beta-blockade.

D. J. Dries, MSE, MD

Reference

1. Herndon DN, Hart DW, Wolf SE, Chinkes DL, Wolfe RR. Reversal of catabolism by beta-blockade after severe burns. *N Engl J Med.* 2001;345:1223-1229.

The effects of prehospital plasma on patients with injury: A prehospital plasma resuscitation

Kim BD, Zielinski MD, Jenkins DH, et al (Mayo Clinic, Rochester, MN)
J Trauma Acute Care Surg 73:S49-S53, 2012

Background.—The prehospital resuscitation of the exsanguinating patient with trauma is time and resource dependent. Rural trauma care magnifies these factors because transportation time to definitive care is increased. To address the early resuscitation needs and trauma-induced coagulopathy in the exsanguinating patient with trauma an aeromedical prehospital thawed plasma—first transfusion protocol was used.

Methods.—Retrospective review of trauma and flight registries between February 1, 2009, and May 31, 2011, was performed. The study population included all patients with traumatic injury transported by rotary wing aircraft who met criteria for massive transfusion protocol.

Results.—A total of 59 patients identified over 28 months met criteria for initiation of aeromedical initiation of prehospital blood product resuscitation. Nine patients received thawed plasma—first protocol compared with 50 controls. The prehospital plasma group was more commonly on warfarin (22 vs. 2%, $p = 0.036$) and had a greater degree of coagulopathy measured by international normalized ratio at baseline (2.6 vs. 1.5, $p = 0.004$) and trauma center arrival (1.6 vs. 1.3, $p < 0.001$). The prehospital plasma group had a predicted mortality nearly three times greater than controls based on Trauma and Injury Severity Score (0.24 vs. 0.66, $p = 0.005$). The use of prehospital plasma resuscitation led to a plasma—red blood cell ratio that more closely approximated a 1:1 resuscitation en route (1.3:1.0 vs. not applicable, $p < 0.001$), at 30 minutes (1.3:1.0 vs. 0.14:1.0, $p < 0.001$), at 6 hours (0.95:1.0 vs. 0.42:1.0, $p < 0.001$), and at 24 hours (1.0:1.0 vs. 0.45:1.0, $p < 0.001$). An equivalent amount of packed red

---

Indications: Blood product administration is indicated for treatment of hemorrhagic shock. Blood products should be administered if an adult patient has 2 of the following after traumatic injury or other evidence of bleeding:

    1) Hypotension (single reading of systolic blood pressure ≤ 90 mm Hg)
    2) Tachycardia (single reading of heart rate ≥ 120)
    3) Penetrating mechanism (i.e. stabbing, gunshot, etc...)
    4) Point of care lactate ≥ 5.0 mg/dL
    5) Point of care International Normalized Ratio (INR) ≥ 1.5

Order of transfusion will be 2 units thawed plasma (A+, A-), followed by up to 4 units pRBCs. Rate of transfusion is determined by the patient's clinical condition and hemodynamic parameters.

For those patients with known anticoagulant use and a stable hemoglobin, 2 units of thawed plasma will be administered followed by close monitoring of hemoglobin levels with i-STAT® to determine if pRBC transfusion is necessary.

FIGURE 1.—Prehospital plasma-first transfusion protocol. (Reprinted from Kim BD, Zielinski MD, Jenkins DH, et al. The effects of prehospital plasma on patients with injury: a prehospital plasma resuscitation. *J Trauma Acute Care Surg.* 2012;73:S49-S53, with permission from Lippincott Williams & Wilkins.)

TABLE 2.—Blood Product Consumption

Variable	Prehospital Plasma Group	Control Group	p
En route			
Plasma, U	2.1	0.0	<0.001
RBC, U	2.5	1.0	<0.001
Crystalloid, L	2.4	1.6	0.211
Plasma/RBC	1.3:1.0	NA	<0.001
Plasma deficit	0.4	1.0	0.323
30 min after injury			
Plasma, U	3.1	0.4	<0.001
RBC, U	3.3	2.4	0.271
Crystalloid, L	2.3	1.7	0.418
Plasma/RBC	1.3:1.0	0.14:1.0	<0.001
Plasma deficit	1.2	2.0	0.378
6 h after injury			
Plasma, U	9.7	5.0	0.012
RBC, U	11.4	10.7	0.812
Crystalloid, L	4.4	6.6	0.077
Plasma/RBC	0.95:1.0	0.42:1.0	<0.001
Plasma deficit	1.7	5.3	0.056
24 h after injury			
Plasma, U	11.5	5.5	0.003
RBC 24, U	12.7	11.4	0.694
Crystalloid, L	6.3	16.4	0.001
Plasma/RBC	1.0:1.0	0.45:1.0	<0.001
Plasma deficit	1.0	5.7	0.043

NA, not applicable.

blood cells were transfused between the groups. Despite more significant hypotension, less crystalloid was used in the prehospital thawed plasma group, through 24 hours after injury (6.3 vs. 16.4 L, $p = 0.001$).

Conclusion.—Use of plasma-first resuscitation in the helicopter system creates a field ready, mobile blood bank, allowing early resuscitation of the patient demonstrating need for massive transfusion. There was early treatment of trauma-induced coagulopathy. Although there was not a survival benefit demonstrated, there was resultant damage control resuscitation extending to 24 hours in the plasma-first cohort (Fig 1, Table 2).

▶ This the first report of a small number of patients examined by Mayo Clinic Air Medical and Trauma practitioners. Patients identified as deserving early administration of blood products received aggressive plasma administration (Fig 1). These patients ultimately had a ratio of plasma to packed red blood cells closest to 1:1 in a small series (Table 2). Use of crystalloids in the patients receiving plasma was also reduced. No pattern of increased complications related to early administration of plasma was reported.

It is important to note that this is a small patient set. We await additional data from the Mayo investigators. Outcome data may be affected by the drop out of more severely injured patients in the plasma group before completion of all data collection creating a "survival bias."[1]

D. J. Dries, MSE, MD

Reference

1. Dries DJ. The contemporary role of blood products and components used in trauma resuscitation. *Scand J Trauma Resusc Emerg Med.* 2010;18:63.

Benchmarking Outcomes in the Critically Injured Trauma Patient and the Effect of Implementing Standard Operating Procedures

Cuschieri J, the Inflammation and Host Response to Injury, Large Scale Collaborative Research Program (Univ of Washington School of Medicine and Harborview Med Ctr, Seattle; et al)

Ann Surg 255:993-999, 2012

Objective.—To determine and compare outcomes with accepted benchmarks in trauma care at 7 academic level I trauma centers in which patients were treated on the basis of a series of standard operating procedures (SOPs).

Background.—Injury remains the leading cause of death for those younger than 45 years. This study describes the baseline patient characteristics and well-defined outcomes of persons hospitalized in the United States for severe blunt trauma.

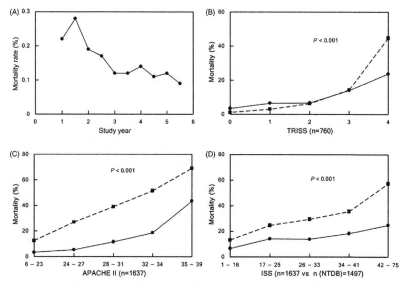

FIGURE 1.—Mortality. Patients divided into quintiles in Panels B, C, and D based underlying score or injury severity. Panel A shows mortality over the entire study period. Observed (solid lines) versus expected (dashed line) outcome for Panel B) mortality by TRISS (P < 0.001), Panel C) mortality by APACHE II (P < 0.001), and Panel D) mortality by NTDB (P < 0.001). (Reprinted from Cuschieri J, the Inflammation and Host Response to Injury, Large Scale Collaborative Research Program, Benchmarking Outcomes in the Critically Injured Trauma Patient and the Effect of Implementing Standard Operating Procedures. *Ann Surg.* 2012;255:993-999, with permission from Lippincott Williams & Wilkins.)

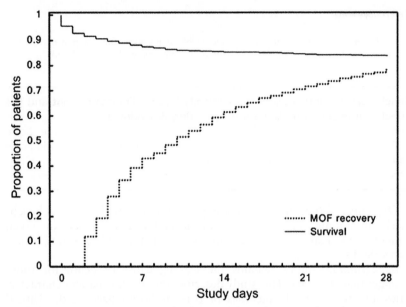

FIGURE 2.—(B) Time to recovery. Panel B shows mortality and time to recovery after severe injury. Kaplan-Meier survival curve and proportion of patients fully recovered from organ dysfunction in the first 28 days after blunt traumatic injury. (Reprinted from Cuschieri J, the Inflammation and Host Response to Injury, Large Scale Collaborative Research Program, Benchmarking Outcomes in the Critically Injured Trauma Patient and the Effect of Implementing Standard Operating Procedures. *Ann Surg.* 2012;255:993-999, with permission from Lippincott Williams & Wilkins.)

Methods.—We followed 1637 trauma patients from 2003 to 2009 up to 28 hospital days using SOPs developed at the onset of the study. An extensive database on patient and injury characteristics, clinical treatment, and outcomes was created. These data were compared with existing trauma benchmarks.

Results.—The study patients were critically injured and were in shock. SOP compliance improved 10% to 40% during the study period. Multiple organ failure and mortality rates were 34.8% and 16.7%, respectively. Time to recovery, defined as the time until the patient was free of organ failure for at least 2 consecutive days, was developed as a new outcome measure. There was a reduction in mortality rate in the cohort during the study that cannot be explained by changes in the patient population.

Conclusions.—This study provides the current benchmark and the overall positive effect of implementing SOPs for severely injured patients. Over the course of the study, there were improvements in morbidity and mortality rates and increasing compliance with SOPs. Mortality was surprisingly low, given the degree of injury, and improved over the duration of the study, which correlated with improved SOP compliance (Figs 1 and 2B).

▶ The Inflammation and Host Response to Injury is a National Institute of General Medical Sciences collaborative project (Glue Grant). This observational, prospective study was conducted at 7 level I trauma centers and patients were enrolled if critically injured by blunt mechanism, were 16 years of age or older, and had shock defined as base deficit 6 meq/L or more and systolic blood pressure less than 90 mm Hg within 60 minutes of arrival to the emergency department and required initiation of blood transfusion within 6 hours of injury.

A series of standard operating procedures (SOPs) were developed by investigators and applied to these patients. In addition to defining SOPs, the authors defined complications.[1] With these data, a contemporary stratified outcome standard for injury has been developed. A snapshot of these data is provided in Figs 1 and 2B.

The authors note steady improvement in SOP compliance during the course of the trial. However, it may be more than compliance, perhaps a Hawthorne effect, that explains the fall in mortality demonstrated on panel A of Fig 1. Despite this concern, data in Figs 1 and 2B represent initial results for a new benchmark regarding outcome of injury and should change our expectations of outcome, particularly with the Acute Physiology and Chronic Health Evaluation II Score and the Injury Severity Score.

D. J. Dries, MSE, MD

Reference

1. Evans HL, Cuschieri J, Moore EE, et al. Inflammation and the host response to injury, a Large-Scale Collaborative Project: patient-oriented research core standard operating room procedures for clinical care IX. Definitions for complications of clinical care of critically injured patients. *J Trauma*. 2009;67:384-388.

Early Platelet Dysfunction: An Unrecognized Role in the Acute Coagulopathy of Trauma

Wohlauer MV, Moore EE, Thomas S, et al (Univ of Colorado Denver; Indiana School of Medicine, Indianapolis; et al)
J Am Coll Surg 214:739-746, 2012

Background.—Our aim was to determine the prevalence of platelet dysfunction using an end point of assembly into a stable thrombus after severe injury. Although the current debate on acute traumatic coagulopathy has focused on the consumption or inhibition of coagulation factors, the question of early platelet dysfunction in this setting remains unclear.

Study Design.—Prospective platelet function in assembly and stability of the thrombus was determined within 30 minutes of injury using whole blood samples from trauma patients at the point of care using thrombelastography-based platelet functional analysis.

Results.—There were 51 patients in the study. There were significant differences in the platelet response between trauma patients and healthy volunteers, such that there was impaired aggregation to these agonists. In trauma patients, the median ADP inhibition of platelet function was 86.1% (interquartile range [IQR] 38.6% to 97.7%) compared with 4.2% (IQR 0 to 18.2%) in healthy volunteers. After trauma, the impairment of

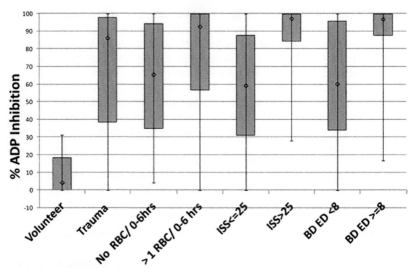

FIGURE 2.—Median percent ADP receptor inhibition in trauma patients compared with healthy volunteers, including stratification according to shock (base deficit [BD]), blood transfusion (RBCs), and tissue injury (Injury Severity Score [ISS]). (Reprinted from Wohlauer MV, Moore EE, Thomas S, et al. Early platelet dysfunction: an unrecognized role in the acute coagulopathy of trauma. *J Am Coll Surg.* 2012;214:739-746, Copyright 2012, with permission from the American College of Surgeons.)

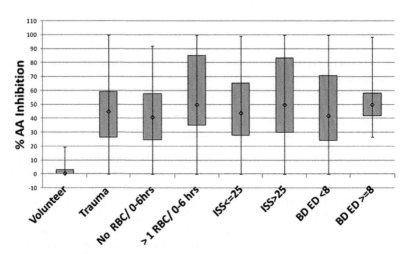

FIGURE 3.—Median percent arachidonic acid (AA) (TXA2) receptor inhibition in trauma patients compared with healthy volunteers, including stratification according to shock (base deficit [BD]), blood transfusion (RBCs), and tissue injury (Injury Severity Score [ISS]). (Reprinted from Wohlauer MV, Moore EE, Thomas S, et al. Early platelet dysfunction: an unrecognized role in the acute coagulopathy of trauma. *J Am Coll Surg.* 2012;214:739-746, Copyright 2012, with permission from the American College of Surgeons.)

platelet function in response to arachidonic acid was 44.9% (IQR 26.6% to 59.3%) compared with 0.5% (IQR 0 to 3.02%) in volunteers (Wilcoxon nonparametric test, $p < 0.0001$ for both tests).

Conclusions.—In this study, we show that platelet dysfunction is manifest after major trauma and before substantial fluid or blood administration. These data suggest a potential role for early platelet transfusion in severely injured patients at risk for postinjury coagulopathy (Figs 2 and 3).

▶ This study adds to a growing volume of recent work demonstrating that shock with soft-tissue injury induces coagulopathy prior to administration of intravenous fluids for hemodilution and prior to blood product administration as part of a balanced resuscitation strategy.[1] We should not be surprised that these investigators have demonstrated platelet dysfunction (Figs 2 and 3). In a large multiinstitutional trauma study, Holcomb and co-workers demonstrated incremental improved outcome in patients receiving massive transfusion in which platelets were administered along with fresh frozen plasma and packed red blood cells.[2] Degree of soft-tissue injury and the presence of acidosis as manifest by base deficit also predict reduced platelet function.[1]

Several patients were on antiplatelet medications at the time of this acute investigation. Remarkably, inhibition to platelet function in stabilizing clot was comparable but not additive to the larger group of trauma patients.

Finally, this study provides additional support for evaluation of platelet function using thrombelastography. This technology is receiving significant attention as a rapid, global assessment of coagulation response in surgical critical illness.[1]

D. J. Dries, MSE, MD

References

1. Dries DJ. The contemporary role of blood products and components used in trauma resuscitation. *Scand J Trauma Resusc Emerg Med.* 2010;18:63.
2. Holcomb JB, Wade CE, Michalek JE, et al. Increased plasma and platelet to red blood cell ratios improves outcome in 466 massively transfused civilian trauma patients. *Ann Surg.* 2008;248:447-458.

The changing pattern and implications of multiple organ failure after blunt injury with hemorrhagic shock
Minei JP, for the Inflammation and the Host Response to Injury Collaborative Research Program (Univ of Texas Southwestern Med Ctr and Parkland Health and Hosp System, Dallas; et al)
Crit Care Med 40:1129-1135, 2012

Objectives.—To describe the incidence of postinjury multiple organ failure and its relationship to nosocomial infection and mortality in trauma centers using evidence-based standard operating procedures.

Design.—Prospective cohort study wherein standard operating procedures were developed and implemented to optimize postinjury care.

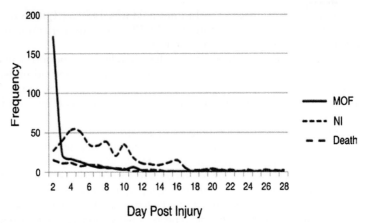

Day Post Injury

FIGURE 1.—Day of onset and frequency of multiple organ failure (*MOF*), nosocomial infection (*NI*), and death. (Reprinted from Minei JP, for the Inflammation and the Host Response to Injury Collaborative Research Program. The changing pattern and implications of multiple organ failure after blunt injury with hemorrhagic shock. *Crit Care Med.* 2012;40:1129-1135, with permission from the Society of Critical Care Medicine and Lippincott Williams & Wilkins.)

Setting.—Seven U.S. level I trauma centers.

Patients.—Severely injured patients (older than age 16 yrs) with a blunt mechanism, systolic hypotension (< 90 mm Hg), and/or base deficit (≥ 6 mEq/L), need for blood transfusion within the first 12 hrs, and an abbreviated injury score ≥ 2 excluding brain injury were eligible for inclusion.

Measurements and Main Results.—One thousand two patients were enrolled and 916 met inclusion criteria. Daily markers of organ dysfunction were prospectively recorded for all patients while receiving intensive care. Overall, 29% of patients had multiple organ failure develop. Development of multiple organ failure was early (median time, 2 days), short-lived, and predicted an increased incidence of nosocomial infection, whereas persistence of multiple organ failure predicted mortality. However, surprisingly, nosocomial infection did not increase subsequent multiple organ failure and there was no evidence of a "second-hit"-induced late-onset multiple organ failure.

Conclusions.—Multiple organ failure remains common after severe injury. Contrary to current paradigms, the onset is only early, and not bimodal, nor is it associated with a "second-hit"-induced late onset. Multiple organ failure is associated with subsequent nosocomial infection and increased mortality. Standard operating procedure-driven interventions may be associated with a decrease in late multiple organ failure and morbidity (Fig 1).

▶ This study is part of the Inflammation and Host Response to Injury Collaborative Project sponsored by the National Institute of General Medical Sciences. Seven trauma centers with evidence-based standard operating procedures enrolled patients in a management protocol featuring goal-directed resuscitation, glycemic control, venous thromboembolism prophylaxis, low tidal volume ventilation, and restrictive transfusion guidelines. Daily markers of organ dysfunction were collected and a Marshall score was determined.[1] Standard definitions for infection were also utilized based on input from the Centers for Disease Control and Prevention.

Although organ dysfunction occurred early after injury, possibly related to resuscitation, a second-hit phenomenon, typically associated with infection, was not observed (Fig 1).[2] Development of multiorgan failure was associated with higher rates of subsequent infection, and persistent multiorgan failure predicts mortality. Although persistence of multiorgan failure predicted development of nosocomial pneumonia, the development of infection, as a second-hit event, was not temporally associated with subsequent development of multiorgan failure.

It is important to note that this is an observational work. A mechanism for these findings has not been proposed. In fact, the results displayed in Fig 1 may reflect the treatment paradigm exercised in these trauma centers.

D. J. Dries, MSE, MD

References

1. Marshall JC, Cook DJ, Christou NV, Bernard GR, Sprung CL, Sibbald WJ. Multiple organ dysfunction score: a reliable descriptor of a complex clinical outcome. *Crit Care Med.* 1995;23:1638-1652.
2. Moore FA, Sauaia A, Moore EE, Haenel JB, Burch JM, Lezotte DC. Postinjury multiple organ failure: a bimodal phenomenon. *J Trauma.* 1996;40:501-510.

Mortality by Decade in Trauma Patients with Glasgow Coma Scale 3
Ley EJ, Clond MA, Hussain ON, et al (Cedars-Sinai Med Ctr, Los Angeles, CA)
Am Surg 77:1342-1345, 2011

The aim of this study was to assess how increasing age affects mortality in trauma patients with Glasgow Coma Scale (GCS) 3. The Los Angeles County Trauma System Database was queried for all patients aged 20 to 99 years admitted with GCS 3. Mortality was 41.8 per cent for the 3306 GCS 3 patients. Mortality in the youngest patients reviewed, those in the third decade, was 43.5 per cent. After logistic regression analysis, patients in the third decade had similar mortality rates to patients in the sixth (adjusted OR, 0.88; CI, 0.68 to 1.14; $P = 0.33$) and seventh decades (adjusted OR, 0.96; CI, 0.70 to 1.31; $P = 0.79$). A significantly lower mortality rate, however, was noted in the fifth decade (adjusted OR, 0.76; CI, 0.61 to 0.95; $P = 0.02$). Conversely, significantly higher mortality rates were noted in the eighth (adjusted OR, 1.93; CI, 1.38 to 2.71; $P = 0.0001$) and combined ninth/tenth decades (adjusted OR, 2.47; CI, 1.71 to 3.57; $P < 0.0001$). Given the high survival in trauma patients with GCS 3 as well as continued improvement in survival compared with historical controls, aggressive care is indicated for patients who present to the emergency department with GCS 3.

▶ This report comes from a large urban trauma center with a detailed trauma registry. The authors argue, effectively, that we need to aggressively support the patient presenting with a Glasgow Coma Scale Score of 3. However, it is important to note that there are limits to this work.

Alcohol plays a significant role in presenting Glasgow Coma Scale Score. The impact of alcohol in these patients is not reported. The authors note that Injury Severity Score (ISS) greater than 16 was a predictor for mortality, but the head Abbreviated Injury Score (AIS) greater ≥ 3 was probably not from overlap between AIS and ISS scores. Other predictors of adverse outcome are hypotension and age.

Alcohol can have many adverse effects in the setting of injury. There appears to be a strong correlation between alcohol and prehospital mortality in patients suffering traumatic brain injury. Data regarding the impact of alcohol on in-hospital performance after brain injury are less clear, possibly because of the lack of effective models. Other investigators have proposed that within effective dose ranges, alcohol may provide some protective effects in the setting of brain injury. Adverse long-term effects of alcohol are difficult to doubt.[1,2]

In summary, recognizing that there may be significant confounders in these data, I agree that aggressive care should not be limited in patients presenting with a low Glasgow Coma Scale Score.

D. J. Dries, MSE, MD

References

1. Opreanu RC, Kuhn D, Basson MD. Influence of alcohol on mortality in traumatic brain injury. *J Am Coll Surg.* 2010;210:997-1007.
2. Shahin H, Gopinath SP, Robertson CS. Influence of alcohol on early Glasgow Coma Scale in head-injured patients. *J Trauma.* 2010;69:1176-1181.

The impact of BMI on polytrauma outcome
Hoffmann M, Trauma Registry of the German Society for Trauma Surgery (Univ Hosp Hamburg Eppendorf, Germany; et al)
Injury 43:184-188, 2012

Background.—Varying results have been reported concerning the effect of body mass index (BMI) on polytrauma outcome. Although most studies focus on obesity and its associated preexisting medical diseases as a predictor for increased mortality rates, there is evidence that polytrauma patients with underweight also face an inferior outcome.

Methods.—Records of 5766 trauma patients (minimum 18 years of age, Injury Severity Score ≥ 16, treated from 2004 to 2008) documented in the Trauma Registry of the German Society for Trauma Surgery were subclassified into 4 BMI groups and analysed to assess the impact of BMI on polytrauma outcome.

Results.—Underweight (BMI Group I) as well as obesity (BMI Group IV) in polytraumatized patients are associated with significantly increased mortality by multivariate logistic regression analysis with hospital mortality as the target variable (adjusted odds ratio for BMI Group I, 2.1 (95% CI 1.2–3.8, $p = 0.015$); for BMI Group IV, 1.6 (95% CI 1.1–2.3, $p = 0.009$)). Simple overweight (BMI Group III) does not qualify as a predictor for increased mortality (odds ratio 1.0; 95% CI 0.8–1.3).

Conclusions.—There is a significant correlation between obesity, underweight, and increased mortality in polytraumatized patients. Efforts to promote optimal body weight may reduce not only the risk of chronic diseases but also the risk of polytrauma mortality amongst obese and underweight individuals.

▶ This study utilizes the extensive multicenter German Trauma Registry and evaluates underweight, normal, overweight, and obese patients. Patients who were underweight and those in the obese group had the worst outcomes. This is consistent with a much smaller US study from the University of Michigan. In the Michigan study, patients in the highest weight group and underweight patients had incrementally greater mortality compared with patients who had normal body mass index (BMI) or patients who were obese, as defined by BMI of 25 to 29.9.[1]

The smaller US series points out an increased risk of fractures with higher BMI. The more detailed German study points out an increased risk of sepsis and multiorgan failure with increased weight. Remarkably, the underweight patients in the large German series had a higher mortality rate during the first 24 hours after injury.

The rationale for adverse outcomes in obese patients remains unclear. Other studies point to obesity as a cause for increased procedural complications. The Germans also suggest an increased inflammatory response associated with being overweight. Laboratory data supporting this proposal are not included.

D. J. Dries, MSE, MD

Reference

1. Arbabi S, Wahl WL, Hemmila MR, Kohoyda-Inglis C, Taheri PA, Wang SC. The cushion effect. *J Trauma*. 2003;54:1090-1093.

Ballistic Fractures: Indirect Fracture to Bone
Dougherty PJ, Sherman D, Dau N, et al (Univ of Michigan, Ann Arbor; Wayne State Univ, Detroit, MI)
J Trauma 71:1381-1384, 2011

Background.—Two mechanisms of injury, the temporary cavity and the sonic wave, have been proposed to produce indirect fractures as a projectile passes nearby in tissue. The purpose of this study is to evaluate the temporal relationship of pressure waves using strain gauge technology and high-speed video to elucidate whether the sonic wave, the temporary cavity, or both are responsible for the formation of indirect fractures.

Methods.—Twenty-eight fresh frozen cadaveric diaphyseal tibia (2) and femurs (26) were implanted into ordnance gelatin blocks. Shots were fired using 9- and 5.56-mm bullets traversing through the gelatin only, passing close to the edge of the bone, but not touching, to produce an indirect fracture. High-speed video of the impact event was collected at 20,000 frames/s. Acquisition of the strain data were synchronized with the video at 20,000 Hz. The exact time of fracture was determined by analyzing and comparing the strain gauge output and video.

Results.—Twenty-eight shots were fired, 2 with 9-mm bullets and 26 with 5.56-mm bullets. Eight indirect fractures that occurred were of a simple (oblique or wedge) pattern. Comparison of the average distance of the projectile from the bone was 9.68 mm (range, 3−20 mm) for fractured specimens and 15.15 mm (range, 7−28 mm) for nonfractured specimens (Student's t test, $p = 0.036$).

Conclusions.—In this study, indirect fractures were produced after passage of the projectile. Thus, the temporary cavity, not the sonic wave, was responsible for the indirect fractures.

▶ These authors examine the effect of missiles passing near bone but not making direct contact. It appears that ordnance that cavitates has an increased risk of associated fractures. It is cavitation caused by passage of a missile through tissue that causes fractures rather than the shock wave, occurring over a much shorter time associated with the missile passing through soft tissue. The presence of a comminuted fracture is most consistent with direct impact of the bullet with bone.

A standard gelatin technique is used. This technique for assessing bullet performance was initially developed during World War II. High-speed photography with the transparent gelatin allows a straightforward data analysis.

Only 2 munitions were tested in this study. The first was a 9-mm projectile as a calibration instrument. The second projectile is similar to that used in the current US military rifle, the M16, the most common small arm used at present by US service personnel. I would expect similar results with different projectiles, although the size of the cavity obviously may vary.

One obvious limitation of this study, discussed by the authors in the discussion, is the use of elderly osteopenic bone. Most gunshot fractures occur in males aged 18 to 30 years. Unfortunately, availability of young bone to these investigators was limited. Again, the mode of fracture should remain the same, although the cavity size and forces involved to cause a fracture may vary with the quality of bone.

Finally, it is interesting to consider that body armor, which may cause a bullet to tumble and increase cavitation, could inadvertently increase the risk of indirect fracture.

D. J. Dries, MSE, MD

Hyperfibrinolysis at admission is an uncommon but highly lethal event associated with shock and prehospital fluid administration
Cotton BA, Harvin JA, Kostousouv V, et al (The Univ of Texas Health Science Ctr, Houston; et al)
J Trauma Acute Care Surg 73:365-370, 2012

Background.—Hyperfibrinolysis (HF) has been reported to occur in a range of 2% to 34% of trauma patients. Using rapid thromboelastography (r-TEG), we hypothesized that HF is (1) rarely present at admission on patients with severe injury and (2) associated with crystalloid hemodilution. To further strengthen this hypothesis, we created an in vitro hemodilution model to improve our mechanistic understanding of the early HF.

Methods.—The trauma registry was queried for patients who were our highest-level trauma activations and admitted directly from the scene (October 2009—October 2010). HF was defined as more than 7.5% amplitude reduction 30 minutes after maximal amplitude (LY30). Using r-TEG, we then created an in vitro hemodilution model (0.9% NS) with and without tissue injury (addition of tissue factor and tissue plasminogen activator) to identify crystalloid volumes and injury needed to achieve specific LY30 values.

Results.—Admission r-TEG values were captured on 1996 consecutive admissions. Only 41 patients (2%) had HF at admission r-TEG. The

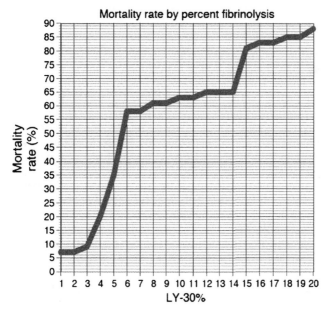

FIGURE.—Increasing mortality with increasing rates of fibrinolysis (LY30). (Reprinted from Cotton BA, Harvin JA, Kostousouv V, et al. Hyperfibrinolysis at admission is an uncommon but highly lethal event associated with shock and prehospital fluid administration. *J Trauma Acute Care Surg.* 2012;73:365-370, with permission from Lippincott Williams & Wilkins.)

groups were similar in demographics. Compared with patients without HF, the HF group had more prehospital crystalloid (1.5 vs. 0.5 L), higher median Injury Severity Score (25 vs. 16), greater admission base deficit (20 vs. 2), and higher mortality (76% vs. 10%); all $p < 0.001$. Controlling for Injury Severity Score and base deficit on arrival, prehospital fluid was associated with a significant increase in likelihood of HF. In fact, each additional liter of crystalloid was associated with a 15% increased odds of HF. The in vitro model found that hemodilution to 15% of baseline and tissue factor + tissue plasminogen activator was required to achieve an LY30 of 50%.

Conclusion.—Although uncommon immediately after injury, HF is associated with prehospital crystalloid administration and shock at admission and is highly lethal. Our in vitro model confirms that tissue injury and significant crystalloid hemodilution result in severe and immediate HF (Fig).

▶ Excessive fibrinolytic activity leads to accelerated clot breakdown and bleeding. Hyperfibrinolysis can be due to anomalies in the fibrinolytic cascade or may be in response to a specific insult. Liver disease, cardiopulmonary bypass, external fibrinolytic agents, sepsis, and obstetric catastrophes may trigger hyperfibrinolysis. Trauma can result in secondary hyperfibrinolysis, possibly through the protein C pathway.[1,2]

These data, obtained from the University of Texas Health Science Center in Houston and the Department of Anesthesiology and Intensive Care Medicine at the trauma center in Salzburg, Austria, suggest that hyperfibrinolysis is an uncommon finding at admission to a hospital, but it is associated with significant mortality. In these trauma centers, patients with hyperfibrinolysis experienced a 76% mortality rate (Fig). Hyperfibrinolysis was associated with higher Injury Severity Score, base deficit, presence of hypotension, and increasing prehospital crystalloid volumes. These data were supported by an in vitro model in which whole blood samples, obtained from healthy volunteers, were diluted with isotonic saline and tissue factor was added to mimic tissue trauma. Tissue plasminogen activator was added to the diluted whole blood samples and fibrinolytic activity measured with thromboelastography.[3] Data from this in vitro model support clinical findings by demonstrating that whole blood dilution was associated with increased fibrinolysis.

This trial is limited by small sample size (41 patients) with hyperfibrinolysis and single-center retrospective data analysis. However, the effectiveness of antifibrinolytic therapy in the recent Corticosteroid Randomisation After Significant Head Injury (CRASH)-2 and Military Application of Tranexamic Acid in Trauma Emergency Resuscitation (MATTERs) trials of tranexamic acid in blunt trauma victims argues in favor of the accuracy and importance of these results.[4,5]

D. J. Dries, MSE, MD

References

1. Brohi K, Cohen MJ, Ganter MT, Matthay MA, Mackersie RC, Pittet JF. Acute traumatic coagulopathy: initiated by hypoperfusion: modulated through the protein C pathway? *Ann Surg.* 2007;245:812-818.
2. Brohi K, Cohen MJ, Ganter MT, et al. Acute coagulopathy of trauma: hypoperfusion induces systemic anticoagulation and hyperfibrinolysis. *J Trauma.* 2008;64: 1211-1217.
3. Levrat A, Gros A, Rugeri L, et al. Evaluation of rotation thrombelastography for the diagnosis of hyperfibrinolysis in trauma patients. *Br J Anaesth.* 2008;100: 792-797.
4. CRASH-2 Trial Collaborators, Shakur H, Roberts I, Bautista R, et al. Effects of tranexamic acid on death, vascular occlusive events, and blood transfusion in trauma patients with significant haemorrhage (CRASH-2): a randomised, placebo-controlled trial. *Lancet.* 2010;376:23-32.
5. Morrison JJ, Dubose JJ, Rasmussen TE, Midwinter MJ. Military Application of Tranexamic Acid in Trauma Emergency Resuscitation (MATTERs) Study. *Arch Surg.* 2012;147:113-119.

The impact of antiplatelet drugs on trauma outcomes

Ferraris VA, Bernard AC, Hyde B, et al (Univ of Kentucky, Lexington)

J Trauma Acute Care Surg 73:492-497, 2012

Background.—Antiplatelet drugs (APDs) are among the most commonly prescribed medications. We wondered whether patients with trauma receiving preinjury APD have worse outcomes.

Methods.—We interrogated our institutional database during a 5-year period to evaluate preoperative risks and trauma outcomes in patients taking APDs before traumatic injury. We used propensity balancing scores to adjust for preoperative risks in assessing outcomes in APD-treated patients.

Results.—During a 5-year period, 1,327 (11.7%) of 11,374 adult patients with trauma took APDs before injury. The yearly use of APD in patients with trauma increased nearly threefold during the study period. Cardiac, pulmonary, and renal comorbidities were significantly more common in APD-treated patients. Multivariate regression indicated that preinjury APDs predicted significantly worse composite morbidity and mortality. After propensity adjustment for preinjury risk factors, APD-treated patients demonstrated significantly increased composite morbidity (39.0 vs. 24.6%, $p = 0.037$) and cardiac complications (23.0 vs. 17.3%, $p = 0.017$) compared with patients without APDs. The type and intensity of APD conferred an incremental risk, with patients taking dual APDs having a significantly worse multivariate risk of adverse outcomes compared with patients taking a single APD.

Conclusion.—APD-treated patients with trauma have significantly more comorbidities compared with those not taking APDs. After adjusting for preoperative risks, APD-treated patients have significantly worse trauma outcomes. Dual APD treatment confers an incremental risk of adverse outcomes compared with single APD preinjury treatment. The number of

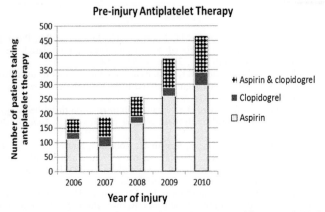

FIGURE 1.—Number of patients with trauma taking APDs. (Reprinted from Ferraris VA, Bernard AC, Hyde B, et al. The impact of antiplatelet drugs on trauma outcomes. *J Trauma Acute Care Surg.* 2012;73:492-497, with permission from Lippincott Williams & Wilkins.)

TABLE 5.—Propensity-Adjusted Outcomes in Patients With and Without APDs Before Trauma

Complication	No APD (n = 790), %	Any Antiplatelet Drug (n = 790), %	p
Mortality rate	8.0	9.4	NS
Respiratory	15.9	16.1	NS
Sepsis	5.3	4.8	NS
Cardiac	13.6	28.0	0.017
Renal	8.2	11.4	0.040
Bleeding	7.7	8.6	NS
CNS	4.6	5.9	NS
Composite morbidity	24.6	39.0	0.037
Length of stay (days ± SD)	7.2 ± 7.8 days	8.5 ± 9.3 days	NS

p, level of significance.

patients with trauma taking APDs increased during the 5-year study period, so we speculate that trauma management of patients taking APDs will occur more commonly in the future (Fig 1, Table 5).

▶ A growing number of patients presenting with various forms of injury receive antiplatelet therapy (Fig 1). Common agents include aspirin and clopidogrel. This report from a Level I trauma center documents the likelihood of preinjury antiplatelet therapy and highlights the problems involved in studying this population.

First, the profile of patients with trauma taking preinjury antiplatelet drugs is vastly different from the trauma population as a whole. Age, the incidence of coronary artery disease, the incidence of diabetes, and other cardiac problems is much higher than the trauma population in general. Common comorbidities such as ethanol use and other drugs are less common in patients receiving antiplatelet agents. Thus, we simply cannot compare 2 patient groups without stratifying for comorbidities (Table 5).

A second remarkable observation is the lack of a clear pattern of bleeding complications.[1,2] Although cardiac and renal complications are increased in patients receiving antiplatelet therapy, bleeding complications are no different when propensity-adjusted outcomes are examined.

With these observations and a detailed analysis, the authors raise important questions. In a patient without frank hemorrhage, should platelet transfusion be given to patients on antiplatelet agents? We now see that the effectiveness of clopidogrel as a platelet inhibitor is inconsistent at best.[1] Unfortunately, these authors did not routinely measure platelet function in the individuals studied. Thus, optimal management of the patient with antiplatelet drugs both at the time of surgery and after injury remains unclear.

D. J. Dries, MSE, MD

References

1. Bansal V, Fortlage D, Lee J, Doucet J, Potenza B, Coimbra R. A new clopidogrel (Plavix) point-of-care assay: rapid determination of antiplatelet activity in trauma patients. *J Trauma*. 2011;70:65-70.
2. Downey DM, Monson B, Butler KL, et al. Does platelet administration affect mortality in elderly head-injured patients taking antiplatelet medications? *Am Surg*. 2009;75:1100-1103.

Hypotension is 100 mm Hg on the battlefield
Eastridge BJ, Salinas J, Wade CE, et al (US Army Inst for Surgical Res, Fort Sam Houston, TX)
Am J Surg 202:404-408, 2011

Background.—Historically, emergency physicians and trauma surgeons have referred to a systolic blood pressure (SBP) of 90 mm Hg as hypotension. Recent evidence from the civilian trauma literature suggests that 110 mm Hg may be more appropriate based on associated acidosis and outcome measures. In this analysis, we sought to determine the relationship between SBP, hypoperfusion, and mortality in the combat casualty.

Methods.—A total of 7,180 US military combat casualties from the Joint Theater Trauma Registry from 2002 to 2009 were analyzed with respect to admission SBP, base deficit, and mortality. Base deficit, as a measure of hypoperfusion, and mortality were plotted against 10-mm Hg increments in admission SBP.

Results.—By plotting SBP, baseline mortality was less than 2% down to a level of 101 to 110 mm Hg, at which point the slope of the curve increased dramatically to a mortality rate of 45.1% in casualties with an SBP of 60 mm Hg or less but more than 0 mm Hg. A presenting SBP of 0 mm Hg was associated with 100% mortality. The data also established a similar effect for base deficit with a sharp increase in the rate of acidosis, which became manifest at an SBP in the range of 90 to 100 mm Hg.

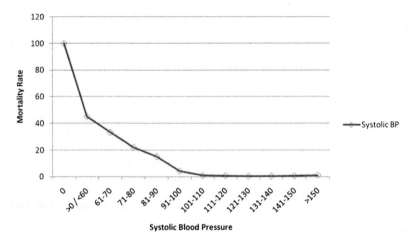

FIGURE 1.—Systolic BP and mortality. (Reprinted from Eastridge BJ, Salinas J, Wade CE, et al. Hypotension is 100 mm Hg on the battlefield. *Am J Surg.* 2011;202:404-408, Copyright 2011, with permission from Elsevier.)

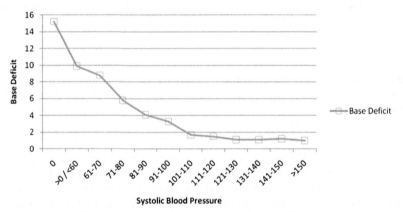

FIGURE 2.—Systolic BP and base deficit. (Reprinted from Eastridge BJ, Salinas J, Wade CE, et al. Hypotension is 100 mm Hg on the battlefield. *Am J Surg.* 2011;202:404-408, Copyright 2011, with permission from Elsevier.)

Conclusions.—This analysis shows that an SBP of 100 mm Hg or less may be a better and more clinically relevant definition of hypotension and impending hypoperfusion in the combat casualty. One utility of this analysis may be the more expeditious identification of battlefield casualties in need of life-saving interventions such as the need for blood or surgical intervention (Figs 1 and 2).

▶ Similar to recent work in the civilian population, this study uses the large military registry developed through data gathered in recent conflicts to identify a threshold systolic blood pressure in which mortality changes and a greater degree of physiologic stress is seen (Figs 1 and 2).[1] The limitation of this study is similar to that in civilian patients, where data are most important (the critically ill patient) and hardest to obtain. Nonetheless, systolic blood pressure is a relatively reproducible parameter. In particular, subjects without an available base deficit (who were excluded in this analysis) may be the specific group where careful data collection is essential but not available.

The authors acknowledge a lack of control over prehospital care and recording of milestones in the management of these patients. Technology used for blood pressure measurement is not standardized. A difference in 10 mm Hg could easily be detected depending on blood pressure measurement technique.[2]

Acknowledging these limitations, I will adjust my systolic blood pressure threshold upward in my initial evaluation of the injured presenting in the emergency department.

D. J. Dries, MSE, MD

References

1. Eastridge BJ, Salinas J, McManus JG, et al. Hypotension begins at 110 mm Hg: redefining "hypotension" with data. *J Trauma*. 2007;63:291-299.
2. Davis JW, Davis IC, Bennink LD, Bilello JF, Kaups KL, Parks SN. Are automated blood pressure measurements accurate in trauma patients? *J Trauma*. 2003;55: 860-863.

Clinical and biomarker profile of trauma-induced secondary cardiac injury
De'Ath HD, Rourke C, Davenport R, et al (Barts and the London NHS Trust, UK)
Br J Surg 99:789-797, 2012

Background.—Secondary cardiac injury has been demonstrated in critical illness and is associated with worse outcomes. The aim of this study was to establish the existence of trauma-induced secondary cardiac injury, and investigate its impact on outcomes in injured patients.

Methods.—Injured adult patients eligible for enrolment in the Activation of Coagulation and Inflammation in Trauma 2 study, and admitted to the intensive care unit between January 2008 and January 2010, were selected retrospectively for the study. Markers of cardiac injury (brain natriuretic peptide (BNP), heart-type fatty acid binding protein (H-FABP) and troponin I) were measured on admission, and after 24 and 72 h in blood samples from injured patients. Individual records were reviewed for adverse cardiac events and death.

Results.—During the study period, 135 patients were enrolled (106 male, 78·5 per cent) with a median age of 40 (range 16—89) years. Eighteen patients (13·3 per cent) had an adverse cardiac event during admission and these events were not associated with direct thoracic injury. The in-hospital mortality rate was higher among the adverse cardiac event cohort: 44 per cent (8 of 18) *versus* 17·1 per cent (20 of 117) (P = 0·008). Raised levels

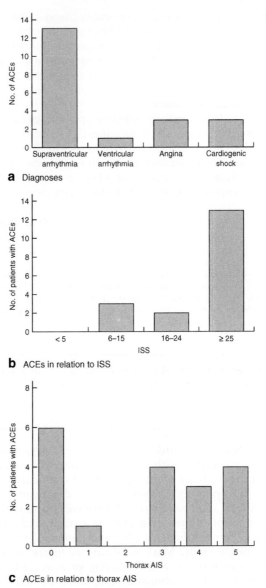

a Diagnoses

b ACEs in relation to ISS

c ACEs in relation to thorax AIS

FIGURE 1.—Adverse cardiac events (ACEs): **a** different diagnoses, **b** in relation to Injury Severity Score (ISS) and **c** in relation to thorax Abbreviated Injury Scale (AIS) score. **b** $P = 0.052$, **c** $P = 0.392$ (χ^2 test for trend). (Reprinted from De'Ath HD, Rourke C, Davenport R, et al. Clinical and biomarker profile of trauma-induced secondary cardiac injury. *Br J Surg.* 2012;99:789-797. British Journal of Surgery Society Ltd. Reproduced with permission. Permission is granted by John Wiley & Sons Ltd on behalf of the BJSS Ltd.)

of H-FABP and BNP at 0, 24 and 72 h, and troponin I at 24 and 72 h, were associated with increased adverse cardiac events. BNP levels were higher in non-survivors on admission (median 550 *versus* 403 fmol/ml; $P = 0 \cdot 022$), after 24 h (794 *versus* 567 fmol/ml; $P = 0 \cdot 033$) and after 72 h (1043 *versus* 753 fmol/ml; $P = 0 \cdot 036$), as were admission troponin I levels.

Conclusion.—Clinical and cardiac biomarker characteristics support the existence of trauma-induced secondary cardiac injury, which is associated with death, and unrelated to direct thoracic injury (Fig 1).

▶ This study echoes work done in American critical care units demonstrating that in the absence of direct thoracic injury, biomarkers of physiologic cardiac insults can be identified and are associated with increased morbidity and mortality.[1,2] Supraventricular tachycardia, as the most common rhythm seen, is a typical reflection of physiologic stress in other patient groups.

This study does not segregate patients based on preexisting cardiac disease. A number of younger patients also had acute cardiac events. In the absence of direct thoracic trauma, this can easily reflect a remote implication of injury (Fig 1).

Obvious limitations of this work are its retrospective nature and lack of consistent and rigorous evaluation for functional cardiac disease. This remains a hypothesis-generating exercise.

D. J. Dries, MSE, MD

References

1. Stewart D, Waxman K, Brown CA, et al. B-type natriuretic peptide levels may be elevated in the critically injured trauma patient without congestive heart failure. *J Trauma.* 2007;63:747-750.
2. Martin M, Mullenix P, Rhee P, Belzberg H, Demetriades D, Salim A. Troponin increases in the critically injured patient: mechanical trauma or physiologic stress? *J Trauma.* 2005;59:1086-1091.

A Systematic Review and Meta-Analysis of Diagnostic Screening Criteria for Blunt Cerebrovascular Injuries

Franz RW, Willette PA, Wood MJ, et al (The Vascular and Vein Ctr at Grant Med Ctr, Columbus, OH; Grant Med Ctr, Columbus, OH; Doctors Hosp, Columbus, OH; et al)
J Am Coll Surg 214:313-327, 2012

Background.—Despite progress in diagnosing and managing blunt cerebrovascular injury (BCVI), controversy remains regarding the appropriate population to screen. A systematic review of published literature was conducted to summarize the overall incidence of BCVI and the various screening criteria used to detect BCVI. A meta-analysis was performed to evaluate which screening criteria may be associated with BCVI. Goals were to confirm inclusion of certain criteria in current screening protocols and possibly eliminate criteria not associated with BCVI.

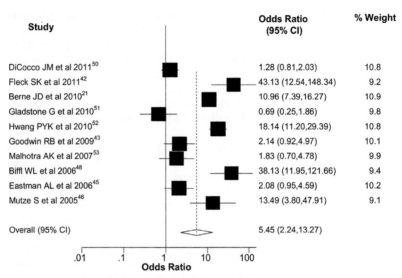

Heterogeneity: Chi^2 = 141.51; df = 9 (p < 0.0001); τ^2 = 1.8498; I^2 = 93.6%
Test for OR = 1: Z = 3.74 (p < 0.0001)

FIGURE 2.—Forest plot demonstrating significant association between cervical spine injury and blunt cerebrovascular injury. (Reprinted from Franz RW, Willette PA, Wood MJ, et al. A systematic review and meta-analysis of diagnostic screening criteria for blunt cerebrovascular injuries. *J Am Coll Surg.* 2012;214:313-327, Copyright 2012, with permission from the American College of Surgeons.)

Study Design.—Studies published between January 1995 and April 2011 using digital subtraction angiography or CT angiography as a diagnostic modality and reporting overall BCVI incidence or prevalence of BCVI for specific screening criteria were examined. Screening criteria were analyzed using a random effects model to determine if an association with BCVI was present.

Results.—The incidence range of BCVI was between 0.18% and 2.70% among approximately 122,176 blunt trauma admissions. The meta-analysis encompassed 418 BCVI and 22,568 non-BCVI patients. Of the 9 screening criteria analyzed, cervical spine (odds ratio [OR] 5.45; 95% CI 2.24 to 13.27; *p* < 0.0001) and thoracic (OR 1.98; 95% CI 1.35 to 2.92; *p* = 0.001) injuries demonstrated a significant association with BCVI.

Conclusions.—Patients with cervical spine and thoracic injuries had significantly greater likelihoods of BCVI compared with patients without these injuries. All patients with either injury should be screened for BCVI. Multivariate logistic regression analysis is needed to elucidate the possible impact of the combined presence of screening criteria, but it was not possible in our study due to limitations in data presentation. Standardized reporting of BCVI data is not established and is recommended to permit future collaboration (Figs 2 and 3).

▶ Cerebrovascular injury secondary to blunt trauma is an infrequent occurrence. Typical presentation includes a period of asymptomatic injury followed by a

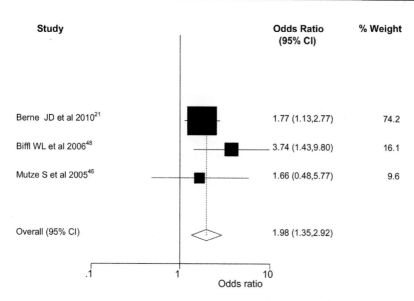

Study   **Odds Ratio (95% CI)**   **% Weight**

Berne JD et al 2010[21]   1.77 (1.13,2.77)   74.2

Biffl WL et al 2006[48]   3.74 (1.43,9.80)   16.1

Mutze S et al 2005[46]   1.66 (0.48,5.77)   9.6

Overall (95% CI)   1.98 (1.35,2.92)

.1   1   10
Odds ratio

Heterogeneity: Chi^2 = 2.00; df = 2 (p = 0.368); τ^2 = 0.000; I^2 = 0.0%
Test for OR=1: Z = 3.47 (p = 0.001)

FIGURE 3.—Forest plot demonstrating significant association between thoracic injury and blunt cerebrovascular injury. (Reprinted from Franz RW, Willette PA, Wood MJ, et al. A systematic review and meta-analysis of diagnostic screening criteria for blunt cerebrovascular injuries. *J Am Coll Surg.* 2012;214:313-327, Copyright 2012, with permission from the American College of Surgeons.)

significant ischemic cerebrovascular insult. In my experience, patients have multiple other injuries and have required mechanical ventilation with sedation and analgesic administration, making serial neurologic examination difficult. If the diagnosis of cerebrovascular injury can be made prior to a catastrophic embolic event, current data suggest that anticoagulant therapy may be effective.

In a previous consensus statement, the Eastern Association for the Surgery of Trauma and the Western Trauma Association suggest a large number of signs, symptoms, and risk factors.[1,2] Clearly, expanding hematoma or other physical examination findings consistent with cervical vascular injury should lead to imaging or operative exploration. A large number of other risk factors, however, have been identified, including facial and skull fractures, depressed Glasgow coma score, close-line—type injury, petrous bone fracture, diffuse axonal injury, and cervical spine fracture. With this large number of injuries, a wide net is cast for blunt cerebrovascular trauma. I suspect that a large number of patients will receive needless evaluation given all of these criteria.

These authors identify 2 key factors that make biomechanical sense in identifying the patient with occult extracranial cerebrovascular injury (Figs 2 and 3). Cervical or thoracic spine fractures imply a significant force was applied and could lead to a significant hyperextension injury, the proposed mechanism of extracranial cerebrovascular trauma. I believe that we can build on these criteria to better understand the natural history of this insult and refine treatment strategies.

Although the meta-analysis here is most impressive, the authors clearly state its limitations. At present, there is no consistent reporting system or diagnostic strategy for blunt cerebrovascular injury. The authors appropriately suggest that CT angiography or digital subtraction angiography is the appropriate modality at present. These are not used consistently nor are reporting criteria for these injuries consistently use in the studies examined. Thus, the authors have aggregated heterogeneous data to draw these conclusions. Nonetheless, I am impressed and encouraged at these results. Now the clinician encountering a patient with high-risk injures has a workable number of criteria to initiate evaluation with a small number of gold standard studies. With better data and improved interventional radiology techniques, we may better understand the natural history of blunt cerebrovascular injury and refine and improve treatment strategies.

D. J. Dries, MSE, MD

References

1. Biffl WL, Cothren CC, Moore EE, et al. Western Trauma Association critical decisions in trauma: screening for and treatment of blunt cerebrovascular injuries. *J Trauma*. 2009;67:1150-1153.
2. Bromberg WJ, Collier BC, Diebel LN, et al. Blunt cerebrovascular injury practice management guidelines: the Eastern Association for the Surgery of Trauma. *J Trauma*. 2010;68:471-477.

Base deficit as a marker of survival after traumatic injury: Consistent across changing patient populations and resuscitation paradigms
Hodgman EI, Morse BC, Dente CJ, et al (Emory Univ School Medicine, Atlanta, GA)
J Trauma Acute Care Surg 72:844-851, 2012

Background.—Damage control resuscitation (DCR) has improved outcomes in severely injured patients. In civilian centers, massive transfusion protocols (MTPs) represent the most formal application of DCR principles, ensuring early, accurate delivery of high fixed ratios of blood components. Recent data suggest that DCR may also help address early trauma-induced coagulopathy. Finally, base deficit (BD) is a long-recognized and simple early prognostic marker of survival after injury.

Methods.—Outcomes of patients with admission BD data resuscitated during the DCR era (2007–2010) were compared with previously published data (1995–2003) of patients cared for before the DCR era (pre-DCR). Patients were considered to have no hypoperfusion (BD, >-6), mild (BD, -6 to -14.9), moderate (BD, -15 to -23.9), or severe hypoperfusion (BD, <-24).

Results.—Of 6,767 patients, 4,561 were treated in the pre-DCR era and 2,206 in the DCR era. Of the latter, 218 (9.8%) represented activations of the MTP. DCR patients tended to be slightly older, more likely victims of penetrating trauma, and slightly more severely injured as measured by trauma scores and BD. Despite these differences, overall survival was

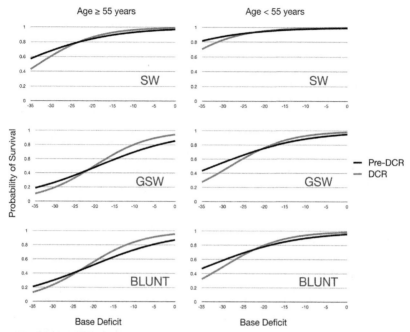

FIGURE 2.—Survival for all groups is essentially unchanged for all BD values. This is true for both young patients and older patients and regardless of mechanism of injury. Pre-DCR, historic controls; DCR, current era patients. (Reprinted from Hodgman EI, Morse BC, Dente CJ, et al. Base deficit as a marker of survival after traumatic injury: consistent across changing patient populations and resuscitation paradigms. *J Trauma Acute Care Surg.* 2012;72:844-851, with permission from Lippincott Williams & Wilkins.)

unchanged in the two eras (86.4% vs. 85.7%, $p = 0.67$), and survival curves stratified by mechanism of injury were nearly identical. Patients with severe BD who were resuscitated using the MTP, however, experienced a substantial increase in survival compared with pre-DCR counterparts.

Conclusion.—Despite limited adoption of formal DCR, overall survival after injury, stratified by BD, is identical in the modern era. Patients with severely deranged physiology, however, experience better outcomes. BD remains a consistent predictor of mortality after traumatic injury. Predicted survival depends more on the energy level of the injury (stab wound vs. nonstab wound) than the mechanism of injury (blunt vs. penetrating) (Fig 2).

▶ These data come from the expansive records of one of the major trauma centers in the United States. Base deficit, an important marker of tissue ischemia, appears to be a valuable means to stratify severity of injury.[1] This argument is solidified in the largest patient review on this subject that I have recently seen.

Within these data there are a number of other important observations. First, much of the trauma literature in resuscitation is focused on application of massive transfusion protocols.[2,3] As these authors point out, massive transfusion strategies are probably necessary in 10% or less of patients presenting to major trauma centers. While overall survival in the large patient dataset is unchanged over many years, where the massive transfusion protocol is used, mortality has been dramatically reduced. In the small group of patients with massive transfusion in the setting of significant base deficit, survival was tripled (19% vs > 60%) in patients sustaining blunt injury and improved in patients sustaining penetrating trauma as well (47% vs 71%). Where the physiologic insult was less severe as demonstrated by a small base deficit, survival was unchanged across the extended time spectrum for this review.

This work clearly identifies a critical role for hypoperfusion in adverse trauma outcomes and, secondarily, early traumatic coagulopathy. This finding parallels a carefully written preclinical trial published in the same issue of the *Journal of Trauma and Acute Care Surgery.*[4] However, patients with more significant tissue injury also had poorer outcome across the range of base deficits studied. Patients with multisystem blunt trauma or gunshot wounds, in which more energy is imparted to the patient, did worse than patients with trauma secondary to stab wounds.[1]

The 2 widely acknowledged metabolic predictors of physiologic stress are base deficit, as featured here, and lactate. While many centers use lactate to stratify metabolic stress, lactate determination until now has been slowed by the requirement for a time-consuming laboratory assay. As bedside lactate determination becomes available, I believe that studies similar to this may be possible for injured patients and allow stratification of lactate levels as a means to discern the metabolic stress of injury.

D. J. Dries, MSE, MD

References

1. Tremblay LN, Feliciano DV, Rozycki GS. Assessment of initial base deficit as a predictor of outcome: mechanism of injury does make a difference. *Am Surg.* 2002;68:689-694.
2. Larson CR, White CE, Spinella PC, et al. Association of shock, coagulopathy, and initial vital signs with massive transfusion in combat casualties. *J Trauma.* 2010; 69:S26-S32.
3. Cotton BA, Dossett LA, Haut ER, et al. Multicenter validation of a simplified score to predict massive transfusion in trauma. *J Trauma.* 2010;69:S33-S39.
4. Doran CM, Doran CA, Woolley T, et al. Targeted resuscitation improves coagulation and outcome. *J Trauma Acute Care Surg.* 2012;72:835-843.

Use of computed tomography in the initial evaluation of anterior abdominal stab wounds

Berardoni NE, Kopelman TR, O'Neill PJ, et al (Maricopa Med Ctr, Phoenix, AZ)
Am J Surg 202:690-696, 2011

Background.—The purpose of this study was to assess the ability of computed tomography (CT) to facilitate initial management decisions in patients with anterior abdominal stab wounds.

Methods.—A retrospective review was conducted of patients with anterior abdominal stab wounds who underwent CT over 4.5 years. Any

TABLE 1.—Positive Findings on CT (n = 30) and Initial Management Plans

Radiographic Finding	Number of Scans with Positive Findings	Management Plan Nonoperative (n = 10)	Management Plan Operative (n = 20)
SOI	10*	5	5
Hepatic	9	5	4
Splenic	1	0	1
Renal	1	0	1
Active blush	3	1	2
Pneumoperitoneum	7	1	6
Minimal	2	1	1
Free fluid without SOI	12	2	10
Isolated minimal	3	3	0
Mesenteric changes	8	0	8
Omental hematoma	1	1	0
Hollow viscous wall changes	6	0	6
Diaphragm abnormality	1	0	1

*One scan with both splenic and renal injuries.

TABLE 2.—Results on CT and Correlation of Intraoperative Findings

Patient	CT Suspicious for HVI	CT Suspicious for SOI	CT Suspicious for Other	Intraoperative HVI	Intraoperative SOI	Vascular Injury	Diaphragm Injury	Pancreas Injury	Mesenteric or Omental Injury
1	Y			Y					
2		Y			Y		Y		
3	Y		Retrogastric hematoma	Y	Y			Y	
4		Y			Y		Y		
5	Y		Intra-abdominal blush	Y	Y				
6	Y	Y		Y*	Y		Y		
7	Y			Y*					Y
8	Y			Y					
9	Y			Y					
10	Y		Diaphragm irregularity	Y			Y		
11	Y			Y					
12	Y			Y					Y
13		Y		Y*	Y		Y		Y
14		Y			Y		Y		

*Serosal injury only.

abnormality suspicious for intra-abdominal injury was considered a positive finding on CT.

Results.—Ninety-eight patients met the study's inclusion criteria. Positive findings on CT were noted in 30 patients (31%), leading to operative intervention in 67%. Injuries were confirmed in 95% of cases, but only 70% were therapeutic. Ten patients had nonoperative management despite positive findings on CT, including 5 patients with solid organ injuries. One patient underwent operative intervention for clinical deterioration, with negative findings. No computed tomographic evidence of injury was noted in the remaining 68 patients (69%), but 1 patient was noted to have a splenic injury while undergoing operative evaluation of the diaphragm. All remaining patients were treated nonoperatively with success.

Conclusions.—In patients with anterior abdominal stab wounds, CT should be considered to facilitate initial management decisions, as it has the ability to delineate abnormalities suspicious for injury (Tables 1 and 2).

▶ This role for computed tomography (CT) is particularly important in a busy trauma center, in which the time and resources wasted on negative laparotomy must be conserved. In my experience, oral and rectal contrast is unnecessary to effectively perform an abdominal examination with CT. In addition, the use of anesthesia or the time involved in hospitalization for observation can be avoided with negative abdominal CT. Wound tracks can be examined, particularly in obese patients, to determine the course of the abdominal wall stab wound.

Statistics provided in this article strongly support this technique. Abdominal CT in this setting has 96% sensitivity, 97% specificity, 93% positive predictive value, and 99% negative predictive value. None of these patients had operative intervention delayed by the use of CT. Like these authors, we have been able to discharge patients from the emergency department if responsible follow-up is available, with negative CT findings and a very brief period of observation. Longer follow-up, a problem in trauma studies, is needed to confirm the absence of diaphragm injury, which is a tough diagnosis with any imaging strategy (Tables 1 and 2).

Overall, I believe that abdominal CT is a valuable modality in this application, and the patient admitted with abdominal CT to evaluate an abdominal wall stab wound has been effectively screened for problems related to the stab while in the emergency department. If such a patient is admitted to the intensive care unit because of other concerns, the intensivist may be confident that appropriate initial testing has been done.

D. J. Dries, MSE, MD

Complications following thoracic trauma managed with tube thoracostomy
Menger R, Telford G, Kim P, et al (Hosp of the Univ of Pennsylvania, Philadelphia)
Injury 43:46-50, 2012

Introduction.—Tube thoracostomy is a common procedure used to treat traumatic chest injuries. Although the mechanism of injury traditionally does not alter chest tube management, complication rates may vary depending on the severity of injury. The purpose of this study was to investigate the incidence of and risk factors associated with chest tube complications (CTCs) following thoracic trauma.

TABLE 4.—Multivariate Analysis for Chest Tube Complications

| | Chest Tube Management Complications | | |
	OR	95%CI	P-Value
ICU length of stay in days	0.96	0.91, 1.01	0.15
Hospital length of stay in days	1.03	1.00, 1.07	0.07
Chest AIS ≥4 vs. ≤3	2.61	1.13, 6.01	0.02
Extrathoracic injury	2.11	0.80, 5.57	0.13

Methods.—A retrospective chart review of all trauma patients (≥ 16 years old) admitted to an urban level 1 trauma centre (1/2007—12/2007) was conducted. Patients who required chest tube (CT) therapy for thoracic injuries within 24 h of admission and survived until CT removal were included. CTCs were defined as a recurrent pneumothorax or residual haemothorax requiring CT reinsertion within 24 h after initial tube removal or addition of new CT > 24 h after initial placement. Variables including demographic data, mechanism, associated injuries, initial vital signs, chest abbreviated injury score (AIS), injury severity score (ISS), Glasgow coma score (GCS) and length of stay (LOS) and CT-specific variables (e.g. indication, timing of insertion, and duration of therapy) were compared using the chi square test, Mann—Whitney test, and multivariate analysis.

Results.—154 patients were included with 22.1% ($n = 34$) developing a CTC. On univariate analysis, CTCs were associated with longer ICU and hospital LOS ($p = 0.02$ and $p < 0.001$), increased chest AIS ($p = 0.01$), and the presence of an extrathoracic injury ($p = 0.047$). Results of the multivariate analysis indicated that only increased chest AIS (OR 2.49; $p = 0.03$) was a significantly independent predictor of CTCs.

Conclusions.—CTCs following chest trauma are common and are associated with increased morbidity. The severity of the thoracic injury, as measured by chest AIS, should be incorporated into the development of CT management guidelines in order to decrease the incidence of CTCs (Table 4).

▶ Complications associated with chest tube placement are infrequently reported. These data, from a major US trauma center, document that chest tube placement is not a benign procedure. Unfortunately, the risk of complications is increased in the setting of increasing chest injury (Table 4). The authors are appropriate to note, as has been previously reported, that the use of mechanical ventilation is not associated with chest tube—related complications. In fact, a large series of chest drain removal procedures from the University of New Mexico documents the absence of adverse effects with mechanical ventilation.[1] Limitations to this study are noted on review of the report. Perhaps most important is that consistent data regarding chest tube placement are not available. Thus, tube malposition or iatrogenic injury could have contributed to complications noted. Given the vast experience of this team with management of injury, however, I must agree that the risk of chest drain complications is best predicted by the severity of primary chest injuries.

D. J. Dries, MSE, MD

Reference

1. Tawil I, Gonda JM, King RD, Marinaro JL, Crandall CS. Impact of positive pressure ventilation on thoracostomy tube removal. *J Trauma*. 2010;68:818-821.

Fracture stabilisation in a polytraumatised African population—A comparison with international management practice
Grey B, Rodseth RN, Muckart DJJ (Univ of KwaZulu-Natal, Congella, South Africa; Inkosi Albert Luthuli Central Hosp, Durban, South Africa)
Injury 43:219-222, 2012

Introduction.—Fracture management in polytrauma patients has favoured early definitive fracture fixation with some authors advocating a staged management approach in these potentially unstable patients. We aimed to investigate the timing of surgical fracture stabilisation in polytrauma patients with significant orthopaedic injuries in a Level 1 trauma unit in South Africa (RSA) and to compare its performance with Level 1 trauma units in the USA and Europe.

Materials and Methods.—A retrospective review was performed extracting polytrauma patients with a New Injury Severity Score (NISS) ≥ 15, with significant pelvic or long bone fractures managed surgically. We compared these data with recently published data from the USA and Europe.

Results.—Over a 3 year period pedestrian (46.3%) and motor vehicle or motorcycle accidents (40.7%) were the predominant mechanisms of injury in the 123 eligible patients. Compared to international data, patients were significantly younger (32.41 years (SD 13.4) vs. USA 44.1 years (SD 16.39) and Germany 41.2 years (SD 15.35), $p < 0.001$); and had a higher NISS score (RSA 31.93 (10.3), USA 27.4 (8.65), Germany 29.4 (6.88), $p = 0.007$). Less definitive fixation took place in the first 24 h (RSA 37.4%, USA 57.1%, Germany 65.6%, $p < 0.001$), but overall definitive fixation took place earlier (RSA 3.6 days (SD 4.39), USA 5.5 days (SD 4.2), Germany 6.6 days (SD 8.7), $p = 0.001$).

TABLE 2.—Fracture Management in the First 24 h

Orthopaedic Management	RSA ($n = 123$)	USA ($n = 77$)	Germany ($n = 93$)	p Value
Primary definitive fixation (%)	46 (37.4)	44 (57.1)	61 (65.6)	<0.001*
Non-invasive: traction or backslab (%)	34 (27.6)	7 (9.1%)	1 (1.1%)	<0.001*
Temporising external fixation (%)	12 (9.8)	19 (24.8)	21 (22.6)	0.005*
Definitive external fixation (%)	36 (29.3)	7 (9.1)	10 (10.8)	<0.001*

RSA, Republic of South Africa; USA, United States of America.
*Statistically significant.

Conclusion.—In a developing country when compared to international trauma centres, less primary definitive fixation was performed in the first 24 h (Table 2).

▶ These authors demonstrate that in the setting of South African trauma practice, where prehospital times can be significant, timing to definitive fracture fixation could be delayed when compared with International First World trauma centers.

Patients were examined with early fracture stabilization (48 hours, between 48 and 96 hours, and after 96 hours). Notably, trauma victims who were received directly from the scene had fixation within 24 hours in 70% of cases. Unfortunately, many patients do not come directly from the scene in South Africa.

Table 2 suggests that South African practice makes greater use of definitive external fixation for fracture control (Table 2). We are not given data to suggest whether this improves outcome. There is no overt reason why patients need to have later conversion to an intramedullary nail system or other internal fixation if appropriate bony alignment is obtained with external fixators.

Early definitive (internal) fixation of fractures within 24 hours has been reported as a preferred treatment in multitrauma patients resulting in reduction of acute respiratory distress syndrome, intensive care unit utilization, and fat embolization.[1] Unfortunately, we are not given data about the incidence of these complications with different fracture management strategies. We will continue to follow the natural experiment between external and internal fixation as definitive fracture treatment with interest.

Two other observations may be made. First, the definition of polytrauma is unclear.[2] Polytrauma is not specified in this article other than with presentation of Injury Severity Scores. Second, noting that the South African patient population had a greater burden of injury, external fixation as a more-rapid and less-invasive orthopedic intervention may be most appropriate.

D. J. Dries, MSE, MD

References

1. Seibel R, LaDuca J, Hassett JM, et al. Blunt multiple trauma (ISS 36), femur traction, and the pulmonary failure-septic state. *Ann Surg.* 1985;202:283-295.
2. Butcher N, Balogh ZJ. AIS>2 in at least two body regions: a potential new anatomical definition of polytrauma. *Injury.* 2012;43:196-199.

Factor IX complex for the correction of traumatic coagulopathy
Joseph B, Amini A, Friese RS, et al (Univ of Arizona College of Medicine, Tucson)
J Trauma Acute Care Surg 72:828-834, 2012

Background.—Damage control resuscitation advocates correction of coagulopathy; however, options are limited and expensive. The use of prothrombin complex concentrate (PCC), also known as factor IX complex, can quickly accelerate reversal of coagulopathy at relatively low cost. The

270 / Critical Care Medicine

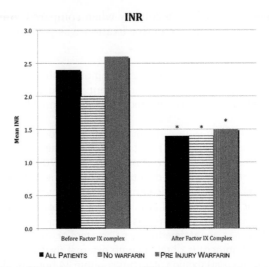

FIGURE 2.—Mean INR before and after factor IX complex administration by groups. *p < 0.05. (Reprinted from Joseph B, Amini A, Friese RS, et al. Factor IX complex for the correction of traumatic coagulopathy. *J Trauma Acute Care Surg.* 2012;72:828-834, with permission from Lippincott Williams & Wilkins.)

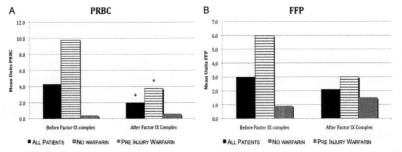

FIGURE 3.—(A) Mean PRBCs transfused before and after factor IX complex administration by groups. *p < 0.05. (B) Mean FFP transfused before and after factor IX complex administration by groups. *p < 0.05. (Reprinted from Joseph B, Amini A, Friese RS, et al. Factor IX complex for the correction of traumatic coagulopathy. *J Trauma Acute Care Surg.* 2012;72:828-834, with permission from Lippincott Williams & Wilkins.)

purpose of this study is to describe our experience in the use of factor IX complex in coagulopathic trauma patients.

Methods.—All patients receiving PCC at our Level I trauma center over a two-year period (2008−2010) were reviewed. PCC was used at the discretion of the trauma attending for treatment of coagulopathy, reversal of coumadin, and when recombinant factor VIIa was indicated.

Results.—Forty-five trauma patients received 51 doses of PCC. Sixty-two per cent were male and mean Injury Severity Score was 23 (± 14.87). Standard dose was 25 units per kg and mean cost per patient was $1,022 ($504−3,484). Fifty-eight per cent of patients were on warfarin before admission. Mean international normalized ratio (INR) was decreased after PCC administration ($p = 0.001$). Packed red blood cell transfusion was also reduced after factor IX complex ($p = 0.018$). Mean INR was reduced in both the nonwarfarin ($p = 0.001$) and warfarin ($p = 0.001$) groups. Packed red blood cell transfusion was less in the nonwarfarin group ($p = 0.002$) however was not significant in the warfarin group. Subsequent thromboembolic events were observed in 3 of the 45 patients (7%). Mortality was 16 of 45 (36%).

Conclusion.—PCC rapidly and effectively treats coagulopathy after traumatic injury. PCC therapy leads to a significant correction in INR in all trauma patients, regardless of coumadin use, and concomitant reduction in blood product transfusion. PCC should be considered as an effective tool to treat acute coagulopathy of trauma. Further prospective studies examining the safety, efficacy, cost, and outcomes comparing PCC and recombinant factor VIIa are needed (Figs 2 and 3).

▶ Driven by shock and high-volume tissue injury, traumatic coagulopathy is a marker for poor outcome that may be found even before patients arrive in the emergency department.[1] Aggressive administration of a balanced package of coagulation factors and red blood cells is currently thought to be the optimal management strategy.[2,3] This article is an early report with replacement of fresh frozen plasma as an agent for management of coagulopathy with a factor IX complex containing all vitamin K—dependent coagulation factors (factor II, factor VII, factor IX, and factor X). Although the authors address use of this material in the management of traumatic coagulopathy, there are really 2 small patient groups studied here. The first comprises approximately 20 patients with blunt traumatic mechanism and traumatic coagulopathy, as just described. The second group comprises elderly patients with traumatic brain injury typically associated with warfarin use.

Each patient group saw reduction in the international normalized ratio with administration of the factor IX complex (Fig 2). Use of packed red blood cells and fresh frozen plasma was also reduced (Fig 3). Cost of factor IX complex was significant but less than historic costs of recombinant factor VIIa, the previously studied hemostatic agent for treatment of coagulopathy after trauma.[4] There is no obvious pattern of significant thromboembolic complications, and patient groups are far too small to make any statement regarding mortality.

Products such as factor IX complex may be most valuable in patients with intolerance of volume administration associated with fresh frozen plasma and the need for rapid correction of coagulopathy after injury. A typical patient is elderly with isolated brain injury and concomitant warfarin use. For the typical young trauma patient with previous good health, factor IX complex may be significantly more expensive than administration of fresh frozen plasma where the plasma will be well tolerated by the patient.

This article provides initial safety data and weak support for larger trials of this material where impact on mortality and significant morbidity can be critically assessed.

D. J. Dries, MSE, MD

References

1. Dries DJ. The contemporary role of blood products and components used in trauma resuscitation. *Scand J Trauma Resusc Emerg Med*. 2010;18:63.
2. Brohi K, Singh J, Heron M, Coats T. Acute traumatic coagulopathy. *J Trauma*. 2003;54:1127-1130.
3. Hess JR, Brohi K, Dutton RP, et al. The coagulopathy of trauma: a review of mechanisms. *J Trauma*. 2008;65:748-754.
4. Boffard KD, Riou B, Warren B, et al. Recombinant factor VIIa as adjunctive therapy for bleeding control in severely injured trauma patients: two parallel randomized, placebo-controlled, double-blind clinical trials. *J Trauma*. 2005;59: 8-15.

Autotransfusion of hemothorax blood in trauma patients: is it the same as fresh whole blood?
Salhanick M, Corneille M, Higgins R, et al (Univ of Texas Health Science Ctr, San Antonio, TX)
Am J Surg 202:817-822, 2011

Background.—Autotransfusable shed blood has been poorly characterized in trauma and may have similarities to whole blood with additional benefits.

Methods.—This was a prospective descriptive study of adult patients from whom ≥50 mL of blood was drained within the first 4 hours after chest tube placement. Pleural and venous blood samples were analyzed for coagulation, hematology, and electrolytes.

Results.—Twenty-two subjects were enrolled in 9 months. The following measured coagulation factors of hemothorax were significantly depleted compared with venous blood: international normalized ratio (> 9 in contrast to 1.1, $P < .001$), activated partial thromboplastin time (> 180 in contrast to 28.5 seconds, $P < .001$), and fibrinogen (< 50 in contrast to 288 mg/dL, $P < .001$). The mean hematocrit (26.4 in contrast to 33.9), ($P = .003$), hemoglobin (9.3 in contrast to 11.8 g/dL, $P = .004$), and platelet count (53 in contrast to 174 K/μL, $P < .001$) of hemothorax were significantly lower than venous blood. A hemothorax volume of 726 mL was calculated to be equivalent to 1 U of red blood cells.

Conclusions.—Hemothorax blood contains significantly decreased coagulation factors and has lower hemoglobin when compared with venous blood (Tables 1 and 2).

▶ The authors demonstrate a deterioration of coagulation factors in blood obtained from a chest collection system. One concern in this study is the collection at 4 hours after chest drain placement. It is unclear whether contact with the pleura or contact with the chest drain system depleted fibrinogen and other clotting factors (Tables 1 and 2). Clearly, red cells from a chest collection system do not have the age-related complications, which may be seen with transfusion of packed red cells.[1] We must understand, however, that we are not returning

TABLE 1.—Hematology Profile

Parameter	Pleural Blood (SD)	Venous Blood (SD)	*P* Value
Hematocrit (%)	26.4 (9.5)	33.9 (8.4)	.003*
Hemoglobin (g/dL)	9.2 (3.1)	11.7 (2.9)	.004*
Platelet (K/μL)	53.0 (40.9)	174.4 (81.7)	<.001*
WBC (K/μL)	9.8 (7.3)	11.0 (4.7)	.47*

SD = standard deviation.
*Signed rank test.

TABLE 2.—Coagulation Profile

Parameter	Pleural Blood (Median)	Venous Blood (SD) (Median)	*P* Value
INR	>9	1.1	<.001*
aPTT (s)	>180	28.5	<.001*
Fibrinogen (mg/dL)	<50	288	<.001*
D-dimer (ng/mL)	>7,360†	—	—
Factor V (% of normal)	<5†	—	—
Factor VIII (% of normal)	64.7 (42.1)	—	—
Thrombin time	>120	—	—

SD = standard deviation.
*Wilcoxon Test.
†Twenty-one of 22 subjects had immeasurably high D-dimer, and the only subject with measurable D-dimer had a concentration of 3,584 ng/mL.

fresh, normal blood to the patient. This simple study makes me question whether large amounts of shed blood should be replaced in patients where the risk of coagulopathy is real.[2,3]

D. J. Dries, MSE, MD

References

1. Dries DJ. The contemporary role of blood products and components used in trauma resuscitation. *Scand J Trauma Resusc Emerg Med.* 2010;18:63.
2. Rizoli SB, Scarpelini S, Callum J, et al. Clotting factor deficiency in early trauma-associated coagulopathy. *J Trauma.* 2011;71:S427-S434.
3. Aird WC. Coagulation. *Crit Care Med.* 2005;33:S485-S487.

Are Certain Fractures at Increased Risk for Compartment Syndrome After Civilian Ballistic Injury?
Meskey T, Hardcastle J, O'Toole RV (Univ of Maryland School of Medicine, Baltimore)
J Trauma 71:1385-1389, 2011

Background.—Compartment syndrome after ballistic fracture is uncommon but potentially devastating. Few data are available to help guide

TABLE 1.—Rate of Compartment Syndrome for Ballistic Fractures of All Bones

Bone	No. of Fractures	Fractures + Compartment Syndrome, N (%)	p	Risk Factor
Femur	159	4 (2.6)	1.0	0.9
Tibia	79	9 (11.4)	<0.001	4.1
Fibula	69	8 (11.6)	<0.001	4.2
Radius	64	2 (3.1)	1.0	1.1
Ulna	56	2 (3.6)	0.7	1.3
Carpal	23	1 (4.3)	0.3	1.6
Humerus	110	0 (0)	0.06	0
Metacarpal	51	0 (0)	0.6	0
Phalanx (finger)	40	0 (0)	0.62	0
Ilium	69	0 (0)	0.25	0
Scapula	59	0 (0)	0.41	0
Metatarsal	14	0 (0)	1	0
Sacrum	17	0 (0)	1	0
Clavicle	23	0 (0)	1	0
Phalanx (toe)	12	0 (0)	1	0
Patella	8	0 (0)	1	0
Pubic ramus	18	0 (0)	1	0
Ischium	7	0 (0)	1	0
Acetabulum	26	0 (0)	1	0
Calcaneus	12	0 (0)	1	0
Tarsal	8	0 (0)	1	0
Talus	7	0 (0)	1	0
Symphysis pubis	4	0 (0)	1	0
Pelvis	3	0 (0)	1	0
Total	938	26 (2.8)		

clinicians regarding risk factors for developing compartment syndrome after ballistic fractures. Our primary hypothesis was that ballistic fractures of certain bones would be at higher risk for development of compartment syndrome.

Methods.—A retrospective review at a Level I trauma center from 2001 through 2007 yielded 650 patients with 938 fractures resulting from gunshots. We reviewed all operative notes, clinic notes, discharge summaries, and data from our prospective trauma database. Cases in which the attending orthopedic surgeon diagnosed compartment syndrome and performed fasciotomy were considered cases with compartment syndrome. We excluded all prophylactic fasciotomies. Univariate analyses were conducted to identify risk factors associated with development of compartment syndrome.

Results.—Twenty-six (2.8%) of the 938 fractures were associated with compartment syndrome. Only fibular (11.6%) and tibial (11.4%) fractures had incidence significantly higher than baseline for all ballistic fractures ($p < 0.001$). Fractures of the proximal third of the fibula were more likely to result in compartment syndrome than fractures of the middle or distal third ($p = 0.03$), as were fractures of the proximal third of the tibia ($p = 0.01$). No other demographic or injury parameters were associated with compartment syndrome.

Conclusion.—Ballistic fractures of the fibula and tibia are at increased risk for development of compartment syndrome over other ballistic fractures. We recommend increased vigilance when treating these injuries, particularly if the fracture is in the proximal aspect of the bone or is associated with vascular injury (Table 1).

▶ These authors review an extensive experience in gunshot wounds associated with extremity fractures. Tibial and fibular fractures, particularly when occurring proximally and in association with vascular injuries, are at the highest risk for compartment syndrome development. As this is a retrospective study, we are not told details regarding the presentation of these fractures and their outcomes. For example, we are not informed about the amputation rate or the degree of disability associated with compartment syndromes in these patients.

The authors also note a significantly lower rate of compartment syndrome in comparison to previous reports of this complication following ballistic fractures. Whether this represents one of the limitations of this retrospective review is unclear. It is also possible that compartments may have been decompressed by vascular surgeons addressing vascular injuries, which frequently accompany fibular and tibial fractures. The authors note that diagnosis was made using clinical criteria in a large number of patients, whereas compartment pressures were measured in only 43% of patients reported (Table 1). Other fractures with associated compartment syndromes include carpal, ulnar, radial, and femoral fractures.

Clearly, the intensivist admitting patients with ballistic fractures of the proximal leg must be aware of the possibility of compartment syndrome.

Unfortunately, the authors did not report Ankle-Brachial Index (ABI) data. A recent study from the Alameda Trauma Center suggests that evaluation of the ABI successfully identified patients who could be safely discharged with extremity gunshot wounds. Unfortunately, the ABI study did not describe the distribution of gunshot wounds studied.[1]

D. J. Dries, MSE, MD

Reference

1. Sadjadi J, Cureton EL, Dozier KC, Kwan RO, Victorino GP. Expedited treatment of lower extremity gunshot wounds. *J Am Coll Surg.* 2009;209:740-745.

AIS > 2 in at least two body regions: A potential new anatomical definition of polytrauma
Butcher N, Balogh ZJ (John Hunter Hosp and Univ of Newcastle, New South Wales, Australia)
Injury 43:196-199, 2012

Background.—The term 'polytrauma' lacks a universally accepted, validated definition. In clinical trials the commonly applied injury severity based anatomical score cut-offs are ISS > 15, ISS > 17 and a recently recommended AIS > 2 in at least two body regions (2 × AIS > 2).

Purpose.—To compare the outcomes of clinically defined polytrauma patients with those defined based on anatomical scores.

TABLE 1.—Outcomes by Anatomical Definition Used

	N	Polytrauma	Death	ICU Admission	MOF
Total	336	44 (13%)	14 (4%) 0.0252–0.0726	85 (25%) 0.2074–0.3030	10 (3%) 0.0144–0.0541
ISS > 15	131	44 (34%)	13 (10%) 0.0539–0.1637	71 (54%) 0.4527–0.6293	10 (8%) 0.0372–0.1359
ISS > 17	102	40 (39%)	11 (11%) 0.0551–0.1848	63 (62%) 0.5161–0.7121	10 (10%) 0.0480–0.1729
2 × AIS > 2	64	37 (58%)	8 (13%) 0.0555–0.2315	43 (67%) 0.5431–0.7841	9 (14%) 0.0664–0.2502 CI 95%

Polytrauma: clinically defined by expert opinion; ICU: Intensive Care Unit; MOF: multiple organ failure.

Material and Methods.—A prospective observational study on all trauma team activation patients over a 7-month period presenting at a level-1 trauma centre were included in the study. The prospective data collection included AIS in each body region, ISS, ICU length of stay (LOS), multiple organ failure (MOF) and mortality.

Results.—336 patients met inclusion criteria (age: 41 ± 20, 74% male, ISS: 15 ± 11, NISS: 19 ± 15, MOF: 3%, mortality: 4%, 25% ICU admission). ISS > 15: 13 deaths (10%), 71 (54%) required ICU admission and 10 (8%) developed MOF. ISS > 17 captured 11 deaths (11%), with 63 (62%) requiring ICU admission and 10 (10%) developing MOF. Defining as (2 × AIS > 2): 8 deaths (13% of the group), with 43 patients requiring ICU admission (67%) and 9 (14%) developing MOF. When examining the performance of these three approaches, the ISS > 15 and the ISS > 17 captured statistically the same amount of clinically defined polytrauma patients ($p = 0.4106$), while the 2 × AIS > 2 definition captured significantly more polytrauma patients than ISS > 15 ($p = 0.0251$) and ISS > 17 ($p = 0.0019$).

Conclusion.—2 × AIS > 2 captured the greatest percentage of the worst outcomes and significantly larger % of the clinically defined polytrauma patients. 2 × AIS > 2 has higher accuracy and precision in defining polytrauma than ISS > 15 and ISS > 17. This simple, retrospectively also reproducible criteria warrants larger scale validation (Table 1).

▶ These authors examine epidemiologic data and initial outcome data in an attempt to find the optimal measure for high-risk patients having multiple injuries. Gold standard in this assessment is the evaluation by a senior trauma surgeon at the end of the first 24 hours. Obviously, head injury can evolve significantly beyond this period.

This use of the Abbreviated Injury Scale is a way to identify polytrauma, but it does not correlate well with mortality as Table 1 indicates. The authors propose using a scale such as this to enroll patients with multisystem injury in studies. However, the gold standard proposed is a subjective assessment. Clearly, we need to study this approach to identify multiple injury with greater rigor prior to embracing it as a reliable means to identify the multiply injured patient.

Perhaps the greatest confounder is traumatic brain injury. Assessment of patients within the first 24 hours using this system will miss some of the severely affected head-injured patients. Studies wishing to avoid head-injured patients may enroll individuals with diffuse axonal injury or frontal injuries in which clinical deterioration is not immediate.[1-3]

In a word, the Injury Severity Score will continue to be an enrollment standard for clinical trials and chart reviews. Limitations of this approach to injury assessment, particularly caused by underrepresentation of traumatic brain injury, are not addressed in the methodology described here. Finally, this provocative article is based on an extremely small sample set and requires more rigorous validation for serious consideration.

D. J. Dries, MSE, MD

References

1. Chelly H, Chaari A, Daoud E, et al. Diffuse axonal injury in patients with head injuries: an epidemiologic and prognosis study of 124 cases. *J Trauma.* 2011;71: 838-846.
2. Calvi MR, Beretta L, Dell'Acqua A, Anzalone N, Licini G, Gemma M. Early prognosis after severe traumatic brain injury with minor or absent computed tomography scan lesions. *J Trauma.* 2011;70:447-451.
3. Peterson EC, Chesnut RM. Talk and die revisited: bifrontal contusions and late deterioration. *J Trauma.* 2011;71:1588-1592.

Military Application of Tranexamic Acid in Trauma Emergency Resuscitation (MATTERs) Study
Morrison JJ, Dubose JJ, Rasmussen TE, et al (US Army Inst of Surgical Res, Fort Sam Houston, TX; US Air Force Med Service, San Antonio, TX; et al)
Arch Surg 147:113-119, 2012

Objectives.—To characterize contemporary use of tranexamic acid (TXA) in combat injury and to assess the effect of its administration on total blood product use, thromboembolic complications, and mortality.

Design.—Retrospective observational study comparing TXA administration with no TXA in patients receiving at least 1 unit of packed red blood cells. A subgroup of patients receiving massive transfusion (≥ 10 units of packed red blood cells) was also examined. Univariate and multivariate regression analyses were used to identify parameters associated with survival. Kaplan-Meier life tables were used to report survival.

Setting.—A Role 3 Echelon surgical hospital in southern Afghanistan.

Patients.—A total of 896 consecutive admissions with combat injury, of which 293 received TXA, were identified from prospectively collected UK and US trauma registries.

Main Outcome Measures.—Mortality at 24 hours, 48 hours, and 30 days as well as the influence of TXA administration on postoperative coagulopathy and the rate of thromboembolic complications.

Results.—The TXA group had lower unadjusted mortality than the no-TXA group (17.4% vs 23.9%, respectively; $P = .03$) despite being more severely injured (mean [SD] Injury Severity Score, 25.2 [16.6] vs 22.5 [18.5], respectively; $P<.001$). This benefit was greatest in the group of patients who received massive transfusion (14.4% vs 28.1%, respectively; $P = .004$), where TXA was also independently associated with survival (odds ratio $= 7.228$; 95% CI, 3.016-17.322) and less coagulopathy ($P = .003$).

Conclusions.—The use of TXA with blood component-based resuscitation following combat injury results in improved measures of coagulopathy and survival, a benefit that is most prominent in patients requiring massive transfusion. Treatment with TXA should be implemented into clinical practice as part of a resuscitation strategy following severe wartime injury and hemorrhage.

► Coagulopathy after trauma is initiated by tissue injury. It may develop without regard to fluid administration and be seen even before patients arrive in the emergency department. Patients with severe tissue injury but no other physiologic derangement are less likely to present with coagulopathy. If shock and tissue injury coexist, severe coagulopathy is a common occurrence. The combination of tissue injury, shock, and coagulopathy has been associated with increased mortality by Dries and others.[1,2]

Hyperfibrinolysis is a direct consequence of the combination of tissue injury and shock. Endothelial injury accelerates fibrinolysis because of direct release of tissue plasminogen activator. Tissue plasminogen activator expression by endothelium is increased in the presence of thrombin. Fibrinolysis is accelerated because of the combined effects of endothelial tissue plasminogen activator release due to ischemia and inhibition of plasminogen activator inhibitor in shock.

The recent CRASH-2 trial demonstrated that an antifibrinolytic therapy improved outcome in a multicenter, multinational trial of patients featuring a large percentage of blunt injuries.[3] The MATTERs trial demonstrates impressive improvement in outcomes with tranexamic acid administration in soldiers with penetrating injury receiving as little as 1 unit of packed red blood cells. With more data from the CRASH-2 database on the way, it is becoming harder to argue against adding antifibrinolytic therapy to our massive transfusion strategy.

While the outcome in this trial is spectacular, it should be noted that patients were not randomly assigned in this retrospective review (Figs 3 and 4 in the original article). Injury was severe with mean Injury Severity Score greater than 20 in each group. We also need to follow the incidence of venous thromboembolic events, as patients receiving tranexamic acid had a greater incidence of these complications.

Combined with massive transfusion protocols, which originated in the military and are now used in civilian trauma practice, the growing volume of data supporting the use of tranexamic acid for the fibrinolytic component of coagulopathy after trauma is the most exciting development in trauma resuscitation in the last decade.

D. J. Dries, MSE, MD

References

1. Dries DJ. The contemporary role of blood products and components used in trauma resuscitation. *Scand J Trauma Resusc Emerg Med.* 2010;18:63.
2. Brohi K, Cohen MJ, Ganter MT, et al. Acute coagulopathy of trauma: hypoperfusion induces systemic anticoagulation and hyperfibrinolysis. *J Trauma.* 2008;64:1211-1217.
3. CRASH-2 Trial Collaborators, Shakur H, Roberts I, Bautista R, et al. Effects of tranexamic acid on death, vascular occlusive events, and blood transfusion in trauma patients with significant haemorrhage (CRASH-2): a randomised, placebo-controlled trial. *Lancet.* 2010;376:23-32.

Critical Role of Activated Protein C in Early Coagulopathy and Later Organ Failure, Infection and Death in Trauma Patients

Cohen MJ, Call M, Nelson M, et al (Univ of California San Francisco, CA; et al)
Ann Surg 255:379-385, 2012

Background.—Recent studies have identified an acute traumatic coagulopathy that is present on admission to the hospital and is independent of iatrogenic causes. We have previously reported that this coagulopathy is due to the association of severe injury and shock and is characterized by a decrease in plasma protein C (PC) levels. Whether this early coagulopathy and later propensity to infection, multiple organ failure and mortality are associated with the activation of PC pathway has not been demonstrated and constitutes the aim of this study.

Methods and Findings.—This was a prospective cohort study of 203 major trauma patients. Serial blood samples were drawn on arrival in the emergency department, and at 6, 12, and 24 hours after admission to the hospital. PT, PTT, Va, VIIIa, PC apC t-PA, and D-dimer levels were assayed. Comprehensive injury, resuscitation, and outcome data were prospectively collected.

A total of 203 patients were enrolled. Patients with tissue hypoperfusion and severe traumatic injury showed a strong activation of the PC which was associated with a coagulopathy characterized by inactivation of the coagulation factors V and VIII and a derepression of the fibrinolysis with high plasma levels of plasminogen activator and high D-dimers. Elevated plasma levels of activated PC were significantly associated with increased mortality, organ injury, increased blood transfusion requirements, and reduced ICU ventilatorfree days. Finally early depletion of PC after trauma is associated with a propensity to posttraumatic ventilator-associated pneumonia.

Conclusions.—Acute traumatic coagulopathy occurs in the presence of tissue hypoperfusion and severe traumatic injury and is mediated by activation of the PC pathway. Higher plasma levels of apC upon admission are predictive of poor clinical outcomes after major trauma. After activation, patients who fail to recover physiologic plasma values of PC have an increased propensity to later nosocomial lung infection (Tables 3-5).

▶ This article is an important extension of seminal work performed by this group to examine the acute coagulopathy of trauma. We now realize that coagulopathy

TABLE 3.—Logistic Regression of Protein C System Effects on Outcome

Predictor	Dependent	OR	CI	P
apC/PC ratio	VAP	2.4	1.6–2.62	0.024
apC/PC ratio	MOF	1.585	1.0–2.5	0.050
apC/PC ratio	ALI	1.894	1.1–3.1	0.01
apC/PC ratio	Mortality	2.1	1.4–3.3	0.0007

apC/PC ratio indicates ratio between plasma levels of activated protein C and protein C zymogen at the admission to the hospital.

TABLE 4.—Activation of Protein C and Hospital Outcome

Predictor	Dependent	B	CI	P
aPC/PC ratio	Ventilator days	5.63	3.49–7.77	<0.0001
aPC/PC ratio	ICU days	5.26	3.23–7.30	<0.0001
aPC/PC ratio	Hospital days	4.17	2.40–5.94	<0.0001

TABLE 5.—Relationship Between Depletion of Protein C Over Time and Outcome

Predictor	Dependent	OR	CI	P
12 hour PC depletion	VAP	.985	0.97–0.99	0.04
Balanced PC response	VAP	Referent		
Moderate depleters	VAP	1.6	0.7–4.1	0.2
PC depleters	VAP	2.7	1.05–6.8	0.04

can occur without hemodilution and can be seen even before patients reach the emergency department. Important factors leading to early coagulopathy after injury are hypoperfusion and volume of injured tissue.

These authors make important observations regarding the contributions of the activated protein C system to coagulopathy after injury. It appears that exaggerated activation of protein C may enhance the coagulopathy after injury. Recognition of this coagulopathy has led to evaluation of equivalent administration of platelets, fresh frozen plasma, and packed red blood cells in patients with significant bleeding after injury.[1]

We also recognize that hemorrhage and tissue injury after trauma affect an immunologic cascade similar to that seen in sepsis. An abundance of preclinical work and some clinical data support depletion of activated protein C as a cofactor for increased infection risk. These authors provide supportive data as they examine ventilator-associated pneumonia in a trauma population. Depletion of activated protein C in the days after injury is associated with increased pneumonia rates (Tables 3-5). Ironically, despite early promise, activated protein C therapy for sepsis has now been withdrawn from the market due to lack of consistent clinical data favoring efficacy.[2]

There are a number of important limitations in this work. Perhaps most important, the authors do not have preinjury samples; thus, they report activated protein C to protein C ratios. Second, thresholds for recognition of depletion of activated protein C are not clear from these data. Thus, we need far more information before a replacement strategy can be considered. Third, some of the statistics in this single-center study do not demonstrate strong associations between the clotting factor levels obtained in the chaotic environment of injury.

D. J. Dries, MSE, MD

References

1. Dries DJ. The contemporary role of blood products and components used in trauma resuscitation. *Scand J Trauma Resusc Emerg Med.* 2010;18:63.
2. Bernard GR, Vincent JL, Laterre PF, et al. Efficacy and safety of recombinant human activated protein C for severe sepsis. *N Engl J Med.* 2001;344:699-709.

Early complementopathy after multiple injuries in humans
Burk A-M, Martin M, Flierl MA, et al (Univ Hosp Ulm, Germany; Lund Univ, Malmö, Sweden; et al)
Shock 37:348-354, 2012

After severe tissue injury, innate immunity mounts a robust systemic inflammatory response. However, little is known about the immediate impact of multiple trauma on early complement function in humans. In the present study, we hypothesized that multiple trauma results in immediate activation, consumption, and dysfunction of the complement cascade and that the resulting severe "complementopathy" may be associated with morbidity and mortality. Therefore, a prospective multicenter study with 25 healthy volunteers and 40 polytrauma patients (mean injury severity score = 30.3 ± 2.9) was performed. After polytrauma, serum was collected as early as possible at the scene, on admission to the emergency room (ER), and 4, 12, 24, 120, and 240 h post-trauma and analyzed for the complement profile. Complement hemolytic activity (CH-50) was massively reduced within the first 24 h after injury, recovered only 5 days after trauma, and discriminated between lethal and nonlethal 28-day outcome. Serum levels of the complement activation products C3a and C5a were

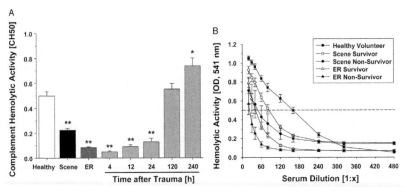

FIGURE 1.—A, Complement function after multiple injuries as assessed by hemolytic serum activity (CH-50) determined from either healthy volunteers (n = 25) or polytraumatized patients (n = 40) with a mean ISS of 30.3 ± 2.9 at several time points after injury. *P < 0.05, **P < 0.01 between trauma group and healthy volunteers. B, Comparison of complement hemolytic serum activity between healthy volunteers, survivors, and nonsurvivors at the scene and at admission to the emergency room (ER). (Reprinted from Burk A-M, Martin M, Flierl MA, et al. Early complementopathy after multiple injuries in humans. *Shock.* 2012;37:348-354, with permission from the Shock Society.)

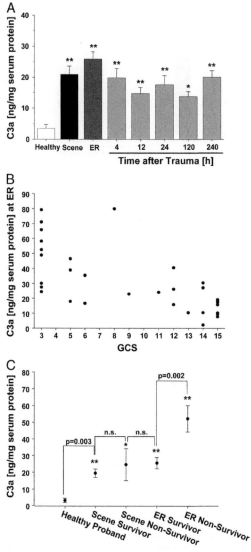

FIGURE 2.—A, Generation of C3a as a function of time after polytrauma. *P < 0.05, **P < 0.01 between trauma group and healthy volunteers. B, Inverse correlation between serum concentration of C3a in the emergency room (ER) and initial severity of traumatic brain injury, as assessed by the Glasgow Coma Scale (GCS). C, Subgroup analysis of serum C3a concentrations at the scene or at admission to the ER obtained from healthy volunteers, survivors, and nonsurvivors. (Reprinted from Burk A-M, Martin M, Flierl MA, et al. Early complementopathy after multiple injuries in humans. *Shock.* 2012;37:348-354, with permission from the Shock Society.)

significantly elevated throughout the entire observation period and corre-lated with the severity of traumatic brain injury and survival. The soluble terminal complement complex SC5b-9 and mannose-binding lectin showed a biphasic response after trauma. Key fluid-phase inhibitors of

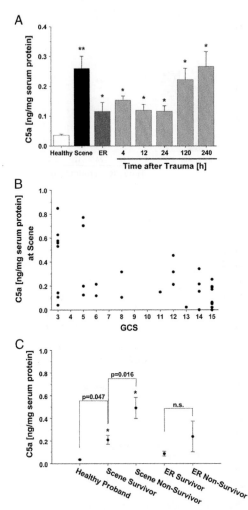

FIGURE 3.—A, Trauma-induced generation of the anaphylatoxin C5a in serum of polytraumatized patients ($n = 40$) versus healthy controls ($n = 25$). $*P < 0.05$, $**P < 0.01$ versus healthy volunteers. B, Inverse correlation of C5a serum concentration at the scene (25.1 ± 1.4 min after injury) and initial Glasgow Coma Scale (GCS), reflecting primary traumatic brain injury. C, Differences in C5a concentrations in serum obtained from polytrauma survivors and nonsurvivors early after injury. (Reprinted from Burk A-M, Martin M, Flierl MA, et al. Early complementopathy after multiple injuries in humans. *Shock.* 2012;37:348-354, with permission from the Shock Society.)

complement, such as C4b-binding protein and factor I, were significantly diminished early after trauma. The present data indicate an almost synchronical rapid activation and dysfunction of complement, suggesting a trauma-induced complementopathy early after injury. These events may participate in the impairment of the innate immune response observed after severe trauma (Figs 1-3).

▶ The complement system is an early and sometimes nonspecific defense against threats to the host. Activation products such as C3a, C5a, and membrane attack complexes play a crucial role in host defense. As noted by these authors, while complement is thought to be present in many of the host responses to stress, there are relatively little data on complement response to trauma.

These data provide evidence of activation and consumption of complement shortly after severe trauma (Figs 1-3). Even at the incident scene, dramatic elevation in complement factors is seen.

Previous studies suggest that increased concentrations of C3a in serum or bronchoalveolar lavage fluid may predict posttraumatic development of acute respiratory distress syndrome.[1,2] This is not borne out in later work or in this study. Notably, this report suggests a correlation between C3a and C5a with severity of traumatic brain injury. However, the number of patients studied was small.

I believe it is premature to draw any clinical conclusions from this work. However, this article adds to the data documenting derangement of blood-borne host defense occurring within minutes after injury and an ebb-and-flow pattern, which seems to parallel that seen with protein C, a more popular target of contemporary studies of posttraumatic coagulopathy.[3]

D. J. Dries, MSE, MD

References

1. Roumen RM, Redl H, Schlag G, et al. Inflammatory mediators in relation to the development of multiple organ failure in patients after severe blunt trauma. *Crit Care Med.* 1995;23:474-480.
2. Zilow G, Joka T, Obertacke U, Rother U, Kirschfink M. Generation of anaphylatoxin C3a in plasma and bronchoalveolar lavage fluid in trauma patients at risk for the adult respiratory distress syndrome. *Crit Care Med.* 1992;20:468-473.
3. Cohen MJ, Call M, Nelson M, et al. Critical role of activated protein C in early coagulopathy and later organ failure, infection and death in trauma patients. *Ann Surg.* 2012;255:379-385.

Tympanic Membrane Rupture in the Survivors of the July 7, 2005, London Bombings
Radford P, Patel HDL, Hamilton N, et al (Barts and the London NHS Trust, UK; et al)
Otolaryngol Head Neck Surg 145:806-812, 2011

Objective.—The goal of this study was to analyze the prevalence of tympanic membrane rupture in the survivors of the London bombings of July 2005 and to assess whether tympanic membrane rupture provides a useful biomarker for underlying primary blast injuries.
Study Design.—Cross-sectional study.

TABLE 1.—Categories of Blast Injury

Class	Mechanism	Common Pathology
Primary	Blast overpressure from high explosives Interacts with air—soft tissue interface in the body	Tympanic membrane rupture Pulmonary barotrauma Gastrointestinal tract rupture or hemorrhage Traumatic brain injury/concussion Traumatic amputation
Secondary	Fragments and debris from the blast or objects affected by the blast (eg, human impact projectiles)	Penetrating injuries affecting any part of the body
Tertiary	The blast wave knocks over or throws victims, causing impact with surrounding solid objects and the floor	Fractures/amputations of limbs Open/closed brain injury
Quaternary	Any other form of injury or exacerbation of existing disease caused by the blast	Burns Exacerbation of respiratory disease Angina, myocardial infarction Crush injuries

TABLE 2.—Data and Analysis

Total survivors, No.	143
Total TMR, No. (%)	69 (48%)
Total primary blast injury (non-TMR), No. (%)	16 (11%)
Total concealed primary blast injury, No. (%)	2 (1.4%)
TMR as a biomarker for other primary blast injuries, %	
Positive predictive value	16
Negative predictive value	92
Sensitivity	65
Specificity	53
TMR as a biomarker for concealed primary blast injury, %	
Positive predictive value	1.4
Negative predictive value	99
Sensitivity	50
Specificity	50

Abbreviation: TMR, tympanic membrane rupture.

Subjects and Methods.—Survivors of the 4 blasts of London bombings on July 7, 2005. Data were gathered from medical records and the London's Metropolitan Police evidence documenting the injuries sustained by 143 survivors of the blasts. All patients with tympanic membrane rupture or primary blast injury were identified. Analysis was made of distance against prevalence of tympanic membrane rupture. Correlation between tympanic membrane rupture and other forms of primary blast injury was then assessed.

Results.—Results from the 143 survivors showed a 48% prevalence of tympanic membrane rupture across all 4 sites. Fifty-one patients had isolated tympanic membrane rupture with no other primary blast injuries.

Eleven patients had tympanic membrane rupture and other primary blast injuries, but only one of these was an initially concealed injury (blast lung).

Conclusions.—Tympanic membrane rupture in survivors of the London bombings on July 7, 2005, had a high prevalence affecting half of patients across a range of distances from the blasts. Tympanic membrane did not act as an effective biomarker of underlying blast lung. In a mass casualty event, patients with isolated tympanic membrane rupture with normal observations and chest radiography can be monitored for a short period and safely discharged with arrangement for ear, nose, and throat follow-up (Tables 1 and 2).

▶ Historically, tympanic membrane rupture has been a marker of significant blast injury.[1,2] These authors demonstrate, with careful data analysis from the recent London train bombings, that a consistent pattern of tympanic membrane rupture related to distance from the blast is not seen and tympanic membrane rupture is not a consistent marker of internal blast injury. This is consistent with other more recent reports on this subject.[3] Thus, whereas patients involved in blast injury must be carefully screened for tympanic membrane rupture, a relationship between this injury and other trauma cannot be clearly made.

An explanation for this finding is included in the excellent introduction to this article. The authors nicely review the categories of blast injury (Table 1). It is important to note that in each case discussed here, blast injury occurred in a closed space. Thus, the classic compression, decompression sequence found when blast injury occurred in an open environment will not be identified. In addition, the authors note position of survivors in the various bombing sites but do not note the location of the dead. Patients wearing earphones or patients shielded by nonsurvivors could be spared tympanic membrane rupture because of headgear or the presence of the bodies of nonsurvivors.

I recommend this article for the careful data summary (Table 2). However, I believe the authors best demonstrate the capricious nature of blast injury, particularly when detonation occurs in a closed space and survivors may be shielded by victims of the blast.

D. J. Dries, MSE, MD

References

1. Leibovici D, Gofrit ON, Shapira SC. Eardrum perforation in explosion survivors: is it a marker of pulmonary blast injury? *Ann Emerg Med.* 1999;34:168-172.
2. Patow CA, Bartels J, Dodd KT. Tympanic membrane perforation in survivors of a SCUD missile explosion. *Otolaryngol Head Neck Surg.* 1994;110:211-221.
3. Harrison CD, Bebarta VS, Grant GA. Tympanic membrane perforation after combat blast exposure in Iraq: a poor biomarker of primary blast injury. *J Trauma.* 2009;67:210-211.

Multiple Organ Failure as a Cause of Death in Patients With Severe Burns
Kallinen O, Maisniemi K, Böhling T, et al (Helsinki Univ Hosp, Finland; Helsinki Univ and HUSLAB, Finland)
J Burn Care Res 33:206-211, 2012

The aim of this study was to investigate the causes of death in patients with burns using both medicolegal autopsy reports and clinical data collected during treatment to specify irreversible organ dysfunctions leading to death. Burn deaths occurring in the Helsinki Burn Center from 1995 to 2005 were identified in the hospital database. The clinical charts and medicolegal autopsy reports were retrieved and compared. The data were evaluated by plastic surgeons specialized in burn care, an intensivist, and a pathologist, with special reference to organ-specific changes in the autopsy reports. From 1999 to 2005, there were 71 burn deaths in the Helsinki Burn Center of which 40% was caused by multiple organ failure (MOF). Death from untreatable burn injury was recorded in 28 patients, whereas other causes were scarce. MOF patients displayed approximately four organ failures on average, ranging from three to eight. All 28 MOF patients were recorded to have acute renal failure, followed by liver damage, of which four patients had acute or chronic liver failure. Sepsis was always affiliated with MOF as a cause of death. In conclusion, careful examination of MOF as a cause of death revealed several organ failures: four organ failures per patient. Acute renal failure was noted in all MOF patients. Sepsis was always affiliated with MOF.

▶ It is encouraging to see this well-written article from Finland regarding burn care, as Finnish articles related to burn care in the English-speaking literature are infrequently encountered. Having a national law mandating autopsy for all patients who die as a result of burn trauma created the ideal database to evaluate. The only unfortunate piece of the puzzle is the small population size of Finland (5.3 million), making this study a small one. The retrospective nature of the study prevents us from drawing conclusions that directly connect cause and effect. However, the association of renal failure in 100% of the burn deaths is noteworthy. Is the renal failure due to unrecognized or undertreated burn shock, is it caused by unresuscitatable burn shock, or does it merely serve as a marker for a lethal injury regardless of treatment modalities? Some of the more interesting findings such as a superior mesenteric artery embolism followed by bowel necrosis and pulmonary embolism may have been noted in the antemortem hospital course and are preventable causes of death. As the authors noted, a larger sample size will be necessary to address these questions.

The National Burn Repository (NBR) of the American Burn Association is moving toward a method whereby members of the organization will be able to query the NBR database and obtain answers to these questions using patient and institutionally deidentified data. Perhaps the authors have already done this, but if not, I would encourage them to do so. If you reside in a state where autopsy is not a legal requirement for patients succumbing to burn injuries, I encourage everyone to attempt to obtain an autopsy. As the authors of this article note, there were some findings that seemed unexpected. Be sure that autopsy discussions are part of your quality improvement program.

B. A. Latenser, MD, FACS

11 Ethics/Socioeconomic/ Administrative Issues

Other

Patient Understanding of Emergency Department Discharge Instructions: Where Are Knowledge Deficits Greatest?

Engel KG, Buckley BA, Forth VE, et al (Northwestern Univ, Chicago, IL; Northwestern Memorial Hosp, Chicago, IL)
Acad Emerg Med 19:1035-1044, 2012

Objectives.—Many patients are discharged from the emergency department (ED) with an incomplete understanding of the information needed to safely care for themselves at home. Patients have demonstrated particular difficulty in understanding post-ED care instructions (including medications, home care, and follow-up). The objective of this study was to further characterize these deficits and identify gaps in knowledge that may place the patient at risk for complications or poor outcomes.

Methods.—This was a prospective cohort, phone interview—based study of 159 adult English-speaking patients within 24 to 36 hours of ED discharge. Patient knowledge was assessed for five diagnoses (ankle sprain, back pain, head injury, kidney stone, and laceration) across the following five domains: diagnosis, medications, home care, follow-up, and return instructions. Knowledge was determined based on the concordance between direct patient recall and diagnosis-specific discharge instructions combined with chart review. Two authors scored each case independently and discussed discrepancies before providing a final score for each domain (no, minimal, partial, or complete comprehension). Descriptive statistics were used for the analyses.

Results.—The study population was 50% female with a median age of 41 years (interquartile range [IQR] = 29 to 53 years). Knowledge deficits were demonstrated by the majority of patients in the domain of home care instructions (80%) and return instructions (79%). Less frequent deficits were found for the domains of follow-up (39%), medications (22%), and diagnosis (14%). Minimal or no understanding in at least one domain was demonstrated by greater than two-thirds of patients and was found in 40% of cases for home care and 51% for return instructions. These deficits occurred less frequently for domains of follow-up (18%), diagnosis (3%), and medications (3%).

Conclusions.—Patients demonstrate the most frequent knowledge deficits for home care and return instructions, raising significant concerns for adherence and outcomes.

▶ Communicating effectively with patients in the emergency department is challenging. This study examined a very key part of communication and understanding during the patient visit—discharge instructions. Previous work by the same authors showed that patients had comprehension deficits across the entire emergency department visit. The current study delved further into comprehension of discharge instructions in particular. A total of 159 patients with 5 common diagnoses were called and interviewed shortly after their visit by trained nurses. Only 70% of patients actually read their instructions. Fortunately, their comprehension was better than those who didn't. A total of 92% of all patients showed a deficit of comprehension in at least 1 area of the instructions and 66% showed a severe deficit, including 11 with a "dangerous" misunderstanding. Home care instructions and "return if worse" instructions showed by far the greatest deficits. This was a nicely done study, although the questions were not validated to see if they really represented patient knowledge, and it is unclear as to the clinical relevance of these misunderstandings/deficits. More than anything, this study serves as a reminder that communication is difficult and that we need to be diligent in reviewing discharge instructions with patients. Whether a better way exists to get the information across to patients (eg, phone texting, email) remains to be determined.

M. D. Zwank, MD

A systematic review of the evidence for telemedicine in burn care: With a UK perspective
Wallace DL, Hussain A, Khan N, et al (Queen Elizabeth Hosp Birmingham, Edgbaston, UK; Univ Hosp of South Manchester, Manchester, UK; Birmingham Children's Hosp, Birmingham, UK)
Burns 38:465-480, 2012

A comprehensive systematic review of telemedicine in burn care was carried out. Studies published between 1993 and 2010 were included. The main outcome measures were the level of evidence, technical feasibility, clinical feasibility, clinical management and cost effectiveness. The search strategy yielded 24 studies, none of which were randomised. There were only five studies with a control group, and in three of these the patients act as their own controls. Four studies performed quantitative cost analysis, and five more provide qualitative cost analysis. All studies demonstrate technical and clinical feasibility. If the significant potentials of telemedicine to assist in the acute triage, management guidance and outpatient care are to be realised, then research needs to be undertaken to provide evidence for such investment.

▶ The improvements in telecommunication have made it possible for health care providers to effectively and efficiently exchange patient information regarding multiple medical conditions, including burns.[1] The addition of visual communication enables the burn specialist to deliver care to rural emergency rooms or those hospitals geographically distant from burn centers. The initial treatment of burn patients requires a complex skill set that receives little emphasis in traditional medical education. Providers must possess knowledge of the typical presentation of burns, be able to determine burn size, calculate fluid needs, and establish a safe airway prior to transfer. Inaccurate initial treatment can have devastating consequences on the subsequent management of the burn patient. As burn care becomes increasingly restricted to larger metropolitan centers, the ability to provide accurate assistance to the transferring center becomes critical. A system enabling visualization of the burn injury and instantaneous feedback to the rural health care worker would improve the initial care of the burn patient. Ultimately, the optimal outcome of the burn patient begins with the earliest stages of assessment and treatment. Let us embrace the current technology and make it an integral part of our practices.

B. A. Latenser, MD, FACS

Reference

1. Holt B, Faraklas I, Theurer L, Cochran A, Saffle JR. Telemedicine use among burn centers in the United States: a survey. *J Burn Care Res.* 2012;33:157-162.

Predictors of health-care needs in discharged burn patients
Liang CY, Wang HJ, Yao KP, et al (Natl Defense Med Ctr, Taipei, Taiwan; Taipei Med Univ, Taiwan; Natl Taiwan Univ, Taipei; et al)
Burns 38:172-179, 2012

Patients' health-care needs are an important issue, but have not been studied in the burn field. The aims of this study were to explore discharged burn patients' health-care needs and related factors. This cross-sectional study used convenience sampling and four questionnaires, including basic information, Mental Status Inventory, Burn Patients' Social Support and Burn Patients' Healthcare Needs for data collection. There were 93 adults, injured on average 45% of total body surface area, who completed the study. Results indicated that the level of psychosocial care needs were higher than physiological needs. The level of physiological care needs changed over time, but psychosocial needs did not change. Self-reported psychosocial needs and physiological care needs correlated with each other. The multiple regressions showed that the most important predictors of overall health-care needs were numbers of visible scarred areas, time since discharge and previous psychiatric history. The findings revealed the burn patients provided clinically useful information and supported further evaluation in the area of care needs for burn patients.

▶ This study of adult burn survivors involves a convenience sample of patients in a plastic surgery clinic in Taipei, Taiwan. The findings are generally not surprising: as time from burn injury extended, the patients reported less impact on their activities of daily living but no decrement in the need for psychosocial support. The presence of scars limited to a location invisible when burn survivors were out in public did not negate the difficulties the patients reported in dealing with the "hidden" scars. Health care practitioners have reported that they do not have adequate training or personnel to help deal with the psychological impact of a burn. Because burns by and large are diseases of the poor, the patient and family may be left without the financial resources to obtain the help they need. According to Benjamin Franklin in *Poor Richard's Almanac*, "an ounce of prevention is worth a pound of cure." Nowhere is that more true than in preventing acute stress disorder within 30 days of the burn injury, or posttraumatic stress disorder when lasting > 30 days after the event. Robust psychological help must be available to the patient and family both during and after acute hospitalization. Personnel with appropriate skill sets to help the patient achieve maximal psychosocial outcomes should be part of every burn center around the world.

B. A. Latenser, MD, FACS

Evaluation of long term health-related quality of life in extensive burns: a 12-year experience in a burn center
Xie B, Xiao S-C, Zhu S-H, et al (The Second Military Med Univ, Shanghai, People's Republic of China)
Burns 38:348-355, 2012

Objectives.—We sought to evaluate the long term health-related quality of life (HRQOL) in patients survived severely extensive burn and identify their clinical predicting factors correlated with HRQOL.

Methods.—A cross-sectional study was conducted in 20 patients survived more than 2 years with extensive burn involving ≥70% total body surface area (TBSA) between 1997 and 2009 in a burn center in Shanghai. Short Form-36 Medical Outcomes Survey (SF-36), Brief Version of Burn Specific Health Scale (BSHS-B) and Michigan Hand Outcome Questionnaire (MHQ) were used for the present evaluation. SF-36 scores were compared with a healthy Chinese population, and linear correlation analysis was performed to screen the clinical relating factors predicting physical and mental component summary (PCS and MCS) scores from SF-36.

Results.—HRQOL scores from SF-36 were significantly lower in the domains of physical functioning, role limitations due to physical problems, pain, social functioning and role limitations due to emotional problems compared with population norms. Multiple linear regression analysis demonstrated that only return to work (RTW) predicted improved PCS.

While age at injury, facial burns, skin grafting and length of hospital stay were correlated with MCS. Work, body image and heat sensitivity obtained the lowest BSHS-B scores in all 9 domains. Improvements of HRQOL could still be seen in BSHS-B scores in domains of simple abilities, hand function, work and affect even after a quite long interval between burns and testing. Hand function of extensive burn patients obtained relatively poor MHQ scores, especially in those without RTW.

Conclusions.—Patients with extensive burns have a poorer quality of life compared with that of general population. Relatively poor physical and psychological problems still exist even after a long period. Meanwhile, a trend of gradual improvements was noted. This information will aid clinicians in decision-making of comprehensive systematic regimens for long term rehabilitation and psychosocial treatment.

▶ Although only 20 of 74 eligible patients completed the survey, this work from the Changhai Hospital in Shanghai has some very noteworthy findings. Similar to burn patients from the United States with major burn injuries, most of these patients sustained burns from flame injuries, and all of them sustained inhalation injuries. Unlike United States burn patients, most of these patients were injured at work. Hands and faces were always involved, and most patients underwent skin grafting to both areas. The length of stay in the burn center associated with the primary event was shorter than for those in the United States, but then only one-fourth of patients were discharged to in-patient rehabilitation centers. One major noteworthy difference is that in this society, the employer is responsible for the economic burden of the burn center stay but not the rehabilitation stay. In a low-income country, going to a rehabilitation center is beyond most workers' means. One of the most interesting findings is that improvements were noted for up to 4 years postburn in the areas of hand function, work, and affect. In the United States, it is common practice to perform an evaluation of patients at 12 months and complete a maximal medical improvement for the employer, indicating the patient has achieved the highest level of wellness he or she can attain postburn. Perhaps burn injury is an area where we should evaluate this practice and see if we are doing this too early. Since return to work (RTW) was the main predictor of how an individual did on health-related quality of life, every effort should be made to optimize the opportunity for the severely burned patient to RTW, even if job retraining is required. Not only will this benefit the patient, but it also benefits the family and decreases the financial burden to society.

B. A. Latenser, MD, FACS

Burn size and survival probability in paediatric patients in modern burn care: a prospective observational cohort study

Kraft R, Herndon DN, Al-Mousawi AM, et al (Univ of Texas Med Branch, Galveston)
Lancet 379:1013-1021, 2012

Background.—Patient survival after severe burn injury is largely determined by burn size. Modern developments in burn care have greatly improved survival and outcomes. However, no large analysis of outcomes in paediatric burn patients with present treatment regimens exists. This study was designed to identify the burn size associated with significant increases in morbidity and mortality in paediatric patients.

Methods.—We undertook a single-centre prospective observational cohort study using clinical data for paediatric patients with burns of at least 30% of their total body surface area (TBSA). Patients were stratified by burn size in 10% increments, ranging from 30% to 100% TBSA, with a secondary assignment made according to the outcome of a receiver operating characteristic (ROC) analysis. Statistical analysis was done with Student's t test, χ^2 test, logistic regression, and ROC analysis, as appropriate, with significance set at $p<0\cdot05$.

Findings.—952 severely burned paediatric patients were admitted to the centre between 1998 and 2008. All groups were comparable in age (mean $7\cdot3$ [SD $5\cdot3$] years, ranging from $6\cdot1$ [$5\cdot1$] years in the 30−39% TBSA group to $9\cdot6$ [$5\cdot4$] years in the 90−100% TBSA group) and sex distribution (628 [66%] boys, ranging from 59% [73/123] in the 60−69% TBSA group to 82% [42/51] in the 90−100% TBSA group). 123 (13%) patients died (increasing from 3% [five of 180] in the 30−39% TBSA group to 55% [28/51] in the 90−100% TBSA group; $p<0\cdot0001$), 154 (16%) developed multiorgan failure (increasing from 6% [ten] in the 30−39% TBSA group to 45% [23] in the 90−100% TBSA group; $p<0\cdot0001$), and 89 (9%) had sepsis (increasing from 2% [three] in the 30−39% TBSA group to 26% [13] in the 90−100% TBSA group; $p<0\cdot0001$). Burn size of 62% TBSA was a crucial threshold for mortality (odds ratio $10\cdot07$, 95% CI $5\cdot56−18\cdot22$, $p<0\cdot0001$).

Interpretation.—We established that, in a modern paediatric burn care setting, a burn size of roughly 60% TBSA is a crucial threshold for postburn morbidity and mortality. On the basis of these findings, we recommend that paediatric patients with greater than 60% TBSA burns be immediately transferred to a specialised burn centre. Furthermore, at the burn centre, patients should be treated with increased vigilance and improved therapies, in view of the increased risk of poor outcome associated with this burn size.

▶ This is quite an interesting study. In reality, it's several studies in one. When taken in a vacuum, the data show a tipping point[1] for mortality with respect to burn size in children: around 60% total body surface area (TBSA) burn. Based on these data, the authors conclude that children with burns greater than 60% TBSA should be transferred to "a specialized burn center"; however, the authors fail to provide their definition of a specialized burn center. Do the authors feel that children with large burns should be treated in burn centers that are verified by the American Burn Association via a process that says successfully verified centers meet or exceed a certain set of standards? Perhaps the authors feel that these severely burned children should be cared for in exclusively pediatric burn centers. Or perhaps the authors feel that only a Shriners Hospital specializing in burn care for children is the appropriate place to care for these children. There are currently 61 verified burn centers, with 17 being designated as adult only and 6 being pediatric only.

There are 91 burn centers contributing deidentified data to the 183 036 patients in the American Burn Association's 2012 National Burn Repository (NBR),[2] and 52 243 are under 16 years of age. Using the 16% mortality rate in this article to create a comparable tipping point to compare with the NBR, we find that in the 0 to 12 months category, the tipping point is 40% to 49% TBSA; at ages 1 to 2 years, the tipping point is 50% to 59% TBSA; at ages 2 to 5 years, the tipping point is also 50% to 59% TBSA; at ages 5 to 15 years, the tipping point is 70% to 79% TBSA. Perhaps patients in this "specialized institution" have already met the survival-of-the-fittest criteria, as they arrive at this burn center some 2 to 4 days postburn, and those destined to die from burn shock in the early period will probably not make it from their referring institution. A superficial analysis does make it seem like burn centers currently caring for the severely burned pediatric patient (who traditionally has a shorter time from burn injury to arrival at a burn center) are caring for burns with roughly the same mortality rates, albeit with slightly worse outcomes for the 0-month-old to 12-month-old severely burned patients.

What would be of great interest is to know the real functional outcome measures for these children between the single institution studied in the article and the larger data pool representing all the children in the NBR. Speaking about mortality rates is really not relevant at this stage of burn care in high-income countries. If patients in this specialized institution have better long-term outcomes than in other burn centers, the authors should have supported their claim with valid data. Until then, I believe burned children are being safely and well cared for in a burn center that is closer to their family, where life goes on.

B. A. Latenser, MD, FACS

References

1. Gladwell M. *The Tipping Point: How Little Things Can Make a Big Difference.* Boston MA, Little Brown; 2000.
2. *2012 National Burn Repository Report of Data from 2002–2011.* 2012. American Burn Association, National Burn Repository®; 2012. Version 8.0.

Impact of Intensive Care Unit Organ Failures on Mortality during the Five Years after a Critical Illness

Lone NI, Walsh TS (Univ of Edinburgh, UK)
Am J Respir Crit Care Med 186:640-647, 2012

Rationale.—The relationship between organ failure during critical illness and long-term survival is uncertain, especially among intensive care unit (ICU) survivors.

Objectives.—To describe the relationship between individual organ failures, total organ failure burden, and mortality during the 5 years after an episode of critical illness.

Methods.—We studied a cohort of sequential admissions to 10 Scottish ICUs (n = 872). Logistic regression was used to explore independent associations between organ failures and mortality over a 5-year time horizon, adjusting for potential confounders.

Measurements and Main Results.—Daily Sequential Organ Failure Assessment scores described organ dysfunction during ICU stay. The sum of the worst scores at any time point during the ICU stay for each organ system except neurological dysfunction was used to calculate total organ failure burden. Mortality was obtained from the national death register. Five-year mortality was 58.2%; 34.4% of deaths occurred within 28 days. In adjusted analyses, cardiovascular (odds ratio [OR], 2.5; 95% confidence interval [CI], 1.8–3.7), liver (OR, 2.3; 95% CI, 1.1–5.0), and respiratory failure (OR, 2.1; 95% CI, 1.3–3.5) were independently associated with 5-year mortality. Organ failure burden was strongly associated with mortality; 81% of patients in the highest tertile died during follow-up (OR, 6.3 relative to lowest tertile; $P < 0.001$). Patients surviving more than 12 months post-ICU were still more likely to subsequently die if they experienced greater organ failure burden in the ICU (OR, 2.4; $P = 0.02$, highest vs. lowest tertile).

Conclusions.—Cardiovascular, respiratory, and liver failures during critical illness strongly predict subsequent 5-year survival. Acute organ failure burden is associated with long-term mortality even among patients who survive up to 1 year after ICU admission.

▶ These authors use the extensive Audit of Transfusion in Intensive Care in Scotland (ATICS) study.[1] Thus, I immediately note that we are seeing data that were collected for another purpose in this article. A second key observation is the elimination of patients with primary neurological diagnoses. In trauma, for example, neurologic outcomes have a significant impact on long-term survival and quality of life. These data on organ failure outcomes clearly do not represent a complete prospective dataset.

Remarkably, hepatic dysfunction has a major outcome effect but data allowing consistent assessment of hepatic insufficiency are missing in multiple patients. This patient population most commonly presented with respiratory failure (more than 82% of subjects).[2]

Finally, the authors point out that intensive care unit bed availability in Scotland is less than in many neighboring countries. This may contribute to a higher acuity patient population in this trial. Unfortunately, no scoring data are available to compare the Scottish experience with the critical care populations in neighboring countries.

The most helpful observation is contained in Fig 3 in the original article. If we examine the "modified" Sequential Organ Failure Assessment score data presented, we can see the stratification of outcome over the years following intensive care unit admission. Despite the limitations given here, development of this dataset is an important step toward confirming the incremental impact of organ failure on long-term outcome after critical illness.[3]

D. J. Dries, MSE, MD

References

1. Walsh TS, Garrioch M, Maciver C, et al; Audit of Transfusion in Intensive Care in Scotland Study Group. Red cell requirements for intensive care units adhering to evidence-based transfusion guidelines. *Transfusion.* 2004;44:1405-1411.
2. Williams TA, Dobb GJ, Finn JC, et al. Determinants of long-term survival after intensive care. *Crit Care Med.* 2008;36:1523-1530.
3. Herridge MS, Tansey CM, Matté A, et al; Canadian Critical Care Trials Group. Functional disability 5 years after acute respiratory distress syndrome. *N Engl J Med.* 2011;364:1293-1304.

Quality of Life/End of Life/Outcome Prediction

Do-not-resuscitate order: a view throughout the world
Santonocito C, Ristagno G, Gullo A, et al (Med School of Catania, Italy; Mario Negri Inst for Pharmacological Res, Milan, Italy; et al)
J Crit Care 28:14-21, 2013

Resuscitation has the ability to reverse premature death. It can also prolong terminal illness, increase discomfort, and consume resources. The do-not-resuscitate (DNR) order and advance directives are still a debated issue in critical care. This review will focus on several aspects, regarding withholding and/or withdrawing therapies and advance directives in different continents. It is widely known that there is a great diversity of cultural and religious beliefs in society, and therefore, some critical ethical and legal issues have still to be solved. To achieve a consensus, we believe in the priority of continuing education and training programs for health care professionals. It is our opinion that a serious reflection on ethical values and principles would be useful to understand the definition of medical professionalism to make it possible to undertake the best way to avoid futile and aggressive care. There is evidence of the lack of DNR order policy worldwide. Therefore, it appears clear that there is a need for standardization. To improve the attitude about the DNR order, it is necessary to achieve several goals such as: increased communication, consensus on law, increased trust among patients and health care systems, and improved standards and quality of care to respect the patient's will and the family's role.

▶ In recent decades, mankind has experienced an unforeseen increase in the development of various methods of life-sustaining treatments and therapies (ie, mechanical ventilation, automated external defibrillation, artificial nutrition and hydration, bypass surgery). Other treatments previously experimented with, such as hemodialysis, defibrillation, and cardiopulmonary resuscitation, have also now reached mainstream. This tremendous progress has provided a growing menu of choices, complicating end-of-life care and decision making. Amid such choices, to protect the autonomy of patients, the implementation of advanced directives (ADs), in which patients explicate end-of-life preferences to be used in situations of incapacitation, have been advised. In theory, these documents appear to be a suitable response to the problem by providing a degree of assurance that an individual's end-of-life wishes are obeyed. Yet, in practice, it has been observed that not only do many patients lack ADs, but also these orders lack standardization in addressing end-of-life care, yielding increased confusion at the end of life.

In their review, Santonocito et al outlined the prevailing ways in which various countries approach withholding life-sustaining care with a specific focus on do-not-resuscitate (DNR) orders. Most countries and cultures around the world remain interested in the discussion of medical treatment options at the end of life. However, the authors have shined light on the fact that conventional attitudes and traditions of particular countries concerning life-sustaining therapy vary widely. This discord is particularly familiar in nations with increasingly diverse populations, such as the United States, which prides itself on being a melting pot of various cultures. This makes the implementation and enforcement of policies and procedures both challenging and disputatious. Santonocito et al suggest that nations standardize a DNR implementation policy to facilitate greater adequacy in obeying individual end-of-life wishes.

Standardization will ideally entail increased communication between the different parties involved (patients, families, religious leaders, providers) in the patient's end-of-life care. For this to succeed, additional ongoing education of physicians is needed to be better prepared for regular discussion of end-of-life issues—both in times of patient sickness and in health. A vital component of this ongoing dialogue will be fostering trust between patients and providers. According to the authors, by directly providing patients with both education about treatment options and psychosocial support, physicians can foster this trust.

The authors identify that increased discussion between patients and providers will result in more individuals documenting their end-of-life wishes. This also will reduce the number of family disputes when relatives are unable to agree on the desires of an ill family member as well as levels of spending at the end of life. The authors fail to acknowledge that end-of-life discussions are very costly to society. These conversations also consume a great deal of time and are very emotionally draining for providers. In the United States (and in many other nations), physicians are not financially reimbursed for these conversations. The goal of fostering ongoing discussion of the end of life will not achieve its potential until this process provides reimbursement for their time to all health care professionals.

J. Weinstock, BS

V. Rajput, MD

Family Factors Affect Clinician Attitudes in Pediatric End-of-Life Decision Making: A Randomized Vignette Study

Ruppe MD, Feudtner C, Hexem KR, et al (Univ of Louisville, KY; The Children's Hosp of Philadelphia, PA)

J Pain Symptom Manage 2012 [Epub ahead of print]

Context.—Conflicts between families and clinicians in pediatric end-of-life (EOL) care cause distress for providers, dissatisfaction for patients' families, and potential suffering for terminally ill children.

Objectives.—We hypothesized that family factors might influence clinician decision making in these circumstances.

Methods.—We presented vignettes concerning difficult EOL decision making, randomized for religious objection to therapy withdrawal and perceived level of family involvement, to clinicians working in three children's hospital intensive care units. Additionally, attitudes about EOL care were assessed.

Results.—Three hundred sixty-four respondents completed the questionnaire, for an overall response rate of 54%. Respondents receiving the "involved family" vignette were more likely to agree to continue medical care indefinitely ($P < 0.0005$). Respondents were marginally more likely to pursue a court-appointed guardian for those patients whose families had nonreligious objections to withdrawal ($P = 0.05$). Respondents who thought that a fear of being sued affected decisions were less likely to pursue unilateral withdrawal (odds ratio 0.8, 95% CI $= 0.6-0.9$). Those who felt personal distress as a result of difficult EOL decision making, thought they often provided "futile" care, or those who felt EOL care was effectively addressed at the institution were less likely to want to defer to the parents' wishes (range of odds ratios $0.7-1$).

Conclusion.—In this randomized vignette study, we have shown that family factors, particularly how involved a family seems to be in a child's life, affect what clinicians think is ethically appropriate in challenging EOL cases. Knowledge of how a family's degree of involvement may affect clinicians should be helpful to the clinical ethics consultants and offer some degree of insight to the clinicians themselves.

▶ End-of-life decision making is a difficult process for patients and families. It is also clearly a taxing experience for clinicians, including doctors and nurses.[1] Clinicians can be unsure of the correct treatment plan, even if the goals of care are agreed upon by all. In the event that there is conflict between clinicians and family regarding appropriate goals of end-of-life care, the distress can be even greater for the clinicians.

In this study, the main result was a higher level of family involvement (as perceived by the clinician) is shown to increase the likelihood of accepting the family decision to continue life-prolonging interventions indefinitely, as opposed to seeking additional resources in an effort to withdraw life-prolonging measures. This is not a surprise, but demonstrating the correlation in a study such as this is important as it brings these influences to light.

One surprising correlation was a tendency for clinicians who feel that end-of-life care is effectively addressed at the institution to be more likely to consider efforts to override a family's decision, such as seeking a court-appointed guardian.

Another result worth noting is the degree of distress that respondents reported. The vast majority either agreed or strongly agreed that "difficulty with end-of-life decision making frequently causes me personal distress," and a similar majority disagreed or strongly disagreed that "in general, end-of-life care decisions are effectively addressed in our hospital." This type of result has been shown in many studies previously, including the landmark Study to Understand Prognoses and Preferences for Outcomes and Risks of Treatments study.[2] This study was considered to be a major catalyst for the hospice movement in the United States. It is discouraging to see that despite recognition and intervention to improve the delivery of end-of-life care, the current study shows a similar trend.

From a methodological standpoint, it would be interesting to learn more about the survey respondents. After reading the vignette, respondents were asked whether they would consider certain interventions, including mediation or ethics consultation, seeking a court-appointed guardian, or seeking a transfer of care. It would be interesting to learn how familiar the respondents were with these options and if they have been involved with any of these processes before.

Many interesting variations could be examined with this clinical vignette method with only minor changes. For instance, it would be interesting to see how clinicians would react if the patient was less clearly terminal, but the family chose to withdraw care.

Communication among doctors, nurses, families, and patients influences the decision-making process in complex ways. Clinicians incorporate an immense amount of new information into complex decisions such as these; however, they also bring a lifetime of past experience and bias. This article reveals an important influence on clinicians' decision making. Recognition of this influence is important in delivering the best possible care to terminally ill children.

P. McMackin, MD

V. Rajput, MD

References

1. Oberle K, Hughes D. Doctors' and nurses' perceptions of ethical problems in end-of-life decisions. *J Adv Nurs.* 2001;33:707-715.
2. A controlled trial to improve care for seriously ill hospitalized patients. The study to understand prognoses and preferences for outcomes and risks of treatments (SUPPORT). The SUPPORT Principal Investigators. *JAMA.* 1995;274:1591-1598.

Withdrawal of care: A 10-year perspective at a Level I trauma center

Sise MJ, Sise CB, Thorndike JF, et al (Scripps Mercy Hosp, San Diego, CA)

J Trauma Acute Care Surg 72:1186-1193, 2012

Background.—Withdrawal or limitation of care (WLC) in trauma patients has not been well studied. We reviewed 10 years of deaths at our adult Level I trauma center to identify the patients undergoing WLC and to describe the process of trauma surgeon-managed WLC.

Methods.—This is a retrospective review of WLC. Each patient was assigned to one of three modes of WLC: care withdrawn, limited or no resuscitation, or organ harvest. Frequency, timing, and circumstances of WLC, including family involvement, ethics committee consultation, palliative care, and hospice, were reviewed.

Results.—From 2000 through 2009, 375 patients died with WLC (54% of all deaths; 93% at ≥ 24 hours). For age ≥ 65 years, 80% were WLC. Overall, 15% had advance directive documents. Traumatic brain or high cervical spine injury was the cause of death in 63%. Factors associated with WLC included age, comorbidities, injury mechanism and severity, and nontrauma activation status. At time of death, 316 (84%) WLC were under trauma surgeon management. In this group, mode of WLC was care withdrawn in 74%, organ harvest in 20%, and limited or no resuscitation in 6%. Rationale for WLC in non-organ harvest patients was poor neurologic prognosis in 86% and futility in 76%. When family was identified, end-of-life discussions with physicians occurred in 100%. Conflicts over WLC occurred in 6.6% and were not associated with any demographic group. Ethics committee was involved in 2.8%. For care-withdrawn patients, median time to death from first WLC order was 6.6 hours. Palliative care and hospice consults (6% and 9%) increased yearly.

Conclusions.—WLC occurred in over 50% of all trauma deaths and exceeded 90% at ≥ 24 hours. Hospice and palliative care were increasingly important adjuncts to WLC. Guidelines for WLC should be developed to ensure quality end-of-life care for trauma patients in whom further care is futile.

Level of Evidence.—III, therapeutic study.

▶ Sise et al provide valuable information on a little-studied topic with their analysis of the withdrawal or limitation of care (WLC) of terminally ill patients at their trauma center. Their study provides insight into where WLC improvements may be made, such as greater utilization of consultation services and suggested areas for further research. They strengthen their stance that further research and education on WLC in the trauma setting is needed simply by showing it is a very common practice and is not without conflict. Ultimately, it seems the authors feel that the trauma community needs to develop a consensus statement and possible guidelines to help optimize end-of-life management and WLC issues in traumatically injured patients. Their study contributes to evidence and insight that would be necessary to form these guidelines.

There have been several other published articles analyzing the use of WLC in the trauma setting. Three similar retrospective studies and 1 large multicenter prospective study found WLC in trauma patients occurs with similar frequency (54%-80%) as reported by Sise et al (54%). Each of these studies found that the most common type of injury in these trauma patients was neurological.[1-4] Two older studies failed to find associations between WLC and age or comorbidity, whereas Sise et al found them to be positively associated. Unlike Sise et al, three prior studies were unable to show an association with race.[1,3,5] Two of these studies found conflicts occurred with a similar frequency as reported by Sise et al.[1,2] A 2010 international survey found variation in physician opinions on delivering end-of-life care by region and religion, which expands on Sise et al's findings of WLC variation between trauma centers.

As revealed in the supplemental discussion with Sise et al's article, guidelines do exist pertaining to WLC. Whether or not these guidelines are adequate for care of the terminally ill trauma patients, however, is not clear and is a point of debate. It is important to consider the potential differences in WLC between the medical, surgical, and trauma patients to help decide whether trauma-specific WLC guidelines are warranted. Sise et al's article does not specifically address these differences, but it does provide the necessary information for such a comparative analysis. Without an analysis documenting the degree and type of differences that exist or a prospective study looking at the use of other societies' WLC guidelines in the trauma setting, it is difficult to make an objective case for developing trauma-specific WLC guidelines. It would not be unreasonable, however, for the American Association for the Surgery of Trauma to develop their guidelines to maintain their position as leaders of their field.

P. Wilse, DO

V. Rajput, MD

References

1. Plaisier BR, Blostein PA, Hurt KJ, Malangoni MA. Withholding/withdrawal of life support in trauma patients: is there an age bias? *Am Surg.* 2002;68:159-162.
2. Trunkey DD, Cahn RM, Lenfesty B, Mullins R. Management of the geriatric trauma patient at risk of death: therapy withdrawal decision making. *Arch Surg.* 2000;135:34-38.
3. Watch LS, Saxton-Daniels S, Schermer CR. Who has life-sustaining therapy withdrawn after injury? *J Trauma.* 2005;59:1320-1326.
4. Cooper Z, Rivara FP, Wang J, MacKenzie EJ, Jurkovich GJ. Withdrawal of life-sustaining therapy in injured patients: variations between trauma centers and non-trauma centers. *J Trauma.* 2009;66:1327-1335.
5. Ball CG, Navsaria P, Kirkpatrick AW, et al. The impact of country and culture on end-of-life care for injured patients: results from an international survey. *J Trauma.* 2010;69:1323-1334.

Palliative Surgery in the Do-Not-Resuscitate Patient: Ethics and Practical Suggestions for Management
Scott TH, Garvin JR (Univ of Pennsylvania, Philadelphia; Hosp of the Univ of Pennsylvania, Philadelphia)
Anesthesiol Clin 30:1-12, 2012

Much has changed in palliative care since 1999 when the senior author of this article published "Anesthesia and Palliative Care," in which he bemoaned the paucity of clinical and training programs, and encouraged anesthesiologists to get more involved. Not only has palliative care in the United States evolved into a well-recognized discipline of its own, with American Council for Graduate Medical Education (ACGME) subspecialty board certification and a rapidly growing number of dedicated fellowship slots, there also has been a concerted effort to educate the public, in addition to professionals, that palliative care is on the same continuum as standard care and demands aggressive symptom management, even when patients choose curative or life-prolonging therapies. Much of this push has been spearheaded by the Center to Advance Palliative Care (CAPC) (http://www.capc.org), a nonprofit organization that has worked tirelessly to promote the benefits of palliative care for alleviation of somatic and existential distress, as well the avoidance of unnecessary medical procedures and costs. The 1999 piece emphasized mostly common sense and compassionate ways in which anesthesiologists can contribute positively to the comfort of this vulnerable population. This article does not restate those points but rather focuses on the complexities and nuances of do-not-resuscitate (DNR) orders when patients present to the operating room (OR).

▶ There are common misunderstandings of medical interventions in the setting of do-not-resuscitate (DNR) status or under hospice care. There is hesitancy on the part of physicians to treat many medical conditions aggressively, even if they are not terminal or fall outside the diagnosis for which a patient is on hospice. Surgery is one of those interventions. However, many patients with DNR orders or under hospice care present for surgery. These surgeries can run the gamut from "routine" to high risk.

Standard living wills do not address the perioperative period. In fact, certain interventions may be specifically prohibited by an individual's living will, which they may not realize are routinely done during surgery. As the author states, "interventions that are considered standard and necessary in the operating room (OR) may be considered 'resuscitation' on the hospital floor." Clearly, clarification of DNR orders is needed.

Such guidelines do exist from the American Society of Anesthesiologists for just this setting.[1] This article presents a straightforward, practical approach to implementing those guidelines and expands on the preoperative evaluation of a patient with a preexisting DNR order. This includes a detailed discussion of the patient's values and wishes in regard to the DNR order and any modifications of exceptions to make in the perioperative period. Specifics of medications, interventions, and time and location when the perioperative period begins and ends as it pertains to any suspension or alteration of the original DNR order are included. It also includes the appointment of a surrogate decision maker regarding the implementation of the modified DNR. There is discussion in the article of the appropriateness of having the anesthesiologist or surgeon (as opposed to a family member or other nonphysician surrogate) act as a proxy making the decisions regarding intraoperative care.

As with any discussion of this type, it can be a time-consuming process if it is to have any significant value. One can gather from the article that this usually occurs in the immediate preoperative area by the anesthesiologist or a delegate of the anesthesiologist. It is, of course, appropriate to address the issue at that time because the anesthesiologist is the one delivering the care in the perioperative period. However, the issue is better addressed well before then. It is also better that a discussion of DNR orders happen with someone with whom the patient has a rapport.[2] In addition to being practical suggestions for anesthesiologists, this article should serve as a call to action for providers seeing these patients in the surgical planning period, such as surgeons, internists, and family practitioners. Addressing the DNR issues well ahead of surgery can alleviate confusion and distress for both patients and providers. It could even prevent last-minute cancellation of surgeries if anesthesiologists have medical or moral objections to some cases. Understandably, the surgeon or primary care doctor may not know the details of perioperative anesthesia care as well as the anesthesiologist. Communication between providers in multidisciplinary format well before the surgery can therefore be beneficial, even though logistically difficult. Even if there is not communication, patient awareness of these decisions can undoubtedly make the discussion with an anesthesiologist easier and more fruitful.

P. McMackin, MD

V. Rajput, MD

References

1. American Society of Anesthesiologists. http://www.asahq.org/For-Members/~/media/ For%20Members/Standards%20and%20Guidelines/2012/CONTINUUM%20OF %20DEPTH%20OF%20SEDATION%20442012.ashx. Accessed January 3, 2013.
2. Downar J, Hawryluck L. What should we say when discussing "code status" and life support with a patient? A Delphi analysis. *J Palliat Med.* 2010;13:185-195.

Law ethics and clinical judgment in end-of-life decisions—How do Norwegian doctors think?

Bahus MK, Steen PA, Førde R (Univ of Oslo, Norway; Univ of Oslo and Oslo Univ Hosp, Norway)
Resuscitation 83:1369-1373, 2012

Aim.—According to Norwegian law, an autonomous patient has the right to refuse life-prolonging treatment. If the patient is not defined as dying, however, health personnel are obliged to instigate life-saving treatment in an emergency situation even against the patient's wishes. The purpose of this study was to investigate how doctors' attitudes and knowledge agree with these legal provisions, and how the statutory provision on emergency situations influences the principle of patient autonomy for severely ill, but not dying, patients.

Method.—A strategic sample of 1175 Norwegian doctors who are specialists in internal medicine, paediatrics, surgery, neurology and neurosurgery received a mail questionnaire about decisions on end-of-life care in hypothetical scenarios. The case presented concerns a 45-year-old autonomous patient diagnosed with end-stage ALS who declines ventilatory treatment. Recipients were randomly selected from the membership roster of the Norwegian Medical Association. 640 (54.5%) responded; of these, 406 had experience with end-of-life decisions.

Results.—56.1% (221/394) stated that ALS patients in such situations can *always* refuse life-prolonging treatment, and 42.4% (167/394) were of the opinion that the patient can *normally* refuse life-prolonging treatment. 1.5% (6/394) stated that the patient cannot refuse life-prolonging treatment.

Conclusions.—The answers indicate that the respondents include patients' refusal in an overall clinical judgement, and interpret patients' right to decline life-saving treatment in different ways. This may reflect the complex legal situation in Norway regarding patient autonomy with respect to the right of severely ill, but not dying, patients' right to decline acute life-saving treatment.

▶ Bahus et al approach the topic of patient autonomy and physicians' roles in emergency situations, specifically as it pertains to amyotrophic lateral sclerosis (ALS) patients and mechanical ventilation in Norway. ALS is particularly complicated because physicians are required to uphold patient autonomy under Norwegian law, but they are also obliged to act in emergency situations when competent patients refuse treatment unless they are considered to be dying.

An approach using the principle of autonomy and respect for persons in terms of ethics can be used to analyze this study. This principle states that the patient or his or her proxy must be involved in determining the treatment course that the patient will undergo. The patient should have the benefits and burdens of each treatment option presented, so that he or she can make an educated decision; however, discussion regarding the patient's wishes should an emergency arise needs to be established and constantly revisited during the course of the patient's disease. In the case of intubation for individuals with ALS, a patient's intentions that have been definitively established before the onset of an emergency situation should be respected. Although the line between law and ethics is sometime blurred, patients retain the right to determine which treatment courses they will receive. To ensure that this happens, it is imperative that physicians approach the topic of end-of-life decisions and wishes for life-sustaining treatments before steep decline of the patient's condition and subsequent necessity for emergent decision-making, namely respiratory failure requiring intubation.

Advance directives and living wills have become increasingly important topics with the continued advancement of medical technology and the ability to prolong life by artificial means. Communication between patients and physicians is paramount to facilitating an open dialogue to address such topics. A study performed by Munroe et al[1] found that the most important factor in determining if an ALS patient will undergo intubation in the setting of respiratory failure is whether end-of-life decisions had been discussed during the course of the patient's treatment and progression of disease. Another investigation by Peretti-Watel et al[2] evaluated nurses' attitudes toward the autonomy of terminally ill patients by presenting a similar vignette about an ALS patient in need of emergent mechanical ventilation. It was found that the 2 factors predictive of the willingness to perform intubation or tracheostomy without patient consent were poor communication and hostility to patients' living wills with the overall conclusion being that insufficient attention is often paid to patients' wishes.

Although it is sometimes difficult to differentiate between legal standards and ethical principles in situations involving end-of-life care, the patient's autonomy and wishes or living will must be upheld. To ensure that this practice becomes commonplace, physicians must continue to partake in open discussions with their patients and surrogate decision makers about code statuses. In many countries where the definition of medical emergency is unclear, measures should be taken to address the details of these terms to reduce confusion in acute situations.

K. Contino, BS
V. Rajput, MD

References

1. Munroe CA, Sirdofsky MD, Kuru T, Anderson ED. End-of-life decision making in 42 patients with amyotrophic lateral sclerosis. *Respir Care.* 2007;52:996-999.
2. Peretti-Watel P, Bendiane MK, Galinier A, et al. District nurses' attitudes toward patient consent: the case of mechanical ventilation on amyotrophic lateral sclerosis patients: results from a French National Survey. *J Crit Care.* 2008;23:332-338.

Religio-ethical discussions on organ donation among Muslims in Europe: an example of transnational Islamic bioethics
Ghaly M (Leiden Univ, The Netherlands)
Med Health Care Philos 15:207-220, 2012

This article analyzes the religio-ethical discussions of Muslim religious scholars, which took place in Europe specifically in the UK and the Netherlands, on organ donation. After introductory notes on fatwas (Islamic religious guidelines) relevant to biomedical ethics and the socio-political context in which discussions on organ donation took place, the article studies three specific fatwas issued in Europe whose analysis has escaped the attention of modern academic researchers. In 2000 the European Council for Fatwa and Research (ECFR) issued a fatwa on organ donation. Besides this "European" fatwa, two other fatwas were issued respectively in the UK by the Muslim Law (Shariah) Council in 1995 and in the Netherlands by the Moroccan religious scholar Muṣṭafā Ben Hamza during a conference on "Islam and Organ Donation" held in March 2006. The three fatwas show that a great number of Muslim religious scholars permit organ donation and this holds true for donating organs to non-Muslims as well. Further, they demonstrate that transnationalism is one of the main characteristics of contemporary Islamic bioethics. In a bid to develop their own standpoints towards organ donation, Muslims living in the West rely heavily on fatwas imported from the Muslim world.

▶ Mohammed Ghaly focuses on the topic of organ donation under Islamic beliefs and culture based on 3 fatwas, which are Islamic religious guidelines. Between 1995 and 2006, 3 international conferences, which resulted in the creation of the aforementioned fatwas, were held to discuss Islam's stand on this practice addressing its various facets: autografts versus allografts, organ donation by living versus cadaveric benefactors, organ types that can be used, and avoiding transplantation of organs that can potentiate genetic information. Common arguments against organ donation within this faith include current scientific study and lack of uniformity of the definition of brain death as well as the belief that God is the owner of the body and people do not have the right to either donate or accept something present from birth. Each fatwa agrees that under the tenets of Islam, both living and cadaveric donations are permitted without mention of whether the donor or recipient is Muslim. Ghaly also concluded that the fatwas are of transnational character, not only as they pertain to organ donation but as it relates to other bioethical issues. Moreover, comment was made on promotion of the fatwas and positive reception of the tenets that they uphold.

An important aspect of organ donation that should be addressed is that of consent. Donors retain the autonomy to designate themselves as organ donors. In the event that they are unable to make such decisions, a proxy or durable power of attorney can step in and provide substituted judgment. In using the principles of beneficence and nonmalfeasance, good should be done and evil should be avoided. In taking an organ from an individual who is considered to be brain dead and transplanting it into another individual, the recipient is then given a chance at life. Distributive justice states that there are limited resources and that they should be shared accordingly. In the setting of organ donation, the list of individuals waiting for a liver, heart, kidney, or other organs continues to grow with many people dying before they are able to receive a transplant.

Organ donation within the Islam religion has been discussed and debated for many decades. According to Adnan Sharif,[1] both living and deceased donor transplantations are compatible with and permitted under the Islam beliefs. He concluded that it is both religion and sociocultural confounders that are involved in the decision-making process for Muslims considering organ donation. Arbour et al[2] hold that organ donation is permissive under the guidelines of Islam even in cases of brain death; however, it is the responsibility of the medical community to ensure that patient and family members fully understand what it means to be brain dead. Moreover, it is suggested that when dealing with end-of-life care in general, culture and faith-based perspective must be understood and respected.

Looking toward the future, it will be important to revisit the beliefs of Islam with the progression of modern medical technology. Additionally, the importance of communication among physicians, patients, and families should continue to be encouraged, as misunderstanding often creates a barrier to participation in such practices.

K. Contino, BS
V. Rajput, MD

References

1. Sharif A. Organ donation and Islam-challenges and opportunities. *Transplantation.* 2012;94:442-446.
2. Arbour R, AlGhamdi HM, Peters L. Islam, brain death, and transplantation: culture, faith, and jurisprudence. *AACN Adv Crit Care.* 2012;23:381-394.

Pediatric ventilation in a disaster: Clinical and ethical decision making
Ytzhak A, Sagi R, Bader T, et al (Israel Defense Forces Med Corps, Tel-Hashomer; et al)
Crit Care Med 40:603-607, 2012

Introduction.—Medical resources may be overwhelmed in a mass disaster situation. Intensive care resources may be limited even further. When the demand for a certain resource, like ventilators, exceeds its availability, caregivers are faced with the task of deciding how to distribute this resource.

Ethical dilemmas arise when a practical decision necessitates ranking the importance of several ethical principles. In a disaster area, the greatest good for the greatest number principle and the goal of equal distribution of resources may take priority over the needs of the individual. Nonetheless, regardless of the interventions available, it is a prime goal to keep the patients' comfort and dignity as much as possible.

Background.—In the mass disaster of the Haiti earthquake of January 2010, The Israeli Defense Forces Medical Corps field hospital was one of the first to respond to the call for help of the Haitian people with surgical and intensive care capabilities. It was the only facility able to ventilate children and neonates in the first week after the earthquake, although this ability was relatively limited.

Special Article.—Five case scenarios that we confronted at the pediatric ward of the field hospital are presented: two children with respiratory compromise due to pulmonary infection, one premature baby with respiratory distress syndrome, an asphyxiated neonate, and a baby with severe sepsis of a probable abdominal origin. In normal circumstances all of them would have been ventilated but with limited resources we raised in each case the question of ventilating or not.

To help in the evaluation of each case we used a decisionsupport tool that was previously developed for ventilator allocation during an influenza pandemic. This tool takes into account several factors, including the illness severity, prognosis, and the expected duration of ventilation.

Conclusions.—Applying ethical priorities to analyze the decision-making problems leads to the understanding that an individualized approach with an ongoing assessment of the patient condition and the availability of resources, rather than a strict predefined decision rule, will give patients a better chance of survival, and will assist in allocating scarce resources.

▶ Health care providers are forced to make difficult resource allocation decisions during disasters. The priority given to certain guiding moral principles must be altered to balance the needs of the individual (autonomy) with those of the community (distributive justice). Multiple aids have been developed specifically to guide care in resource-limited situations.[1] The matrix algorithm to aid in ventilation allocation decision-making discussed by Ytzhak et al was originally proposed by Hick et al in 2007.[1] It was designed to "allow the 'best method or evidence available' to be used" and "... allow(s) better predictive systems to be incorporated without changing the basic framework." The authors' analysis shows that their decision matrix would have given the same recommendations as those ultimately provided by their panel. Despite producing the same outcomes, the authors' conclude that their "individualized patient-centered approach" was able to save lives because it was less rigid than a decision matrix, used ongoing assessments, and considered the "uncertainty factor" of human illness and disaster.

In a 2012 editorial, Szalados discusses the ethical issues surrounding care in disaster medicine. He notes physicians are "not experienced in weighing the greatest good for the greatest number" and are taught to prioritize the needs of their individual patients. This would be particularly true when caring for the pediatric population where "without objective guidelines, heart often wins out over mind ...." Szalados then makes a plea for the development of criteria, stating "... it is becoming increasingly imperative that criteria for allocating scarce resources be well defined ...." He then contrasts the case for objectivity with the authors' experience, describing their decision tool as "analytical and individualized ... not algorithmic or quantitative," yet appearing to successfully allocate scarce resources. Finally, he leaves the issue unresolved, asking "does ethical triage require practical wisdom and an individual moral compass that cannot be distilled into an algorithm?"[2]

In 4 of the 5 cases presented by Ytzhak et al, the decision made in the field was the same as that recommended by the decision aid. In the remaining case, the decision aid did not recommend for or against ventilation; the physician's judgment was to ventilate, and the child ultimately died 3 days later. It is hard to draw any conclusions about 1 method being better than the other with a sample size of only 5. Even so, the decision matrix performed at least as well as the authors' individualized approach.

As discussed by Hick et al, the decision matrix was a dynamic framework to aid physician decision making and not a "strict predefined decision rule" as described by Ytzhak et al. The authors' assertion that because their physician panel did ongoing assessments it was superior to a decision rule is unfair because the decision rule could be reapplied and updated at any time. We can, however, appreciate the importance of what the authors' call the "uncertainty factor" of human illness and disaster where each day can bring dramatic change. It would be beneficial to include this principle in the decision matrix to guarantee its inclusion in physician decision making. Essentially, Ytzhak et al seem to be advocating for ventilation triage decisions to be made by physician panels without the aid of decision matrices or algorithms. We feel, however, that the correct answer is likely to exist, as usual, somewhere in between.

Szalados touched on the incorporation of telemedicine into decision aids given its potential contributions (anonymous objectivity of those monitoring, incorporation of transmitted vital signs, retrieval of medical history).[2] In a recent article, Eyal et al discuss the important ethical differences between "initial triage" when deciding to allocate currently unused resources to a patient and "repeat triage" where a decision to withdrawal care from a patient currently receiving it in favor of a new patient raises many difficult questions. They ultimately conclude that "a degree of priority" must be given to those already receiving treatment.[3] All of these factors should be considered during future decision aid development. Also, as noted by Ytzhak et al, decision aids should be assessed for reproducibility of results between different patients and by different physicians and if consistency is found then prospectively used by future disaster relief groups. Perhaps the most important aspect of disaster relief medicine, however, is to educate hospitals, departments, and, specifically, critical care and emergency department physicians regarding how the paradigm shift during a disaster will swing their responsibility from the individual to the community.

P. Wilse, DO

V. Rajput, MD

References

1. Hick JL, Rubinson L, O'Laughlin DT, et al. Clinical review: allocating ventilators during large-scale disasters—problem, planning, and process. *Crit Care.* 2007;11: 217.
2. Szalados JE. Triaging the fittest: practical wisdom versus logical calculus? *Crit Care Med.* 2012;40:697-698.
3. Eyal N, Firth P; MGY Disaster Relief Ethics Group. Repeat triage in disaster relief: questions from Haiti. *PLoS Curr.* 2012;4:e4fbbdec6279ec.

Use of the Medical Ethics Consultation Service in a Busy Level I Trauma Center: Impact on Decision-Making and Patient Care
Johnson LS, Lesandrini J, Rozycki GS (Emory Univ, Atlanta, GA; Grady Memorial Hosp, Atlanta, GA)
Am Surg 78:735-740, 2012

The purposes of this study were to assess reasons for consultation of the Ethics Consultation Service for trauma patients and how consultations impacted care. We conducted a review of ethics consultations at a Level I trauma center from 2001 to 2010. Data included patient demographics, etiology of injury, and timing/type of the consult, categorized as: shared decision-making, end-of-life, privacy and confidentiality, resource allocation, and professionalism. Consultations were requested on 108 patients (age mean, 46.5 ± 20 years; Injury Severity Score mean, 23 ± 14; length of stay [LOS] mean, 44 ± 44 days), 0.50 per cent of all trauma admissions. Seventy-seven per cent of consultations occurred in the intensive care unit. End of life was the most common consultation (44%) followed by shared decision-making (41%). Average time to consultation was 25 days. Shared decision-making consults occurred much earlier than end-of-life consults as evidenced by a lower consult day/LOS ratio (consult day/LOS = 0.36 ± 0.3 *vs* 0.77 ± 0.3, $P = 0.0001$). Conclusions consisted of: 1) ethics consultation on trauma patients are most commonly for end-of-life and shared decision-making issues; 2) most ethics consultations occur while patients are in the intensive care unit; and 3) earlier ethics consultations are likely to be for shared decision-making issues.

▶ Johnson et al show that ethics consults on their trauma service were a rather infrequent occurrence and typically occurred late in the patient's stay. Characteristics of those receiving consults and the reasons for them were mostly in agreement with the findings of prior studies. Consultation frequency was shown to be increasing since the early 2000s, perhaps because of enhanced education, the Joint Commission mandate for in-hospital mechanisms to address ethical issues, and the freedom and empowerment of nurses and social workers to place such consults. Despite being able to classify the reasons for ethics consults into more than 18 categories, most are related to end-of-life or shared decision-making issues; overall, it was felt that if the patients who ultimately had these "ethical issues" could be identified earlier in their stay, it could "potentially improve care and resource use."

Ethics consultation has been shown to benefit the relationships between families and physicians and decrease resource utilization through improved hospital and intensive care unit (ICU) length of stays and decreased time on mechanical ventilation.[1] Similar improvements have also been realized through the implementation of protocols designed to improve ICU physician communication with families.[2] Success in managing end-of-life situations may hinge more on effective communication by any physician and not just by the ethics consultant. It is clear, however, that extra time and specialized training and experience are required to provide the attention and discussion that families need to appropriately deal with end-of-life situations. Thus, the relative paucity of ethics consults reported by Johnson et al do not necessarily reflect a deficit of care, but may reflect underutilization of a potentially useful service.

Consults, especially those for end-of-life reasons, were placed rather late in the patient's stay (mean time to consult is 25 days). Comparing the mean length of stay of patients receiving end-of-life consults (51.6 days) to similar patients who did not receive consults (19.5 days) suggests that the long length of stay itself likely played a role in precipitating consultation. This would not be surprising given the knowledge that ethics consults have been shown to shorten length of stay and may indicate that a more proactive approach with earlier ethics consultation could be beneficial.

Shared decision-making focuses on assessing a patient's decision-making capacity and then deciding who is to be his or her surrogate decision-maker, the latter of which was actually the most common reason given for ethics consultation in the Johnson et al study (24%). Whether or not an ethics consultation is actually necessary, useful, or an appropriate first step to addressing questions of capacity, however, is not clear. Kontos et al discuss the increasing use of psychiatry consults in determining patient capacity "...despite continued articulation, if not general awareness, that these assessments are not the exclusive province of psychiatry."[3] A study of one ethics consult service showed that after the addition of a palliative care consult service the most common reason for ethics consult changed from "patient capacity in question" to "futility" and "physician opposed to providing life-sustaining treatment."[4] To further complicate the issue, a 2009 study found that 37% of all psychiatry consults for capacity actually had nothing to do with capacity.[5] Although these studies were not specific to the trauma population, they do reveal the inconsistent and inappropriate use of consultants to aid in capacity determination.

The relatively new incorporation of ethical specialists into the hospital system has necessitated these recent studies, such as that by Johnson et al, to characterize and optimize the role of the ethics consult. Additional studies should look to confirm these findings at other trauma centers. If present, they could justify as well as guide efforts to improve the timing, frequency, and quality of ethics consultations for traumatically injured patients.

P. Wilse, DO

V. Rajput, MD

References

1. Schneiderman LJ, Gilmer T, Teezel HD, et al. Effect of ethics consultations on non-beneficial life-sustaining treatments in the intensive care setting: a randomized controlled trial. *JAMA*. 2003;290:1166-1172.
2. Scheunemann LP, McDevitt M, Carson SS, Hanson LC. Randomized, controlled trials of interventions to improve communication in intensive care: a systematic review. *Chest*. 2011;139:543-554.
3. Kontos N, Freudenreich O, Querques J. Beyond capacity: identifying ethical dilemmas underlying capacity evaluation requests. *Psychosomatics*. 2012 Dec 3. [Epub ahead of print].
4. Moeller JR, Albanese TH, Garchar K, et al. Functions and outcomes of a clinical medical ethics committee: a review of 100 consults. *HEC Forum*. 2012;24:99-114.
5. Kornfeld DS, Muskin PR, Tahil FA. Psychiatric evaluation of mental capacity in the general hospital: a significant teaching opportunity. *Psychosomatics*. 2009; 50:468-473.

Denying a Patient's Final Will: Public Safety vs. Medical Confidentiality and Patient Autonomy
Gaertner J, Vent J, Greinwald R, et al (Univ Hosp, Cologne, Germany; et al)
J Pain Symptom Manage 42:961-966, 2011

Especially when caring for patients approaching the end of life, physicians and nursing staff feel committed to fulfilling as many patient desires as possible. However, sometimes a patient's "final will" may threaten public safety. This can lead to severe conflicts, outweighing the physician's obligation and dedication to care for the patient and to respect his autonomy. Yet, public safety can be threatened if confidentiality is not broken. This article provides a concise summary of the medicolegal and ethical fundamentals concerning this difficult situation. If the patient's and others' health and safety are at risk, physicians may (and in some countries must) break medical confidentiality and disclose confidential patient information to the police and other authorities. Physicians should be able to professionally deal with such a conflict in all patients, not only in patients with advanced illness.

▶ When providing care, physicians strive to strike a balance between responsibility for patient well-being and respect for patient autonomy. However, this balance becomes challenging in the setting of palliative care when patients' last wishes come to the forefront. Treatments for end-stage illnesses can severely impair psychosocial functions, resulting in a diminished ability to drive. Oftentimes, patients continue to drive despite warnings with the argument that driving is a last will. When a terminally ill patient's final will jeopardizes both patient and public safety, what is a physician to do?

In this report, Childress and Beauchamp's ethical principles, autonomy, and justice are applied to the issue of unsafe patient driving.[1] Immediately, a conflict arises between patient autonomy and beneficence or obligation to prevent harm. Given that unsafe driving threatens the safety of both the patient and society, this report deems that beneficence outweighs autonomy. This ethical decision brings to light the need to assess conflicts between beneficence and autonomy on a case-by-case basis. In Western practice, autonomy often takes precedence over beneficence when cases apply mainly to individual patient safety.[2] However, when the safety of others comes into play such as in unsafe driving, the balance between autonomy and beneficence tips toward an ethical obligation to protect.

Beyond ethical duties, this report also highlights a physician's legal duties to help guide in decision-making. In the case of unsafe driving, physicians have a legal duty to protect, namely to warn the public of danger their patients may cause. However, this poses a direct conflict with obligations to maintain patient confidentiality. In the United States, the Health Insurance Portability and Accountability Act has a regulation that allows for reporting health information when it is in the public interest.[3] A physician is bound to patient confidentiality unless disclosure is a means to prevent danger as in unsafe driving. Currently, only 6 US states require physicians to report drivers deemed unsafe because of medical conditions.[3] Other states encourage and authorize physicians to report impaired drivers but do not make it mandatory. When reporting is not legally required, a physician's ethical duty to protect public health argues for reporting unsafe drivers if the benefits to the patient and public outweigh patient autonomy.

In the setting of palliative care, the common but difficult decision to revoke patient driving privileges raises conflicts between beneficence and autonomy as well as duty to protect and confidentiality. This report emphasizes that when patients continue to drive unsafely despite warnings, clinicians must be able to judge the extent of potential harm to patient and society and how likely the harm will occur in order to determine whether beneficence and duty to protect outweigh patient autonomy and confidentiality. This raises a need to establish clear practices to assess driving skill and resulting risks. Currently, the American Medical Association has recommended several tests of vision, cognitive function, and motor function to help with decision-making.[3] In the United Kingdom, the Driving and Vehicle Licensing Agency has outlined disease-specific guidelines to assess driving ability.[4] Beyond functional assessment, the next step is for guidelines to focus on patient circumstances, knowledge of available resources, patient education tools, and tactics to maintain physician-patient relationships despite diminished patient autonomy.

Physicians must also be aware of specific laws that help guide in reporting patient information. Many physicians state that they would report unfit drivers, but they fear that this may violate privacy and compromise physician-patient relationships.[5] This calls for increased awareness of state-by-state laws that mandate reporting and positions on protection for reporting physicians. Future focus on guidelines regarding methods to document patient information while minimizing impact on confidentiality breaches may help allay physician concerns.

R. Sharma, BS

V. Rajput, MD

References

1. Beauchamp TL, Childress JF. *Principles of Biomedical Ethics*. 6th ed. New York, NY: Oxford University Press; 2009.
2. Jensen UJ, Mooney G. Changing values: autonomy and paternalism in medicine and health care. In: Jensen UJ, Mooney G, eds. *Changing Values in Medical and Health Care Decision Making*. Chichester, UK: John Wiley and Sons; 1990.
3. "American Medical Association. Physician's Guide to Assessing and Counseling Older Drivers." http://www.amaassn.org/ama/pub/category/10791.html. Accessed January 29, 2013.
4. "DVLA's at a glance guide to the current medical guidelines (for medical professionals)." http://www.dft.gov.uk/dvla/medical/aag.aspx. Accessed January 29, 2013.
5. Marshall SC, Gilbert N. Saskatchewan physicians' attitudes and knowledge regarding assessment of medical fitness to drive. *CMAJ*. 1999;160:1701-1704.

End-of-Life Care Decisions: Importance of Reviewing Systems and Limitations After 2 Recent North American Cases

Burkle CM, Benson JJ (Mayo Clinic, Rochester, MN)

Mayo Clin Proc 87:1098-1105, 2012

Two recent and unfortunate North American cases involving end-of-life treatment highlight the difficulties surrounding medical futility conflicts. As countries have explored the greater influence that patients and their representatives may play on end-of-life treatment decisions, the benefits and struggles involved with such a movement must be appreciated. These 2 cases are used to examine the present systems existing in the United States and Canada for resolving end-of-life decisions, including the difficulty in defining medical futility, the role of medical ethics committees, and controversies involving surrogate decision making.

▶ Burkle and Benson approach the topics of end-of-life care and medical futility through use of 2 recent cases. One involved an elderly gentleman with renal failure, advanced dementia, and respiratory failure for which the wife (later found to not be his legal proxy) demanded dialysis but was thought to be futile by multiple physicians. The other was that of a 13-month-old child with a terminal neurologic disorder found to be in a persistent vegetative state (PVS) but whose parents requested that a tracheostomy be performed so that the child could die at home. The article approaches the definitions of "medical futility" and "meaningful" survival, basically concluding that because the meaning of these terms cannot be established, open communication must exist between the family and medical community. The authors discuss the importance of surrogate decision makers for patients who are unable to decide on their own course of medical treatment. They go on to address a number of guidelines by which medical proxies must abide and alternative means of assigning or firing these individuals in the event that they are not doing that which is in the best interest of the patient. In cases in which disputes between the medical community and patients' families and decision makers cannot be solved by other means, it is the duty of medical ethics committees to become involved.

As science and medical technology continue to advance, there are ever-increasing numbers of ways to sustain life; however, it is here that the terms *meaningful survival* and *medical futility* come into play. Patients in a PVS can be maintained on a ventilator indefinitely, but is this considered to be a meaningful life? Although experts have continued to attempt to arrive at a standard definition for medical futility, it is difficult to make a generalization to every case, yet in many situations, it seems to be rather clear, especially to those physicians who are constantly surrounded by such complex situations.

An important distinguishing point to address here is that of physiologic versus medical futility. Medical futility, as described by Deborah Kasman,[1] is when a particular clinical action, whether it be a drug, surgery, or other intervention, is of no use in attaining a specific goal for a particular patient. On the other hand, physiologic futility holds that there is no physiologic benefit to the patient by providing a particular treatment.

With regard to meaningful life and quality of life, the subtle difference must be highlighted. Rice and Betcher[2] state that quality of life is a subjective term and unique among all individuals. It includes physical, psychological, social, and spiritual domains of well-being. Clark et al[3] hold that meaningful life is rooted in whether an individual can obtain a desired quality of life, which, again, is very subjective in nature.

Sibbald and colleagues[4] questioned a number of individuals actively involved in patient care who worked in intensive care units (ICUs) throughout Canada as to their thoughts on how to define futile care, reasons why they continue to provide it despite believing that it is of no benefit to the patient, and ideas on how to proceed in the future to better allocate ICU resources in the future. They found that many of these physicians, nurses, and respiratory therapists had very similar thoughts about medical futility, including what treatment options should and should not be provided. They were, for the most part, in agreement as to where efforts should be concentrated to limit such care in the future.

Mohindra[5] set out to formulate a conceptual model of medical futility based on a medical factual matrix put forth by David Hume, which uses sheer facts of a particular patient's case to determine whether futility exists. It removed subjectivity from the equation and looks at each patient objectively. He concludes that before determining whether a treatment course is futile, the defined goal of treatment must first be decided on by the patient or proxy and the physician. In accordance with Mohindra's position, Terra and Powell[6] conclude that there must be a defined goal of treatment to determine a particular intervention to be futile; however, they based this conclusion on a principalistic ethical analysis.

Medical futility and meaningful survival are difficult topics to approach from a strictly objective standpoint. Such determination requires open dialogue between medical professionals and the patient or surrogate decision makers. In the case that a surrogate decision maker or health care team is thought to be making decisions that are truly not in the best interest of the patient, it then becomes the responsibility of a medical ethics committee to facilitate the communication and help to clarify the goals of care.

K. Contino, BS

V. Rajput, MD

References

1. Kasman DL. When is medical treatment futile? A guide for students, residents, and physicians. *J Gen Intern Med.* 2004;19:1053-1056.
2. Rice EM, Betcher DK. Evidence base for developing a palliative care service. *Medsurg Nurs.* 2007;16:143-148.
3. Clark D, Ten Have H, Janssens R. Conceptual tensions in European palliative care. In: Ten Have H, Clark D, eds. *The Ethics of Palliative Care: European Perspectives.* Buckingham, UK: Open University Press; 2002:55.
4. Sibbald R, Downar J, Hawryluck L. Perceptions of "futile care" among caregivers in intensive care units. *CMAJ.* 2007;177:1201-1208.
5. Mohindra RK. Medical futility: a conceptual model. *J Med Ethics.* 2007;33:71-75.
6. Terra SM, Powell SK. Is determination of medical futility ethical? *Prof Case Manag.* 2012;17:103-106.

Attitudes Towards End-of-Life Decisions and the Subjective Concepts of Consciousness: An Empirical Analysis

Lotto L, Manfrinati A, Rigoni D, et al (Univ of Padova, Italy; et al)
PLoS One 7:e31735, 2012

Background.—People have fought for their civil rights, primarily the right to live in dignity. At present, the development of technology in medicine and healthcare led to an apparent paradox: many people are fighting for the right to die. This study was aimed at testing whether different moral principles are associated with different attitudes towards end-of-life decisions for patients with a severe brain damage.

Methodology.—We focused on the ethical decisions about withdrawing life-sustaining treatments in patients with severe brain damage. 202 undergraduate students at the University of Padova were given one description drawn from four profiles describing different pathological states: the permanent vegetative state, the minimally conscious state, the locked-in syndrome, and the terminal illness. Participants were asked to evaluate *how dead* or how alive the patient was, and *how appropriate* it was to satisfy the patient's desire.

Principal Findings.—We found that the moral principles in which people believe affect not only people's judgments concerning the appropriateness of the withdrawal of life support, but also the perception of the death status of patients with severe brain injury. In particular, we found that the supporters of the Free Choice (FC) principle perceived the death status of the patients with different pathologies differently: the more people believe in the FC, the more they perceived patients as dead in pathologies where conscious awareness is severely impaired. By contrast, participants who agree with the Sanctity of Life (SL) principle did not show differences across pathologies.

Conclusions.—These results may shed light on the complex aspects of moral consensus for supporting or rejecting end-of-life decisions.

▶ What predicts a layperson's perception of life for a patient with severe neurologic and cognitive dysfunctions and limitations? Lotto and coworkers take on this challenging work by designing a novel tool administered to 200 undergraduates at the University of Padova. Participants were given a description of 4 different pathological states: permanent vegetative state (awake but without awareness of self or environment), minimally conscious state (awake with awareness of self or environment), full locked-in syndrome (awake, aware, but completely and permanently paralyzed), and terminal illness (control scenario, no neurological disability).

After reading the descriptions, participants rated each state on a point scale to describe how alive or dead they felt each patient was. Participants then rated, assuming patients in the scenarios did not wish to continue living in that state, whether they agreed with the patient's desire to withdraw treatment. Finally, participants were asked which of 2 principles they agreed with, the freedom of choice (FC) or autonomy principle, or the sanctity of life (SL) principle.

Unsurprisingly, participants rated persistent vegetative state as that with the "greatest death status." The second-highest rated was the locked-in state, and the third-highest rated was the minimally conscious state. Interestingly, the authors found an interaction between those who allied with free choice and pathology rating; these participants were more likely than their counterparts to rate pathologies with more death status. With further analyses, the authors found that those who endorsed FC rated the minimally conscious and permanent vegetative states as significantly different from terminal illness, whereas those who endorsed the SL principle rated each of the pathologies equally.

In analyzing the decisions to withdraw treatment, authors found those who agreed with FC tended to agree with decisions to withdraw treatment; conversely, those participants who agree with the SL principle tended to disagree with decisions to discontinue support. However, these decisions were not significantly different across pathology, which the authors see as evidence of participants using principles, not pathology, to guide end-of-life decision making.

This study has important limitations. As a small, single-site study in a Southern European country, both internal and external validity are limited. Internal validity is difficult to discern, as we do not know the baseline characteristics of the population beyond gender: religious affiliation and socioeconomic status are unknown. Given the university population, participants are likely middle to upper-middle class, but we may not know for certain. While the authors did not find significant differences in gender, the disproportionate number of females (80%) and small study size suggest insufficient power to detect such differences. The single site being in a Southern European country limits external generalizability, as cultural, religious, and racial differences vary widely between the study location and other regions.

Indeed, we do know that end-of-life decisions are partly a function of location. In 2005, Yaguchi and colleagues[1] surveyed nearly 2000 physicians from 21 countries and found that those in Japan, the United States, Brazil, and Southern Europe (including Italy) were more likely to pursue aggressive resuscitation of a vegetative patient than physicians in Northern Europe, Central Europe, Canada, and Australia. In an objective analysis of intensive care unit end-of-life data across Europe, Sprung and colleagues[2] found that Southern European countries such as Italy used cardiopulmonary resuscitation more and "withdrawing and shortening of the dying process" significantly less than central and Northern European countries. Taken together, this research suggests a profound effect of region on the decision to withdraw life support at the end of life. Even within the United States, wide variation has been seen in end-of-life practices, with the Midwest and Middle Atlantic regions more likely to participate in withdrawal of life support before death than New York.[3]

Lotto has furthered critical care ethics by creating an insightful questionnaire that could one day be used as an educational tool for intensivists and families or primary care physicians and their patients. Further validation is needed before the results can be generalizable.

W. Rafelson, MBA
V. Rajput, MD

References

1. Yaguchi A, Truog RD, Curtis R, et al. International differences in end-of-life attitudes in the intensive care unit: results of a survey. *Arch Intern Med.* 2005;165: 1970-1975.
2. Sprung CL, Cohen SL, Sjokvist P, et al. End-of-life practices in European intensive care units: the Ethicus Study. *JAMA.* 2003;290:790-797.
3. Prendergast TJ, Claessens MT, Luce JM. A national survey of end-of-life care for critically ill patients. *Am J Respir Crit Care Med.* 1998;158:1163-1167.

The role of the principle of double effect in ethics education at US medical schools and its potential impact on pain management at the end of life
Macauley R (Fletcher Allen Health Care, Burlington, VT)
J Med Ethics 38:174-178, 2012

Background.—Because opioids can suppress respiratory drive, the principle of double effect (PDE) has been used to justify their use for terminally ill patients. Recent studies, however, suggest that the risk of respiratory depression in typical end-of-life (EOL) situations may be overstated and that heightened concern for this rare occurrence can lead to inadequate treatment of pain. The purpose of this study is to examine the role of the PDE in medical school ethics education, with specific reference to its potential impact on pain management at EOL.

Method.—After obtaining institutional review board approval, an electronic survey was sent to ethics educators at every allopathic medical school in the USA.

Results.—One-third of ethics educators felt that opioids were 'likely' to cause significant respiratory depression that could hasten death. Educators' opinions of opioid effects did not influence their view of the relevance of the PDE, with approximately 70% deeming it relevant to EOL care. Only 15% of ethics educators believed that associating the PDE with opioid use might discourage clinicians from optimally treating pain, out of concern for respiratory depression.

Conclusion.—This study demonstrates that a significant minority of ethics educators believe, contrary to current evidence, that opioids are 'likely' to cause significant respiratory depression that could hasten death in terminally ill patients. Yet, many of those who do not feel this is likely still rely on the PDE to justify this possibility, potentially (and unknowingly) contributing to clinical misperceptions and underutilisation of opioids at EOL.

▶ Does the principle of double effect (PDE) itself further the misperception that end-of-life pain management is medically and ethically problematic? Macauley tackles these issues in an incisive study on medical ethics education among US allopathic schools. In it, he highlights that the PDE in medical ethics education is often taught in the context of administering opioids, which can have a side effect of respiratory depression and theoretically hasten death. The PDE, Macauley writes, has 4 components:

1. The act itself must be, at worst, morally neutral.
2. The bad effect cannot be the means to the good effect.
3. The good effect must outweigh the bad effect.
4. The agent must only intend the good effect, although the bad effect may be foreseen.

The author argues that opioid administration for palliative care at end of life is often taught in this context: opioid administration is not bad (principle 1); its side effect of respiratory depression is not intended to outweigh pain control (principle 2); pain control at end of life outweighs the negative effect of depressed respiratory drive (principle 3); and the physician administering the opioid intends for pain control, not for a hastened death (principle 4).

In an effort to identify the use of this paradigm, Macauley designed a 12-question survey and invited medical ethics educators—both clinicians and nonclinicians—from all US allopathic schools. Seventy-two respondents representing 59 medical schools responded, half of whom were clinicians. Most respondents were very familiar with the concept of the PDE, the most commonly taught examples of which were opioids for terminally ill patients (72%) and palliative sedation (64%). Most respondents felt that the PDE was useful in justifying opioid use in these scenarios. Surprisingly, about one-third of respondents believed that opioids were likely to cause "significant respiratory depression that could hasten death" (34%). Interestingly, no significant differences were found between clinicians and nonclinicians.

Such findings should surprise us. In medical literature, there is little evidence that palliative opioid administration is directly linked to decreased survival.[1] Macauley himself points to burgeoning research in the field of palliative care that undercuts this basic assumption that opioid administration at end of life hastens death. The work by Portenoy and others[2] points to evidence that opioid toxicity at end of life is minimal. Macauley argues that the PDE justification for opioid use at the end of life is unnecessary and potentially harmful for future physicians who will treat end-of-life patients. However, PDE to justify opioids has been justified by the Supreme Court; as Justice Rehnquist writes: "It is widely recognized that the provision of pain medication is ethically and professionally acceptable even when the treatment may hasten the patient's death if the medication is intended to alleviate pain and severe discomfort, not to cause death."[3] The PDE has been applied to many controversial issues, including the idea of "just war" during the 2002 Afghanistan War.[4] His standpoint is buttressed by the American College of Critical Care Medicine, as they wrote in their 2008 guidelines for end-of-life care, "Some have argued that the doctrine of double effect is not necessary, since studies suggest that the use of sedatives and analgesics at the end of life does not actually hasten death."[5]

Macauley's work carries some limitations. While the PDE-opioid link has been clearly established, its effect on trainees is not. His work could be grounded not only by surveying educators but students and trainees as well. Moreover, some in the medical ethics community still maintain that teaching the PDE in the context of pharmacotherapy is still useful. The American College of Critical Care Medicine argues the PDE is still helpful for "justifying those individual cases where the drugs clearly appear to hasten death but are necessary to control symptoms."[3] Ethicists can obviate the opiophobia by teaching the PDE in the context of highly potent benzodiazepines and anesthetics, rather than opioids. What is needed, perhaps, is not to discard the concept of the PDE in medical ethics, but rather to support education to students, trainees, and physicians on evidence-based pain management at the end of life.

W. Rafelson, MBA

V. Rajput, MD

References

1. Sykes N, Thorns A. Sedative use in the last week of life and the implications for end-of-life decision making. *Arch Intern Med.* 2003;163:341-344.
2. Portenoy RK, Sibirceva U, Smout R, et al. Opioid use and survival at the end of life: a survey of a hospice population. *J Pain Symptom Manage.* 2006;32:532-540.
3. U.S. Supreme Court. Vacco v. Quill. *Wests Supreme Court Report.* 1997;117: 2293-2312.
4. Leaning J. Was the Afghan conflict a just war? *BMJ.* 2002;324:353-355.
5. Truog RD, Campbell ML, Curtis JR, et al. Recommendations for end-of-life care in the intensive care unit: a consensus statement by the American College of Critical Care Medicine. *Crit Care Med.* 2006;36:953-963.

Death and legal fictions

Shah SK, Truog RD, Miller FG (Natl Insts of Health, Bethesda, MD; Children's Hosp, Boston, MA)
J Med Ethics 37:719-722, 2011

Advances in life-saving technologies in the past few decades have challenged our traditional understandings of death. Traditionally, death was understood to occur when a person stops breathing, their heart stops beating and they are cold to the touch. Today, physicians determine death by relying on a diagnosis of 'total brain failure' or by waiting a short while after circulation stops. Evidence has emerged, however, that the conceptual bases for these approaches to determining death are fundamentally flawed and depart substantially from the established biological conception of death. We argue that the current approach to determining death consists of two different types of unacknowledged legal fictions. These legal fictions were developed for practices that are largely ethically legitimate but need to be reconciled with the law. The considerable debate over the determination of death in the medical and scientific literature has not informed the public that vital organs are being procured from still-living donors and it seems unlikely that this information can remain hidden for long. Given the instability of the status quo and the difficulty of making the substantial legal changes required by complete transparency, we argue for a second-best policy solution: acknowledging the legal fictions involved in determining death to move in the direction of greater transparency. This may someday result in more substantial legal change to directly confront the challenges raised by life-sustaining and life-preserving technologies without the need for fictions.

▶ Shah et al describe the current medico-legal paradigm for determining death in the United States as flawed and in need of repair. They discuss how the 1981 Uniform Definition of Death Act and the 2008 definition of "whole brain death" from the President's Council on Bioethics do not allow those who satisfy neurological criteria for brain death and many of those whose organs are ultimately harvested to be legally defined as dead. To accommodate this technical discrepancy between the law and current practice, the authors believe we unwittingly use legal principles known as "fictions," which they describe as "false statements to serve a particular legal purpose." We agree with the authors that, according to the legal definitions given here, many organ donors are not "dead." We also agree that despite this discrepancy our current methods of organ procurement are morally justifiable. It is not clear to us, however, whether the divergence between the law and our actions is or will likely ever be of practical or substantial significance, as feared by the authors. Nor is it clear that the use of "legal fictions" in this case amounts to much more than a hypothetical legal argument that could be used to defend current organ procurement practices in court should they be challenged on these grounds.

In 2007 Epstein,[1] wrote about legal fictions in medical ethics in an effort to "break the silence," acknowledging the subject "has rarely invoked the intellectual interest it begs." The author categorized and briefly discussed 18 legal fictions he believed to exist, several involving end-of-life situations. For example, he argued that someone in an irreversible coma does not actually have any "interests." So, when we justify withdrawal of care from them by saying it was in their best interests, we are not actually correct (because they have no interests) and thus we are using a false statement (it is in the their best interest) to serve a legal purpose (justify withdrawal of care to allow circulatory failure). Epstein also discussed how withdrawal of life-sustaining treatment is not truly different from active euthanasia, that respecting a patient's wishes to refuse life-saving interventions is not legally different from physician-assisted suicide, and that hastening a patient's death is not entirely unmotivated by a desire to bring about his or her death. Because these common actions all are legally based on statements that can be argued to be untrue they also are examples of legal fictions.

In 2012, Cogan[2] discussed the concerns of English law surrounding mechanical ventilation in patients simply to keep their organs viable for future harvesting. In 1995, the Exeter Protocol, which advocated family-consented mechanical ventilation of deeply comatose patients to keep them "alive" until their organs could be harvested, was declared unlawful. Since then, the author has argued that the legal climate surrounding principles such as "best interest" have changed, and that the Exeter Protocol would probably now be considered legal. The author also makes the important point that regardless of their legality, these actions must be acceptable to the professionals carrying them out and by the public at large. This illustrates the similarity between European and American efforts to define death. The specifics may be different, but clearly both regions are struggling to analyze and modify their legal code against a backdrop of dynamic public attitudes, sluggish politico-legal systems, and persistently advancing medical and bioethical fields in a way that supports the generally accepted and morally permissible action of organ procurement and donation.

Freeman and Bernat's 2012 article Ethical Issues in Organ Transplantation[3] describes the current neurological determination of brain death as "now...accepted throughout the world." They note, however, that organ donation after the circulatory determination of death is ripe with controversy because of the difficulty in determining when exactly it is that death has occurred. The authors believe we can define permanent cessation of circulatory function as arrest that has occurred long enough in a patient with do not resuscitate orders that auto-resuscitation (the heart spontaneously restarting on its own) will not occur. Because auto-resuscitation has not been shown to occur in closely monitored intensive care patients after 1 to 2 minutes of asystole and the patient will not be externally resuscitated in the future, these patients can then be pronounced as dead and their organs harvested. Shah et al contend that because this patient could potentially be resuscitated (if not for the do-not-resuscitate order), his or her death state is only irreversible by choice and not physiologically irreversible. Because Shah et al feel that death should be irreversible by definition; they describe the distinction between permanent and irreversible circulatory arrest as a "conceptual sleight-of-hand invoked solely to legitimate organ donation." This is where they believe we invoke the principle of "anticipatory fiction" whereby a death that has not yet occurred (the dying donor) is pronounced dead on the grounds that death will imminently occur in the future and to delay the pronouncement would cause harm (by violating the wishes of the donor and risking the quality of the organs).

Shah et al contribute valuable insight to the ongoing debate over how we define death, particularly in the context of organ donation. Interestingly, despite their efforts to demonstrate the inadequacy of our current legal definitions of death and the potential legal and moral implications of continuing to harvest organs under our current paradigm, they do feel current organ donation actions to be morally and legally justified. Essentially, they want to raise awareness of the disparity between what they believe our laws currently allow and what we actually do. They hope that by admitting this disconnect we will facilitate a greater discussion that would temper any possible public backlash while sowing the seeds for eventual legal reforms. In this way, we will allow what is legally permissible to catch up and synchronize with the morally permissible actions we already undertake.

W. Philip, DO
V. Rajput, MD

References

1. Epstein M. Legal and institutional fictions in medical ethics: a common, and yet largely overlooked, phenomenon. *J Med Ethics.* 2007;33:362-364.
2. Cogan J. Elective ventilation for organ donation: law, policy and public ethics. *J Med Ethics.* 2012 Dec 7. [Epub ahead of print].
3. Freeman RB, Bernat JL. Ethical issues in organ transplantation. *Prog Cardiovasc Dis.* 2012;55:282-289.

The Ethics and Reality of Rationing in Medicine

Scheunemann LP, White DB (Univ of North Carolina Hosps, Chapel Hill; Univ of Pittsburgh Med Ctr, PA)
Chest 140:1625-1632, 2011

Rationing is the allocation of scarce resources, which in health care necessarily entails withholding potentially beneficial treatments from some individuals. Rationing is unavoidable because need is limitless and resources are not. How rationing occurs is important because it not only affects individual lives but also expresses society's most important values. This article discusses the following topics: (1) the inevitability of rationing of social goods, including medical care; (2) types of rationing; (3) ethical principles and procedures for fair allocation; and (4) whether rationing ICU care to those near the end of life would result in substantial cost savings.

▶ Does rationing occur in the United States? Scheunemann and others argue yes and use the example of critically ill adults to argue that "microallocation"— physicians allocating scarce resources among many patients—occurs regularly. He points to a recent survey in which only 60% of intensivists responded that they provide all patients with every beneficial therapy, without regard to its cost. Intensivists make microallocation decisions daily: deciding which patient to see first, who to see for the most time, and, of course, which patients to transfer in and which to transfer out when the intensive care unit (ICU) is full. About 15% of patients attempted to be transferred to the ICU are denied, a significant minority of whom are solely denied because of bed shortage.

This is a launching pad for the authors' discussion on rationing in medical care in the United States. They argue that ICU physicians should be well versed in the discussion on medical rationing, because it is a regular occurrence. The authors focus on macroallocation decisions, or rationing on a societal level to fairly allocate resources such as organs and Medicaid dollars. The authors outline 4 types of principles that are used in the process to decide who should receive the scarce resource:

1. Utilitarianism: maximize quality-adjusted life years
2. Egalitarianism: lottery system or "first come, first served"
3. Prioritarianism: favor the worst-off, with preference to the young
4. Rule of rescue: save those from imminent death

Scheunemann and others deftly bring examples of macroallocation decisions in the history of US health policy. For example, under utilitarianism, the authors write how the state of Oregon, facing severe budget shortfalls in the 1990s, offered limited health coverage to the poor. Using quality-adjusted life years (QALY) to justify which treatments ought to be covered, the Oregon Health Plan favored preventive, primary care services over advanced, costly treatments. The authors expose the unforgiving nature of utilitarianism, as seen when a poor Oregon boy who needed a bone marrow transplant was denied because of QALY considerations. Whereas in the United Kingdom citizens accept QALY considerations as a necessary part of rationing, as seen in the National Institute of Clinical Effectiveness, in the United States such decisions are fraught with difficulty.

On the other hand, egalitarianism is an attempt to fairly allocate resources by using a waiting list; participants are seen either in order (first-come, first-served) or by a lottery system. The difficulty with first-come, first-served systems, as seen in the United Network for Organ Sharing, is the ability for well-connected individuals to more quickly be listed, and listed multiple times, than those who are poorer and not as well connected.

Prioritarianism is a concept that is often interpreted as allowing as many people as possible to achieve a normal life span. In 2008, writing in the *Lancet*, Persad and colleagues[1] wrote a similar review of principles of rationing, and advocated for an alternative "complete lives system," which favors those in the earlier stages of life, as well as incorporating prognosis. Scheunemann incorporates this theory somewhat in his discussion of prioritarianism but notes that it is typically blind to prognosis; he argues that a multiprinciple rationale, such as the one Emanuel argues for, is optimal.

Finally, the rule of rescue—the one that clinicians are probably most familiar with—entails our impulse to save those facing imminent death, regardless of the cost or prognosis. The authors argue that this is likely the least cost-effective principle, yet it is with this one that physicians are most familiar. A patient "codes" and the physician diverts all resources to that patient. Can we balance the need to save someone from imminent death with the fear of delivering futile care?

Surprisingly, the authors argue that despite critical care consuming nearly 1% of US gross domestic product, more than 80% of critical care costs are fixed, and so denying end-of-life care that is seen as futile may only save 20% of projected costs. In the staunch battle, perhaps regulating fixed costs as priority may be a way to avoid rationing; before the hospital opens a new ICU wing or heart hospital, perhaps a state commission on health care costs can regulate whether such expansion is justified for the population. While the authors do not touch on this, in an era of escalating costs of care, rationing fixed costs may be just as important, and more palatable, than rationing variable costs.

So which principle do ICU physicians agree most with? In 2011, Kohn and colleagues[2] surveyed a thousand ICU clinicians, asking which of 2 patients to give a theoretical last ICU bed to: a gravely ill patient with little chance of surviving or a deceased or near-death patient for whom ICU care would help others through organ donation. More than one-third of ICU clinicians argued that the scarce ICU resources should be allocated to a patient unlikely to benefit from them, overlooking the societal benefits of organ transplant. The authors argue that a significant number of ICU clinicians adhere to the rule of rescue.[2] We believe that the rule of rescue is inherent in medical training and has an indelible effect on physicians' practice patterns more than any other principle.

Scheunemann and others make an attempt to convince the reader that ICU physicians participate in microallocation of resources and should be abreast of all the principles of allocation. However, most clinicians would argue they see patients in order from most to least sick and that principles such as egalitarianism and utilitarianism, while applicable in macroallocation, are unjustifiable for individual practice patterns. Using QALY analysis, a lottery, or first-come first-served system in daily practice, rather than seeing the sickest first, is difficult for the reader to imagine. The similarities between micro- and macroallocation, while intriguing, need more investigation.

W. Rafelson, MBA

V. Rajput, MD

References

1. Persad G, Wertheimer A, Emanuel EJ. Principles for allocation of scarce medical interventions. *Lancet.* 2009;373:423-431.
2. Kohn R, Rubenfeld GD, Levy MM, Ubel PA, Halpern SD. Rule of rescue or the good of the many? Analysis of physicians' and nurses' preferences for allocating ICU beds. *Intensive Care Med.* 2011;37:1210-1217.

Early Withdrawal of Life Support in Severe Burn Injury
Pham TN, Otto A, Young SR, et al (Univ of Washington, Seattle)
J Burn Care Res 33:130-135, 2012

Despite many advances in modern burn care, deaths still occur in the burn intensive care unit. For patients with severe burns, providers may advocate to withdraw life support early during hospitalization when the extent of injury makes survival highly unlikely or when the patient's condition deteriorates during resuscitation. Our regional burn center has implemented a stepwise withdrawal protocol since 2001 in an effort to standardize symptoms palliation at the end of life. In this study, the authors evaluated the frequency of early withdrawal and the protocol impact on end-of-life processes of care in burn patients who died within 72 hours of hospitalization. A 13-year review of all burn patients aged ≥18 years admitted to our burn center to identify all patients who died within 72 hours of hospitalization was performed. Patients were dichotomized to the periods before (1995 to mid-2001) and after implementation of standardized withdrawal protocol (mid-2001 to 2007). Descriptive analyses were performed to compare end-of-life care processes between the two periods. A total of 4374 adult patients with acute burns were admitted during the 13-year study period, of which 252 (6%) died during hospitalization. Of the patients who died within 72 hours, 106 (84%) had withdrawal of life support compared with 20 (16%) who died with ongoing life support. Higher mean TBSA distinguished patients who died by withdrawal (61 vs 48%, $P = .06$). Since mid-2001, all 61 patients who had life support withdrawn were by protocol. Implementation of the protocol has led to more frequent use of opioid infusion (98 vs 87%, $P = .07$) and benzodiazepine infusion (95 vs 49%, $P < .01$), without hastening time to death (median 5.0 vs 5.5 hours, $P = .70$). The large majority of early burn deaths at our regional center occur via withdrawal of life support. Implementation of a protocolized withdrawal has resulted in more consistent provision of analgesia and sedation without hastening death. Burn centers should consider using a protocol for withdrawal of life support to improve consistency in end-of-life symptoms palliation.

▶ Compared with the patient with a protracted illness or progressively debilitating disease when death is near, the anticipated death resulting from an overwhelming burn injury is a sudden event. The patient and family in this situation do not have the opportunity to plan in advance or discuss all treatment options in a leisurely manner. The authors note the significant advances made in their burn center after instituting an end-of-life protocol. Those advances came in the way of the percent of patients receiving opioid and benzodiazepine infusions, being liberated from the ventilator, and patients or families being offered spiritual counseling and support.

Processes not changed after instituting an end-of-life protocol include the median time from withdrawal decision to death. I agree with the authors' conclusions that use of a protocol does not hasten demise, but it may improve the patient's experience. However, using a protocol is not a substitute for family meetings and supportive communications for the patient and his or her loved ones. Most academic medical centers have palliative care services that may enhance the support not only for the patient and family but for the care providers as well.

In this day and age of the protocol-driven approach to patient care, it is disheartening to consider that patients who are not anticipated to survive their injuries will die without being provided the optimal opportunity for a dignified, pain-free transition between life and death. The authors recommend that end-of-life symptom palliation should be performed for burn patients according to a protocol. I believe the protocol(s) should be generalized to every patient population, where we can provide symptom relief for the patient, comfort to the family, and knowledge for the care providers that we have provided a comfortable and dignified experience to the best of our abilities.

B. A. Latenser, MD, FACS

Does Admission During Morning Rounds Increase the Mortality of Patients in the Medical ICU?

Bisbal M, Pauly V, Gainnier M, et al (Aix-Marseille Université, France; et al)
Chest 142:1179-1184, 2012

Background.—Early optimization of treatment is crucial when admitting patients to the ICU and could depend on the organization of the medical team. The aim of this retrospective bservational study was to determine whether admissions during morning rounds are independently associated with hospital mortality in a medical ICU.

Methods.—The 3,540 patients admitted from May 2000 to April 2010 to the medical ICU of Sainte Marguerite Hospital in Marseille, France, were divided into two groups based on the time of admission. The non-morning rounds group was admitted between 1:00 PM and 7:59 AM, and the morning rounds group was admitted between 8:00 AM and 12:59 PM. Hospital mortality (crude and adjusted) was compared between the two groups.

Results.—The 583 patients (16.5%) admitted during morning rounds were older and sicker upon admission compared with those patients admitted during non-morning rounds. The crude hospital mortality was 35.2% (95% CI, 31.4-39.1) in the group of patients admitted during morning rounds and 28.0% (95% CI, 26.4-29.7) in the other group ($P < .001$). An admission during morning rounds was not independently associated with hospital death (adjusted hazard ratio, 1.10; 95% CI, 0.94-1.28; $P = .24$).

Conclusions.—Being admitted to the medical ICU during morning rounds is not associated with a poorer outcome than afternoon and night admissions. The conditions of the patients admitted during morning rounds were more severe, which underlines the importance of the ICU team's availability during this time. Further studies are needed to evaluate if the presence of a specific medical team overnight in the wards would be able to improve patients' outcome by preventing delayed ICU admission.

▶ Several studies have examined the relationship between time of admission to the intensive care unit (ICU) and outcome. Concern has been raised that patients admitted during off hours and weekends have poorer outcomes than those admitted during the daytime, which are high staffing periods, when the onsite intensivist is likely to be immediately available. This study, conducted in a French unit, examines outcome of patients admitted in the morning during rounds when a coverage gap could occur as opposed to those admitted at other times.[1] Although the morning admission group had a poorer outcome, predictors of increased morbidity were present.

Morning admissions had higher organ failure scores and were at risk for delayed transfer to the ICU, which has been associated with higher mortality in previous work.[2]

Limitations of this work include inability to generalize the staffing model used in this hospital to other ICUs and inclusion of a study cohort limited to a medical unit.

D. J. Dries, MSE, MD

References

1. Afessa B, Gajic O, Morales IJ, et al. Association between ICU admission during morning rounds and mortality. *Chest.* 2009;136:1489-1495.
2. Chalfin DB, Trzeciak S, Likourezos A, Baumann BM, Dellinger RP; DELAY-ED Study Group. Impact of delayed transfer of critically ill patients from the emergency department to the intensive care unit. *Crit Care Med.* 2007;35:1477-1483.

Refusal of Intensive Care Unit Admission Due to a Full Unit: Impact on Mortality

Robert R, for the Association des Réanimateurs du Centre Ouest Group (CHU de Poitiers, France; et al)
Am J Respir Crit Care Med 185:1081-1087, 2012

Rationale.—Intensive care unit (ICU) beds are a scarce resource, and patients denied intensive care only because the unit is full may be at increased risk of death.

Objective.—To compare mortality after first ICU referral in admitted patients and in patients denied admission because the unit was full.

Methods.—Prospective observational multicenter cohort study of consecutive patients referred for ICU admission during two 45-day periods, conducted in 10 ICUs.

Measurements and Main Results.—Of 1,762 patients, 430 were excluded from the study, 116 with previously denied admission to another ICU and 270 because they were deemed too sick or too well to benefit from ICU admission. Of the remaining 1,332 patients, 1,139 were admitted, and 193 were denied admission because the unit was full (65 were never admitted, 39 were admitted after bumping of another patient, and 89 were admitted on subsequent referral). Crude Day 28 and Day 60 mortality rates in the nonadmitted and admitted groups were 30.1 versus 24.3% ($P = 0.07$) and 33.3 versus 27.2% ($P = 0.06$), respectively. Day 28 mortality adjusted on age, previous disease, Glasgow scale score less than or equal to 8, shock, creatinine level greater than or equal to 250 μmol/L, and prothrombin time greater than or equal to 30 seconds was nonsignificantly higher in patients refused ICU admission only because of a full unit compared with patients admitted immediately. Patients admitted after subsequent referral had higher mortality rates on Day 28 ($P = 0.05$) and Day 60 ($P = 0.04$) compared with directly admitted patients.

Conclusions.—Delayed ICU admission due to a full unit at first referral is associated with increased mortality.

▶ We typically assume appropriate decision making in referral of patients to the critical care unit.[1,2] Indirectly, the authors test this assumption by examining outcomes of patients referred to the intensive care unit (ICU) but declined because of a full unit. Some data are required to put this study in context. For example, the time from first referral until ICU admission was 80 minutes. In 128 patients admitted after initial refusal because of a full unit, median time to admission was 195 minutes. Patients admitted in response to a second ICU referral were admitted at 309 minutes. Although these time differences are statistically significant, the overall difference is nowhere near as long as I might expect. In addition, it is important to notice that the percentage of patients refused admission because the unit was full varied across the participating units from 1% to 61% (median 31%; Fig 2 in the original article).

An obvious strength of this study is the attention paid to triage criteria. Patients were considered for this study but excluded if they were felt by investigators to be too well to benefit from critical care referral. In addition, patients who were too sick to benefit were also excluded.

In this article, which I believe reflects the state of the art, I was impressed that the authors note poor compliance with triage recommendations and policies in hospitals. In fact, compliance with triage recommendations is poorer in patients refused because the unit is full. The authors admit that the young patient with a severe condition is more likely to be admitted even if another individual is bumped.

This study is an important start to answer an important question. The crude ICU refusal rate was more than 20%.[3] However, it is unclear how many patients were refused admission simply because of previous inappropriate ICU admissions. We are simply told that units were full. Clearly, additional work needs to be done on development of appropriate and consistently applied ICU admission criteria. Then, refusal of ICU admission can be better assessed.

D. J. Dries, MSE, MD

References

1. Guidelines for intensive care unit admission, discharge, and triage. Task Force of the American College of Critical Care Medicine, Society of Critical Care Medicine. *Crit Care Med.* 1999;27:633-638.
2. Capuzzo M, Moreno RP, Alvisi R. Admission and discharge of critically ill patients. *Curr Opin Crit Care.* 2010;16:499-504.
3. Azoulay E, Pochard F, Chevret S, et al. Compliance with triage to intensive care recommendations. *Crit Care Med.* 2001;29:2132-2136.

The Epidemiology of Intensive Care Unit Readmissions in the United States
Brown SES, Ratcliffe SJ, Kahn JM, et al (Perelman School of Medicine at the Univ of Pennsylvania, Philadelphia; Univ of Pittsburgh Med Ctr, PA)
Am J Respir Crit Care Med 185:955-964, 2012

Rationale.—The incidence of intensive care unit (ICU) readmissions across the United States is unknown.

Objectives.—To determine incidence of ICU readmissions in United States hospitals, and describe the distribution of time between ICU discharges and readmissions.

Methods.—This retrospective cohort study used 196,202 patients in 156 medical and surgical ICUs in 106 community and academic hospitals participating in Project IMPACT from April 1, 2001, to December 31, 2007. We used mixed-effects logistic regression, adjusting for patient and hospital characteristics, to describe how ICU readmission rates differed across patient types, ICU models, and hospital types.

Measurements and Main Results.—Measurements consisted of 48- and 120-hour ICU readmission rates and time to readmission. A total of 3,905 patients (2%) were readmitted to the ICU within 48 hours, and 7,171 (3.7%) within 120 hours. In adjusted analysis, there was no difference

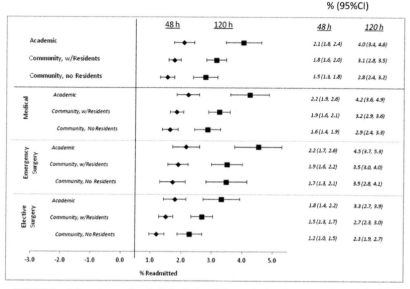

FIGURE 1.—Adjusted rates of readmission by hospital organization. Percent readmitted after 48 and 120 hours. Rates represent predicted probabilities of intensive care unit readmission after adjusting for patient, intensive care unit, and hospital characteristics. CI = confidence interval. (Reprinted from Brown SES, Ratcliffe SJ, Kahn JM, et al. The epidemiology of intensive care unit readmissions in the United States. *Am J Respir Crit Care Med.* 2012;185:955-964, with permission from the American Thoracic Society.)

in ICU readmissions across patient types or ICU models. Among medical patients, those in academic hospitals had higher odds of 48- and 120-hour readmission than patients in community hospitals without residents (1.51 [95% confidence interval, 1.12—2.02] and 1.63 [95% confidence interval, 1.24—2.16]). Median time to ICU readmission was 3.07 days (interquartile range, 1.27—6.58). Closed ICUs had the longest times to readmission (3.55 d [interquartile range, 1.42—7.50]).

Conclusions.—Approximately 2% and 4% of ICU patients discharged to the ward are readmitted within 48 and 120 hours, within a median time of 3 days. Medical patients in academic hospitals are more likely to be readmitted than patients in community hospitals without residents. ICU readmission rates could be useful for policy makers and investigations into their causes and consequences (Figs 1-3).

▶ This is a massive epidemiologic dataset. Subjects enrolled come from the Project IMPACT dataset. Thus, this is not a randomized or systematically obtained selection of intensive care unit (ICU) patients. The authors also acknowledge that burn, cardiac, or coronary patients are not included in this analysis.

In addition to the data sample provided in the abstract, the authors note that among patients admitted to an ICU, 8.6% died during their initial ICU stay, with

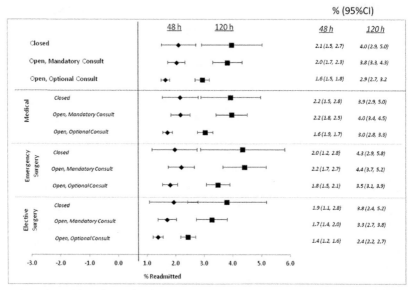

FIGURE 2.—Adjusted rates of readmission by intensive care unit (ICU) model. Percent readmitted after 48 and 120 hours. Rates represent predicted probabilities of ICU readmission after adjusting for patient, ICU, and hospital characteristics. CI = confidence interval. (Reprinted from Brown SES, Ratcliffe SJ, Kahn JM, et al. The epidemiology of intensive care unit readmissions in the United States. *Am J Respir Crit Care Med*. 2012;185:955-964, with permission from the American Thoracic Society.)

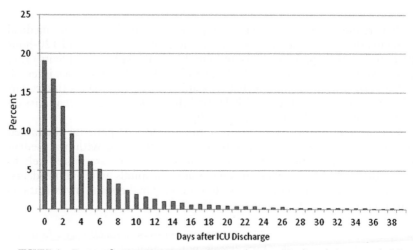

FIGURE 3.—Days to first intensive care unit (ICU) readmission. Unadjusted time to readmission across all ICU, hospital, and patient types, calculated from the time of discharge to the time of ICU readmission. Does not include readmissions to ICUs other than that from which the patient was initially discharged. (Reprinted from Brown SES, Ratcliffe SJ, Kahn JM, et al. The epidemiology of intensive care unit readmissions in the United States. *Am J Respir Crit Care Med*. 2012;185:955-964, with permission from the American Thoracic Society.)

5% dying in hospital subsequent to ICU discharge. When patients who are never readmitted to the ICU are compared with those readmitted within 48 hours, early readmission patients had a 20.7% hospital mortality and only 36.6% of patients were discharged home. Median length of hospital stay was 8 days in patients without ICU readmission in 48 hours versus 15 days in the early readmission group.

Not surprisingly, respiratory insufficiency and other forms of organ failure are more common in patients readmitted to the ICU. Although the majority of patients are readmitted soon after discharge from ICU, we see differences in types of practice with respect to timing of critical care readmission (Fig 3). What we cannot tell is differing degree of acuity or patient characteristics in hospitals of different types (Figs 1 and 2).

Among other interesting observations made, afternoon and evening discharge were important risk factors for ICU readmission in the multivariate analyses conducted.[1] This is consistent with prior work and suggests that patients discharged at these times are more likely moved from the ICU to create room for other patients. Perhaps these individuals were less well prepared for their initial ICU discharge.

In all, these compendia of data is an excellent tool for hypothesis generation.[2-4] As ICU expenditures continue to grow, we must make optimal use of this valuable resource.

D. J. Dries, MSE, MD

References

1. Renton J, Pilcher DV, Santamaria JD, et al. Factors associated with increased risk of readmission to intensive care in Australia. *Intensive Care Med.* 2011;37: 1800-1808.
2. Pronovost PJ, Angus DC, Dorman T, Robinson KA, Dremsizov TT, Young TL. Physician staffing patterns and clinical outcomes in critically ill patients: a systematic review. *JAMA.* 2002;288:2151-2162.
3. McMillan TR, Hyzy RC. Bringing quality improvement into the intensive care unit. *Crit Care Med.* 2007;35:S59-S65.
4. Kim MM, Barnato AE, Angus DC, Fleisher LA, Kahn JM. The effect of multidisciplinary care teams on intensive care unit mortality. *Arch Intern Med.* 2010;170: 369-376.

A systematic review of silver-containing dressings and topical silver agents (used with dressings) for burn wounds

Aziz Z, Abu SF, Chong NJ (Univ of Malaya, Kuala Lumpur, Malaysia)
Burns 38:307-318, 2012

Silver preparations are commonly used for burns, but evidence of their effectiveness remains poorly defined. The aim of the study was to evaluate the effectiveness of silver-containing dressings and topical silver for preventing infection and promoting healing in burns wounds through a meta-analysis of the available evidence. The Cochrane Central Register of Controlled Trials and relevant databases were searched. Drug companies and experts in this field were also contacted. Randomised controlled trials (RCTs) of silver dressings or topical silver (used with dressings) compared with non-silver dressings were eligible for inclusion. We identified 14 RCTs involving 877 participants. One small trial of a silver-containing dressing showed significantly better healing time compared to the control [MD −3.6; 95% CI −4.94 to −2.26 for partial thickness burns and MD −3.9; 95% CI −4.54 to −3.26 for superficial burns]. Topical silver showed significantly worse healing time compared to the non-silver group [WMD 3.96; 95% CI 2.41−5.51] and showed no evidence of effectiveness in preventing wounds infection [WMD 2.48; 95% CI 0.39−15.73]. Our review suggests that silver-containing dressings and topical silver were either no better or worse than control dressings in preventing wound infection and promoting healing of burn wounds.

▶ This article attempts to evaluate the role of topical silver in burn care. Silver in some form, whether nanocrystalline, bound to another agent, or released on contact, has become the *sine qua non* of topical wound care in high-income countries. Multiple companies provide silver-containing dressings, each one touting that theirs is the best. Many debates have raged over the past decade about the most desirable form in which to provide silver to the burn wound, and I think it has resulted in a draw. What these authors have attempted to do is use a more scientific approach to examine the literature regarding silver in general, regardless of the delivery method. As the authors have pointed out, there are many studies, including randomized controlled trials. Upon drilling into these studies, we find most of the studies to be flawed, either because of small size, study bias, sponsorship by a company making a silver-containing burn wound dressing, or different definitions. The studies could not be combined to evaluate the data on a number of points. Although it is tempting to say that silver makes a difference in a wound (and this is my bias), so this study neither supports nor refutes the impact of silver in burn wound dressings.

B. A. Latenser, MD, FACS

Pathogenic alteration in severe burn wounds
Fu Y, Xie B, Ben D, et al (Second Military Med Univ, Shanghai, China)
Burns 38:90-94, 2012

The present study aims to define the trend of time related changes with local bacterial alteration of bacterial resistance in severe burns in our burn center during a 12-year period. Retrospective analysis of microbiological results on severely burned wounds between 1998 and 2009 was carried out. A study of 3615 microbial isolates was performed. *Staphylococcus aureus* was the most commonly isolated pathogen (38.2%) followed by *A. baumannii* (16.2%), *Streptococcus viridans* (11.4%), *Pseudomonas aeruginosa* (10.4%), *coagulase-negative staphylococci* (CNS, 9.2%). The species ratios of *S. aureus* and *A. baumannii* increased significantly from

1st to 8th week of hospitalization, while those of *Streptococcus viridans*, *P. aeruginosa* and *coagulase-negative staphylococci* decreased during the same period. Bacterial resistance rates were compared between the periods 1998–2003 and 2004–2009. Vancomycin remained as the most sensitive antibiotic in *S. aureus* including methicillin-resistant *S. aureus* (*MRSA*). It was very likely that the majority of infections caused by *Streptococcus viridans*, *P. aeruginosa* and *coagulase-negative staphylococci* occurred in the early stage of burn course and the majority of infections caused by *A. baumannii* occurred 4 weeks after admission. The use of different antibiotics was probably the major contributor to these trends.

▶ The authors have examined a phenomenon that burn care providers have known for a long time. That is, the pathogens in a burn wound change over time, both within an individual burn patient, and within the large context of the burn center. It is relatively easy to track the individual bacterial isolates but more difficult to assess the meaning of those findings. As the authors noted, by the end of the hospital stay, a positive wound culture rarely translated into a real burn wound infection. The authors used wound cultures as the basis for their study. Given the absence of quantitative wound cultures, I will assume these samples were wound swabs, which have not been shown to correlate with burn wound infections. In 2007, the American Burn Association (ABA) published the results of their consensus conferment to define sepsis and infection in burns. That publication clearly defines the distinctions between burn wound colonization, infection, and invasive infection.[1] Although alluded to, the authors did not really address fungal wound cultures and infections, something that would have enhanced the global burn knowledge base. There is a very small sample size for this large burn center over an extended period. I think all these factors dilute the impact of the findings. I would refer interested readers to the ABA's Consensus Conference findings instead.

B. A. Latenser, MD, FACS

Reference

1. Greenhalgh DG, Saffle JR, Holmes JH, et al. American Burn Association consensus conference to define sepsis and infection in burns. *J Burn Care Res.* 2007;28:776-790.

12 Pharmacology/ Sedation-Analgesia

Anticoagulation management around percutaneous bedside procedures: Is adjustment required?
Barton CA, McMillian WD, Osler T, et al (Fletcher Allen Health Care, Burlington, VT; Univ of Vermont, Colchester)
J Trauma 72:815-820, 2012

Background.—Percutaneous endoscopic gastrostomy (PEG) and percutaneous dilatational tracheostomy (PDT) are frequently performed bedside in the intensive care unit. Critically ill patients frequently require anticoagulant (AC) and antiplatelet (AP) therapies for myriad indications. There are no societal guidelines proffering strategies to manage AC/AP therapies periprocedurally for bedside PEG or PDT. The aim of this study is to evaluate the management of AC/AP therapies around PEG/PDT, assess periprocedural bleeding complications, and identify risk factors associated with bleeding.

Methods.—A retrospective, observational study of all adult patients admitted from October 2004 to December 2009 receiving a bedside PEG or PDT was conducted. Patients were identified by procedure codes via an in-hospital database. A medical record review was performed for each included patient.

Results.—Four hundred fifteen patients were included, with 187 PEGs and 352 PDTs being performed. Prophylactic anticoagulation was held for approximately one dose before and two doses or less after the procedure. There was wide variation in patterns of holding therapy in patients receiving anticoagulation via continuous infusion. There were 19 recorded minor bleeding events, 1 (0.5%) with PEG and 18 (5.1%) with PDT, with no hemorrhagic events. No association was found between international normalized ratio, prothrombin time, or activated partial thromboplastin time values and bleed risk ($p = 0.853$, 0.689, and 0.440, respectively). Platelet count was significantly lower in patients with a bleeding event ($p = 0.006$).

Conclusions.—We found that while practice patterns were quite consistent in regard to the management of prophylactic anticoagulation, it varied widely in patients receiving therapeutic anticoagulation. It seems that prophylactic anticoagulation use did not affect bleed risk with PEG/PDT.

▶ Percutaneous dilatational tracheostomy and percutaneous endoscopic gastrostomy are common procedures in the critical care unit.[1] This study examines a pattern of practice for use of prophylactic anticoagulation involving antiplatelet agents and other anticoagulants during the time of these procedures. We see that routine limitation of these agents when given for prophylaxis is unnecessary unless long-acting antiplatelet agents are administered. Of laboratory data suggesting increased risk for periprocedural bleeding, only thrombocytopenia (platelet count less than 50 000) is indicative of increased risk. There are insufficient data to comment on patients who receive therapeutic anticoagulation when procedures are performed.

There are several important limitations in this work. Perhaps most important is the potential for significant limitation of data quality in this retrospective chart review. Laboratory data were obtained only by convenience. Thus, a potentially valuable pattern of laboratory results could have been missed. The only criteria to identify procedures of interest was the detection of procedural codes in administrative datasets.

In summary, brief periprocedural limitation of prophylactic anticoagulation and short-acting antiplatelet agents is reasonable for bedside procedures. Carefully constructed prospective data collection is essential to confirm other observations made. Finally, the severity of any bleeding complication is not quantified.

D. J. Dries, MSE, MD

Reference

1. Goldman RK. Minimally invasive surgery. Bedside tracheostomy and gastrostomy. *Crit Care Clin.* 2000;16:113-130.

Hydroxyethyl Starch or Saline for Fluid Resuscitation in Intensive Care
Myburgh JA, for the CHEST Investigators and the Australian and New Zealand Intensive Care Society Clinical Trials Group (George Inst for Global Health, Sydney, New South Wales, Australia; et al)
N Engl J Med 367:1901-1911, 2012

Background.—The safety and efficacy of hydroxyethyl starch (HES) for fluid resuscitation have not been fully evaluated, and adverse effects of HES on survival and renal function have been reported.

Methods.—We randomly assigned 7000 patients who had been admitted to an intensive care unit (ICU) in a 1:1 ratio to receive either 6% HES with a molecular weight of 130 kD and a molar substitution ratio of 0.4 (130/0.4, Voluven) in 0.9% sodium chloride or 0.9% sodium chloride (saline) for all fluid resuscitation until ICU discharge, death, or 90 days after randomization. The primary outcome was death within 90 days. Secondary outcomes included acute kidney injury and failure and treatment with renal-replacement therapy.

Results.—A total of 597 of 3315 patients (18.0%) in the HES group and 566 of 3336 (17.0%) in the saline group died (relative risk in the HES group, 1.06; 95% confidence interval [CI], 0.96 to 1.18; $P = 0.26$). There was no significant difference in mortality in six predefined subgroups. Renal-replacement therapy was used in 235 of 3352 patients (7.0%) in the HES group and 196 of 3375 (5.8%) in the saline group (relative risk, 1.21; 95% CI, 1.00 to 1.45; $P = 0.04$). In the HES and saline groups, renal injury occurred in 34.6% and 38.0% of patients, respectively ($P = 0.005$), and renal failure occurred in 10.4% and 9.2% of patients, respectively ($P = 0.12$). HES was associated with significantly more adverse events (5.3% vs. 2.8%, $P < 0.001$).

Conclusions.—In patients in the ICU, there was no significant difference in 90-day mortality between patients resuscitated with 6% HES (130/0.4) or saline. However, more patients who received resuscitation with HES were treated with renal-replacement therapy. (Funded by the National Health and Medical Research Council of Australia and others; CHEST ClinicalTrials.gov number, NCT00935168.)

▶ This is another major study from the Australian and New Zealand critical care study group evaluating survival and renal response to use of a standard starch as opposed to normal saline in resuscitation (Fig 2 in the original article). Renal insufficiency has been seen in smaller studies with a high concentration of starch. However, this study uses a lower concentration of starch and a similar concern arises.[1-3] Patients receiving the Voluven (starch) solution required less fluid in the course of resuscitation but received up to 50 mL/kg of the starch solution per day, a relatively large dose. The starch group also received more blood products than the saline group in this resuscitation study. Could some of these outcomes relate to use of transfusion?

Creatinine levels were significantly increased and urine output decreased in the patients receiving starch as opposed to saline during the first 7 days of this trial (Fig 3 in the original article). The other lesser-adverse event was pruritus and rash. This finding may be associated with increased accumulation of starch within the reticuloendothelial system. A similar mechanism may contribute to kidney and hepatic injury.

An important limitation is the lack of standard criteria for initiation of renal replacement therapy. Renal replacement was initiated at the discretion of attending clinicians. Thus, a key adverse outcome was subjectively determined. Nonetheless, the volume of concerning data related to the use of starch solutions in the setting of critical illness continues to grow.

D. J. Dries, MSE, MD

References

1. Finfer S, Liu B, Taylor C, et al. Resuscitation fluid use in critically ill adults: an international cross-sectional study in 391 intensive care units. *Crit Care.* 2010; 14:R185.

2. Schortgen F, Lacherade JC, Bruneel F, et al. Effects of hydroxyethylstarch and gelatin on renal function in severe sepsis: a multicentre randomised study. *Lancet.* 2001;357:911-916.

3. Perner A, Haase N, Guttormsen AB, et al. Hydroxyethyl starch 130/0.42 versus Ringer's acetate in severe sepsis. *N Engl J Med.* 2012;367:124-134.

Early Intensive Care Sedation Predicts Long-Term Mortality in Ventilated Critically Ill Patients
Shehabi Y, Sedation Practice in Intensive Care Evaluation (SPICE) Study Investigators and the ANZICS Clinical Trials Group (Univ of New South Wales, Randwick, Australia; et al)
Am J Respir Crit Care Med 186:724-731, 2012

Rationale.—Choice and intensity of early (first 48 h) sedation may affect short- and long-term outcome.

Objectives.—To investigate the relationships between early sedation and time to extubation, delirium, and hospital and 180-day mortality among ventilated critically ill patients in the intensive care unit (ICU).

Methods.—Multicenter (25 Australia and New Zealand hospitals) prospective longitudinal (ICU admission to 28 d) cohort study of medical/surgical patients ventilated and sedated 24 hours or more. We assessed administration of sedative agents, ventilation time, sedation depth using Richmond Agitation Sedation Scale (RASS, four hourly), delirium (daily), and hospital and 180-day mortality. We used multivariable Cox regression to quantify relationships between early deep sedation (RASS, -3 to -5) and patients' outcomes.

Measurements and Main Results.—We studied 251 patients (mean age, 61.7 ± 15.9 yr; mean Acute Physiology and Chronic Health Evaluation [APACHE] II score, 20.8 ± 7.8), with 21.1% (53) hospital and 25.8% (64) 180-day mortality. Over 2,678 study days, we completed 14,736 RASS assessments. Deep sedation occurred in 191 (76.1%) patients within 4 hours of commencing ventilation and in 171 (68%) patients at 48 hours. Delirium occurred in 111 (50.7%) patients with median (interquartile range) duration of 2 (1–4) days. After adjusting for diagnosis, age, sex, APACHE II, operative, elective, hospital type, early use of vasopressors, and dialysis, early deep sedation was an independent predictor of time to extubation (hazard ratio [HR], 0.90; 95% confidence interval [CI], 0.87–0.94; $P < 0.001$), hospital death (HR, 1.11; 95% CI, 1.02–1.20; $P = 0.01$), and 180-day mortality (HR, 1.08; 95% CI, 1.01–1.16; $P = 0.026$) but not delirium occurring after 48 hours ($P = 0.19$).

Conclusions.—Early sedation depth independently predicts delayed extubation and increased mortality, making it a potential target for interventional studies.

▶ This multicenter prospective observational trial was conducted in multiple intensive care units in Australia and New Zealand. Management during the initial 48 hours of intubation was emphasized. Common agents used include midazolam (55%) and propofol (56%) in these patients. Approximately 20% of patients received both of these agents. Fentanyl and morphine were also used in greater than 40% of patients. When patients had longer intensive care unit (ICU) stay, midazolam was used more frequently than propofol.[1,2] When patients were lightly sedated so that assessment for delirium was possible, 31% of patients assessed in the first 24 hours of the study were positive for delirium, whereas 24% of patients were delirious at least 1 of the first 2 days of this trial. The proportion of patients with delirium increased with increasing ICU stay with more than 67% of patients staying in ICU longer than 14 days experiencing at least 1 day of delirium (Fig 2 in the original article).

In this observational trial, clinicians prescribed sedation targets for less than 25% of all Richmond Agitation Sedation Scale assessments. Only one third of these assessments met the prescribed sedation target. Deliberate cessation of all sedatives and analgesics occurred in approximately 13% of patients during the first 24 hours and 23% of patients during study day 2. Routine sedation interruption was rarely practiced (approximately 3% of all study days).[3,4]

This study extends early work demonstrating a relationship between sedation depth and clinical outcomes (Fig 4 in the original article). It is sobering to realize that in a group of ICUs participating in a study consortium, monitored practice frequently deviates significantly from proposed norms.[5,6] Given the observational nature of this work, however, confounders such as dynamic changes in illness severity, presence or absence of shock or sepsis, or individual patient variability could not be measured. Nonetheless, we must recognize that the risk associated with delirium begins at the time of intubation.

D. J. Dries, MSE, MD

References

1. Jackson DL, Proudfoot CW, Cann KF, Walsh T. A systematic review of the impact of sedation practice in the ICU on resource use, coasts and patient safety. *Crit Care*. 2010;14:R59.
2. Patel SB, Kress JP. Sedation and analgesia in the mechanically ventilated patient. *Am J Respir Crit Care Med*. 2012;185:486-497.
3. Sessler CN, Gosnell MS, Grap MJ, et al. The Richmond Agitation-Sedation Scale: validity and reliability in adult intensive care unit patients. *Am J Respir Crit Care Med*. 2002;166:1338-1344.
4. Ely EW, Inouye SK, Bernard GR, et al. Delirium in mechanically ventilated patients: validity and reliability of the Confusion Assessment Method for the Intensive Care unit (CAM-ICU). *JAMA*. 2001;286:2703-2710.
5. Ely EW, Shintani A, Truman B, et al. Delirium as a predictor of mortality in mechanically ventilated patients in the intensive care unit. *JAMA*. 2004;291:1753-1762.
6. Kress JP, Pohlman AS, O'Connor MF, Hall JB. Daily interruption of sedative infusions in critically ill patients undergoing mechanical ventilation. *N Engl J Med*. 2000;342:1471-1477.

Dexmedetomidine vs Midazolam or Propofol for Sedation During Prolonged Mechanical Ventilation: Two Randomized Controlled Trials

Jakob SM, for the Dexmedetomidine for Long-Term Sedation Investigators (Bern Univ Hosp and Univ of Bern, Switzerland; et al)
JAMA 307:1151-1160, 2012

Context.—Long-term sedation with midazolam or propofol in intensive care units (ICUs) has serious adverse effects. Dexmedetomidine, an α_2-agonist available for ICU sedation, may reduce the duration of mechanical ventilation and enhance patient comfort.

Objective.—To determine the efficacy of dexmedetomidine vs midazolam or propofol (preferred usual care) in maintaining sedation; reducing duration of mechanical ventilation; and improving patients' interaction with nursing care.

Design, Setting, and Patients.—Two phase 3 multicenter, randomized, double-blind trials carried out from 2007 to 2010. The MIDEX trial compared midazolam with dexmedetomidine in ICUs of 44 centers in 9 European countries; the PRODEX trial compared propofol with dexmedetomidine in 31 centers in 6 European countries and 2 centers in Russia. Included were adult ICU patients receiving mechanical ventilation who needed light to moderate sedation for more than 24 hours (midazolam, n=251, vs dexmedetomidine, n=249; propofol, n=247, vs dexmedetomidine, n=251).

Interventions.—Sedation with dexmedetomidine, midazolam, or propofol; daily sedation stops; and spontaneous breathing trials.

Main Outcome Measures.—For each trial, we tested whether dexmedetomidine was noninferior to control with respect to proportion of time at target sedation level (measured by Richmond Agitation-Sedation Scale) and superior to control with respect to duration of mechanical ventilation. Secondary end points were patients' ability to communicate pain (measured using a visual analogue scale [VAS]) and length of ICU stay. Time at target sedation was analyzed in per-protocol population (midazolam, n=233, vs dexmedetomidine, n=227; propofol, n=214, vs dexmedetomidine, n=223).

Results.—Dexmedetomidine/midazolam ratio in time at target sedation was 1.07 (95% CI, 0.97-1.18) and dexmedetomidine/propofol, 1.00 (95% CI, 0.92-1.08). Median duration of mechanical ventilation appeared shorter with dexmedetomidine (123 hours [IQR, 67-337]) vs midazolam (164 hours [IQR, 92-380]; $P = .03$) but not with dexmedetomidine (97 hours [IQR, 45-257]) vs propofol (118 hours [IQR, 48-327]; $P = .24$). Patients' interaction (measured using VAS) was improved with dexmedetomidine (estimated score difference vs midazolam, 19.7 [95% CI, 15.2-24.2]; $P<.001$; and vs propofol, 11.2 [95% CI, 6.4-15.9]; $P<.001$). Length of ICU and hospital stay and mortality were similar. Dexmedetomidine vs midazolam patients had more hypotension (51/247 [20.6%] vs 29/250 [11.6%]; $P = .007$) and bradycardia (35/247 [14.2%] vs 13/250 [5.2%]; $P<.001$).

Conclusions.—Among ICU patients receiving prolonged mechanical ventilation, dexmedetomidine was not inferior to midazolam and propofol in maintaining light to moderate sedation. Dexmedetomidine reduced duration of mechanical ventilation compared with midazolam and improved patients' ability to communicate pain compared with midazolam and propofol. More adverse effects were associated with dexmedetomidine.

Trial Registration.—clinicaltrials.gov Identifiers: NCT00481312, NCT00479661 (Fig 2, Table 3).

▶ This article brings dexmedetomidine into the mainstream for use with ventilated patients.[1] The most important finding with dexmedetomidine is shown in Table 3. Compared to propofol and midazolam, dexmedetomidine allowed a

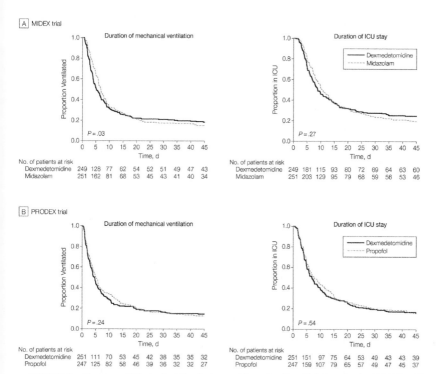

FIGURE 2.—Duration of Mechanical Ventilation and Intensive Care Unit Stay. In the MIDEX trial (midazolam vs dexmedetomidine), the median duration of mechanical ventilation was, for dexmedetomidine, 123 hours (interquartile range [IQR], 67-337 hours) and, for midazolam, 164 hours (IQR, 92-380 hours) (Gehan-Wilcoxon $P = .03$). The median length of stay in the intensive care unit (ICU) from randomization until the patient was medically fit for discharge was, for dexmedetomidine, 211 hours (IQR, 115-831 hours) and, for midazolam, 243 hours; Gehan-Wilcoxon $P = .27$). In the PRODEX trial (propofol vs dexmedetomidine), the median duration of mechanical ventilation was, for dexmedetomidine, 97 hours (IQR, 45-257 hours) and, for propofol, 118 hours (IQR, 48-327 hours) (Gehan-Wilcoxon $P = .24$). The median length of stay in the ICU from randomization until the patient was medically fit for discharge was, for dexmedetomidine, 164 hours (IQR, 90-480 hours) and, for propofol, 185 hours (93-520 hours; Cox's proportional hazards test $P = .54$). Study drugs were given for a maximum of 336 hours in both trials. (Reprinted from Jakob SM, for the Dexmedetomidine for Long-Term Sedation Investigators. Dexmedetomidine vs midazolam or propofol for sedation during prolonged mechanical ventilation: two randomized controlled trials. *JAMA.* 2012;307:1151-1160. Copyright (2012) American Medical Association. All rights reserved.)

TABLE 3.—Patients' Arousability, Ability to Communicate Pain, and Ability to Cooperate With Nursing Care

	Adjusted Mean Estimate (95% CI)		P Value[a]	Estimate of Difference (95% CI)
	Dexmedetomidine	Preferred Usual Care		
Dexmedetomidine vs midazolam (MIDEX)	(n = 249)	(n = 251)		
Total VAS score[b]	49.7 (45.5 to 53.8)	30.0 (25.9 to 34.1)	<.001	19.7 (15.2 to 24.2)
Can the patient communicate pain?	46.3 (41.7 to 50.9)	24.2 (19.7 to 28.8)	<.001	22.1 (17.1 to 27.1)
How arousable is the patient?	58.2 (53.7 to 62.6)	40.7 (36.3 to 45.1)	<.001	17.5 (12.7 to 22.3)
How cooperative is the patient?	44.8 (40.3 to 49.2)	25.1 (20.8 to 29.5)	<.001	19.7 (14.8 to 24.5)
Dexmedetomidine vs propofol (PRODEX)	(n = 251)	(n = 247)		
Total VAS score[b]	51.3 (46.9 to 55.7)	40.1 (35.7 to 44.6)	<.001	11.2 (6.4 to 15.9)
Can the patient communicate pain?	49.3 (44.5 to 54.2)	35.4 (30.5 to 40.4)	<.001	13.9 (8.7 to 19.1)
How arousable is the patient?	59.1 (54.7 to 63.4)	47.8 (43.4 to 52.3)	<.001	11.2 (6.5 to 16.0)
How cooperative is the patient?	47.2 (42.3 to 52.2)	38.0 (33.0 to 43.0)	<.001	9.2 (3.9 to 14.5)

Abbreviation: VAS, visual analogue scale.
[a]Analysis of covariance with effects for treatment, country, and baseline values.
[b]A higher score represents a better outcome.

greater degree of interaction with the patient.[2,3] Beginning with a greater degree of interaction, it is not surprising that a statistical improvement in ventilator weaning is noted (Fig 2). The authors also demonstrate that, contrary to initial utilization, dexmedetomidine may be employed for extended periods after admission to an intensive care unit (ICU) with mechanical ventilation or after surgical procedures.

It is important to note the exclusion criteria in this trial. Patients with neurologic dysfunction and patients requiring resuscitation (a significant portion of trauma and surgical ICU practice) were excluded. Like propofol, and to a lesser degree midazolam, dexmedetomidine has adverse hemodynamic effects manifest as bradycardia and hypotension. The most important benefit of this agent seen in my practice is the ability to maintain the use of the drug, titrated simply to a level of sedation, whether the patient is ventilated or not.

The authors claim that varied approaches to ventilator weaning are accounted for in the large study population and the randomization process. Although this may be true from a statistical standpoint, a weaning protocol featuring midazolam or propofol, to be most effective, must be executed differently from weaning when dexmedetomidine is used. In my opinion, effective weaning can be done with any of these agents in appropriately selected patients.[4] The clinician must be skilled in use of the medication used. Finally, I note that the mean age of patients in each group from these 2 trials is approximately 65 years. Behavior of patients with these medications varies with age. For example, benzodiazepines are less effective in the elderly.[5] A young trauma population will metabolize and respond to these agents differently from patients in other age brackets.

D. J. Dries, MSE, MD

References

1. Tan JA, Ho KM. Use of dexmedetomidine as a sedative and analgesic agent in critically ill adult patients: a meta-analysis. *Intensive Care Med.* 2010;36:926-939.
2. Kress JP, Pohlman AS, O'Connor MF, Hall JB. Daily interruption of sedative infusions in critically ill patients undergoing mechanical ventilation. *N Engl J Med.* 2000;342:1471-1477.
3. Ely EW, Inouye SK, Bernard GR, et al. Delirium in mechanically ventilated patients: validity and reliability of the confusion assessment method for the intensive care unit (CAM-ICU). *JAMA.* 2001;286:2703-2710.
4. Roberts R, Ruthazer R, Chi A, et al. Impact of a national propofol shortage on duration of mechanical ventilation at an academic medical center. *Crit Care Med.* 2012;40:406-411.
5. Pandharipande P, Shintani A, Peterson J, et al. Lorazepam is an independent risk factor for transitioning to delirium in intensive care unit patients. *Anesthesiology.* 2006;104:21-26.

Article Index

Chapter 1: Airways/Lungs

Early alveolar and systemic mediator release in patients at different risks for ARDS
after multiple trauma   1

Association Between Use of Lung-Protective Ventilation With Lower Tidal
Volumes and Clinical Outcomes Among Patients Without Acute Respiratory
Distress Syndrome: A Meta-analysis   2

Measurement of forces applied during Macintosh direct laryngoscopy compared
with GlideScope® videolaryngoscopy   4

Difficult airway management in the emergency department: GlideScope
videolaryngoscopy compared to direct laryngoscopy   5

A Comparison of the C-MAC Video Laryngoscope to the Macintosh Direct
Laryngoscope for Intubation in the Emergency Department   6

Early Administration of Systemic Corticosteroids Reduces Hospital Admission
Rates for Children With Moderate and Severe Asthma Exacerbation   7

Burns, inhalation injury and ventilator-associated pneumonia: Value of routine
surveillance cultures   9

Review of Burn Injuries Secondary to Home Oxygen   10

Chapter 2: Cardiovascular

Hypothermia in Comatose Survivors From Out-of-Hospital Cardiac Arrest: Pilot
Trial Comparing 2 Levels of Target Temperature   13

High prevalence of corrected QT interval prolongation in acutely ill patients is
associated with mortality: Results of the QT in Practice (QTIP) Study   14

Effectiveness of the LUCAS device for mechanical chest compression after cardiac
arrest: systematic review of experimental, observational and animal studies   16

Effects of fluid resuscitation with synthetic colloids or crystalloids alone on shock
reversal, fluid balance, and patient outcomes in patients with severe sepsis:
A prospective sequential analysis   17

2-Hour Accelerated Diagnostic Protocol to Assess Patients With Chest Pain
Symptoms Using Contemporary Troponins as the Only Biomarker: The ADAPT
Trial   20

Ultrafiltration in Decompensated Heart Failure with Cardiorenal Syndrome   21

Long-Term Prognosis Following Resuscitation From Out of Hospital Cardiac
Arrest: Role of Percutaneous Coronary Intervention and Therapeutic Hypothermia   23

Prevalence of acute myocardial infarction in patients with presumably new left
bundle-branch block   26

Bedside Monitoring to Adjust Antiplatelet Therapy for Coronary Stenting   30

Rivaroxaban in Patients with a Recent Acute Coronary Syndrome   34

Intraaortic Balloon Support for Myocardial Infarction with Cardiogenic Shock 38

Fast-track practice in cardiac surgery: results and predictors of outcome   43

The Cardiopulmonary Effects of Vasopressin Compared With Norepinephrine in
Septic Shock   45

Percutaneous Coronary Intervention at Centers With and Without On-Site
Surgery: A Meta-Analysis   47

Pulmonary Embolism: The Weekend Effect   48

Usefulness of Preemptive Anticoagulation in Patients With Suspected Pulmonary
Embolism: A Decision Analysis   50

Creation and Validation of a Simple Venous Thromboembolism Risk Scoring Tool
for Thermally Injured Patients: Analysis of the National Burn Repository   52

Chapter 3: Hemodynamics and Monitoring

Comparison of hemodynamic measurements from invasive and noninvasive
monitoring during early resuscitation   55

Comparison of hemodynamic measurements from invasive and noninvasive
monitoring during early resuscitation   56

The Deleterious Effect of Admission Hyperglycemia on Survival and Functional
Outcome in Patients With Intracerebral Hemorrhage   58

Multimodality Monitoring for Cerebral Perfusion Pressure Optimization in
Comatose Patients With Intracerebral Hemorrhage   59

Accuracy of an expanded early warning score for patients in general and trauma
surgery wards   60

Chapter 4: Infectious Disease

Linezolid in Methicillin-Resistant *Staphylococcus aureus* Nosocomial Pneumonia:
A Randomized, Controlled Study   63

Hospital Admission Decision for Patients With Community-Acquired Pneumonia:
Variability Among Physicians in an Emergency Department   64

Cerium nitrate treatment prevents progressive tissue necrosis in the zone of stasis
following burn   66

The prevalence of genes encoding leukocidins in *Staphylococcus aureus* strains
resistant and sensitive to methicillin isolated from burn patients in Taleghani
hospital, Ahvaz, Iran   67

Prevalence and Outcomes of Antimicrobial Treatment for *Staphylococcus aureus*
Bacteremia in Outpatients with ESRD   68

Prospective Observational Study Comparing Three Different Treatment Regimes in
Patients with *Clostridium difficile* Infection   70

Performance of *Candida* Real-time Polymerase Chain Reaction, β-D-Glucan Assay,
and Blood Cultures in the Diagnosis of Invasive Candidiasis   71

The Frequency of Autoimmune N-Methyl-D-Aspartate Receptor Encephalitis
Surpasses That of Individual Viral Etiologies in Young Individuals Enrolled in the
California Encephalitis Project   72

Chlorhexidine Bathing to Reduce Central Venous Catheter-associated Bloodstream
Infection: Impact and Sustainability   74

Fidaxomicin Versus Vancomycin for *Clostridium difficile* Infection: Meta-Analysis of Pivotal Randomized Controlled Trials   75

Variability of antibiotic concentrations in critically ill patients receiving continuous renal replacement therapy: A multicentre pharmacokinetic study   76

Estimated global mortality associated with the first 12 months of 2009 pandemic influenza A H1N1 virus circulation: a modelling study   77

Impact of Treatment Strategy on Outcomes in Patients with Candidemia and Other Forms of Invasive Candidiasis: A Patient-Level Quantitative Review of Randomized Trials   79

Concurrent Use of Warfarin and Antibiotics and the Risk of Bleeding in Older Adults   80

Procalcitonin usefulness for the initiation of antibiotic treatment in intensive care unit patients   81

Limiting Severe Outcomes and Impact on Intensive Care Units of Moderate-Intermediate 2009 Pandemic Influenza: Role of Infectious Diseases Units   83

Validation of a Clinical Score for Assessing the Risk of Resistant Pathogens in Patients With Pneumonia Presenting to the Emergency Department   84

Effect of Empirical Treatment With Moxifloxacin and Meropenem vs Meropenem on Sepsis-Related Organ Dysfunction in Patients With Severe Sepsis: A Randomized Trial   86

The utility of procalcitonin in critically ill trauma patients   88

Comparison of Oligon catheters and chlorhexidine-impregnated sponges with standard multilumen central venous catheters for prevention of associated colonization and infections in intensive care unit patients: A multicenter, randomized, controlled study   90

Association between systemic corticosteroids and outcomes of intensive care unit—acquired pneumonia   93

Infections Caused by Multidrug Resistant Organisms Are Not Associated with Overall, All-Cause Mortality in the Surgical Intensive Care Unit: The 20,000 Foot View   96

Chapter 5: Postoperative Management

Pilot Implementation of a Perioperative Protocol to Guide Operating Room—to—Intensive Care Unit Patient Handoffs   99

Comparative Effectiveness of Preventative Therapy for Venous Thromboembolism After Coronary Artery Bypass Graft Surgery   101

Variability in Surgeons' Perioperative Practices May Influence the Incidence of Low-Output Failure After Coronary Artery Bypass Grafting Surgery   103

Temporary biventricular pacing decreases the vasoactive-inotropic score after cardiac surgery: A substudy of a randomized clinical trial   105

Standardized postoperative handover process improves outcomes in the intensive care unit: A model for operational sustainability and improved team performance   107

Institutional Factors Beyond Procedural Volume Significantly Impact Center Variability in Outcomes After Orthotopic Heart Transplantation   110

Advanced care nurse practitioners can safely provide sole resident cover for level three patients: impact on outcomes, cost and work patterns in a cardiac surgery programme 113

Frequency, characteristics, and outcomes of pediatric patients readmitted to the cardiac critical care unit 115

Blood Transfusion and the Risk of Acute Kidney Injury After Transcatheter Aortic Valve Implantation 116

In Vivo Molecular Imaging of Murine Embryonic Stem Cells Delivered to a Burn Wound Surface via Integra® Scaffolding 119

Association Between Hospital Intraoperative Blood Transfusion Practices for Surgical Blood Loss and Hospital Surgical Mortality Rates 120

Acute abdomen in pregnancy requiring surgical management: a 20-case series 122

Postoperative Complications in Patients With Obstructive Sleep Apnea 123

Haloperidol prophylaxis decreases delirium incidence in elderly patients after noncardiac surgery: A randomized controlled trial 126

Rates and patterns of death after surgery in the United States, 1996 and 2006 128

Physical Fitness in People After Burn Injury: A Systematic Review 131

Outcomes and Predictors in Burn Rehabilitation 132

Chapter 6: Sepsis/Septic Shock

Prognostic Value of Incremental Lactate Elevations in Emergency Department Patients With Suspected Infection 135

Can changes in arterial pressure be used to detect changes in cardiac index during fluid challenge in patients with septic shock? 136

Multiplex polymerase chain reaction pathogen detection in patients with suspected septicemia after trauma, emergency, and burn surgery 137

Advances in Mesenchymal Stem Cell Research in Sepsis 138

A multicenter trial to compare blood culture with polymerase chain reaction in severe human sepsis 140

Diagnostic value of positron emission tomography combined with computed tomography for evaluating patients with septic shock of unknown origin 141

Early goal-directed therapy (EGDT) for severe sepsis/septic shock: which components of treatment are more difficult to implement in a community-based emergency department? 142

Antibiotic strategies in severe nosocomial sepsis: Why do we not de-escalate more often? 144

Etomidate is associated with mortality and adrenal insufficiency in sepsis: A meta-analysis 145

Severe Sepsis and Septic Shock in Pregnancy 148

The effectiveness of hypertonic saline and pentoxifylline (HTS−PTX) resuscitation in haemorrhagic shock and sepsis tissue injury: Comparison with LR, HES, and LR−PTX treatments 150

Transfusion of packed red blood cells is not associated with improved central venous oxygen saturation or organ function in patients with septic shock   151

Dopamine versus norepinephrine in the treatment of septic shock: A meta-analysis   153

Red blood cell transfusions are associated with lower mortality in patients with severe sepsis and septic shock: A propensity-matched analysis   155

Red blood cell transfusions are associated with lower mortality in patients with severe sepsis and septic shock: A propensity-matched analysis   156

Initial resuscitation guided by the Surviving Sepsis Campaign recommendations and early echocardiographic assessment of hemodynamics in intensive care unit septic patients: A pilot study   159

Fever Control Using External Cooling in Septic Shock: A Randomized Controlled Trial   161

Fever Control Using External Cooling in Septic Shock: A Randomized Controlled Trial   163

Physical and Mental Health in Patients and Spouses After Intensive Care of Severe Sepsis: A Dyadic Perspective on Long-Term Sequelae Testing the Actor–Partner Interdependence Model   164

An evaluation of the diagnostic accuracy of the 1991 American College of Chest Physicians/Society of Critical Care Medicine and the 2001 Society of Critical Care Medicine/European Society of Intensive Care Medicine/American College of Chest Physicians/American Thoracic Society/Surgical Infection Society sepsis definition   166

Septic Shock Attributed to *Candida* Infection: Importance of Empiric Therapy and Source Control   168

Effect of Bedside Ultrasonography on the Certainty of Physician Clinical Decisionmaking for Septic Patients in the Emergency Department   170

C1-esterase inhibitor infusion increases survival rates for patients with sepsis   172

An evaluation of the diagnostic accuracy of the 1991 American College of Chest Physicians/Society of Critical Care Medicine and the 2001 Society of Critical Care Medicine/European Society of Intensive Care Medicine/American College of Chest Physicians/American Thoracic Society/Surgical Infection Society sepsis definition   174

Chapter 7: Metabolism/Gastrointestinal/Nutrition/Hematology-Oncology

Fibrinogen function after severe burn injury   177

Five-Year Outcomes after Oxandrolone Administration in Severely Burned Children: A Randomized Clinical Trial of Safety and Efficacy   178

Red blood cell transfusion is associated with increased rebleeding in patients with nonvariceal upper gastrointestinal bleeding   180

Outcome of Patients Who Refuse Transfusion After Cardiac Surgery: A Natural Experiment With Severe Blood Conservation   182

Impact of Blood Product Transfusion on Short and Long-Term Survival After Cardiac Surgery: More Evidence   183

Red Blood Cell Transfusion: A Clinical Practice Guideline From the AABB   185

Is fresh-frozen plasma clinically effective? An update of a systematic review of randomized controlled trials   187

Bacterial Sepsis after Living Donor Liver Transplantation: The Impact of Early Enteral Nutrition   188

Chapter 8: Neurologic: Traumatic and Non-traumatic

Continuous electroencephalography monitoring for early prediction of neurological outcome in postanoxic patients after cardiac arrest: a prospective cohort study   191

Implementation of Adapted PECARN Decision Rule for Children With Minor Head Injury in the Pediatric Emergency Department   192

Cognitive and Neurologic Outcomes after Coronary-Artery Bypass Surgery   194

Timing of neuroprognostication in postcardiac arrest therapeutic hypothermia   196

Acute lung injury in critical neurological illness   197

Magnesium for aneurysmal subarachnoid haemorrhage (MASH-2): a randomised placebo-controlled trial   198

Anemia and brain oxygen after severe traumatic brain injury   199

Will Delays in Treatment Jeopardize the Population Benefit From Extending the Time Window for Stroke Thrombolysis?   200

Decompressive Hemicraniectomy in Patients With Supratentorial Intracerebral Hemorrhage   201

Tight glycemic control increases metabolic distress in traumatic brain injury: A randomized controlled within-subjects trial   202

Placebo-Controlled Trial of Amantadine for Severe Traumatic Brain Injury   204

Factors influencing intracranial pressure monitoring guideline compliance and outcome after severe traumatic brain injury   205

A Randomized Trial of Tenecteplase versus Alteplase for Acute Ischemic Stroke   206

Poststroke delirium incidence and outcomes: Validation of the Confusion Assessment Method for the Intensive Care Unit (CAM-ICU)   207

Delirium in Acute Stroke: A Systematic Review and Meta-Analysis   209

A Randomized and Blinded Single-Center Trial Comparing the Effect of Intracranial Pressure and Intracranial Pressure Wave Amplitude-Guided Intensive Care Management on Early Clinical State and 12-Month Outcome in Patients With Aneurysmal Subarachnoid Hemorrhage   210

An evaluation of three measures of intracranial compliance in traumatic brain injury patients   211

Cardiac and central vascular functional alterations in the acute phase of aneurysmal subarachnoid hemorrhage   213

Closure or Medical Therapy for Cryptogenic Stroke with Patent Foramen Ovale   214

Midlevel practitioners can safely place intracranial pressure monitors   216

A Trial of Intracranial-Pressure Monitoring in Traumatic Brain Injury   217

Blast-related mild traumatic brain injury is associated with a decline in self-rated health amongst US military personnel   219

Performance of the Canadian CT Head Rule and the New Orleans Criteria for Predicting Any Traumatic Intracranial Injury on Computed Tomography in a United States Level I Trauma Center   221

Chapter 9: Renal

Predicting Acute Kidney Injury Among Burn Patients in the 21st Century: A Classification and Regression Tree Analysis   223

Body mass index and acute kidney injury in the acute respiratory distress syndrome   224

Association Between a Chloride-Liberal vs Chloride-Restrictive Intravenous Fluid Administration Strategy and Kidney Injury in Critically Ill Adults   226

Chapter 10: Trauma and Overdose

Embolization for Multicompartmental Bleeding in Patients in Hemodynamically Unstable Condition: Prognostic Factors and Outcome   229

Debunking the survival bias myth: Characterization of mortality during the initial 24 hours for patients requiring massive transfusion   230

Debunking the survival bias myth: Characterization of mortality during the initial 24 hours for patients requiring massive transfusion   232

Stress-Induced Hyperglycemia, Not Diabetic Hyperglycemia, Is Associated With Higher Mortality in Trauma   235

Long-Term Propranolol Use in Severely Burned Pediatric Patients: A Randomized Controlled Study   237

The effects of prehospital plasma on patients with injury: A prehospital plasma resuscitation   239

Benchmarking Outcomes in the Critically Injured Trauma Patient and the Effect of Implementing Standard Operating Procedures   241

Early Platelet Dysfunction: An Unrecognized Role in the Acute Coagulopathy of Trauma   243

The changing pattern and implications of multiple organ failure after blunt injury with hemorrhagic shock   245

Mortality by Decade in Trauma Patients with Glasgow Coma Scale 3   247

The impact of BMI on polytrauma outcome   248

Ballistic Fractures: Indirect Fracture to Bone   249

Hyperfibrinolysis at admission is an uncommon but highly lethal event associated with shock and prehospital fluid administration   251

The impact of antiplatelet drugs on trauma outcomes   253

Hypotension is 100 mmHg on the battlefield   255

Clinical and biomarker profile of trauma-induced secondary cardiac injury   257

A Systematic Review and Meta-Analysis of Diagnostic Screening Criteria for Blunt Cerebrovascular Injuries   259

Base deficit as a marker of survival after traumatic injury: Consistent across changing patient populations and resuscitation paradigms ... 262

Use of computed tomography in the initial evaluation of anterior abdominal stab wounds ... 264

Complications following thoracic trauma managed with tube thoracostomy ... 266

Fracture stabilisation in a polytraumatised African population—A comparison with international management practice ... 268

Factor IX complex for the correction of traumatic coagulopathy ... 269

Autotransfusion of hemothorax blood in trauma patients: is it the same as fresh whole blood? ... 272

Are Certain Fractures at Increased Risk for Compartment Syndrome After Civilian Ballistic Injury? ... 273

AIS > 2 in at least two body regions: A potential new anatomical definition of polytrauma ... 275

Military Application of Tranexamic Acid in Trauma Emergency Resuscitation (MATTERs) Study ... 278

Critical Role of Activated Protein C in Early Coagulopathy and Later Organ Failure, Infection and Death in Trauma Patients ... 280

Early complementopathy after multiple injuries in humans ... 282

Tympanic Membrane Rupture in the Survivors of the July 7, 2005, London Bombings ... 285

Multiple Organ Failure as a Cause of Death in Patients With Severe Burns ... 288

Chapter 11: Ethics/Socioeconomic/Administrative Issues

Patient Understanding of Emergency Department Discharge Instructions: Where Are Knowledge Deficits Greatest? ... 291

A systematic review of the evidence for telemedicine in burn care: With a UK perspective ... 292

Predictors of health-care needs in discharged burn patients ... 293

Evaluation of long term health-related quality of life in extensive burns: a 12-year experience in a burn center ... 294

Burn size and survival probability in paediatric patients in modern burn care: a prospective observational cohort study ... 296

Impact of Intensive Care Unit Organ Failures on Mortality during the Five Years after a Critical Illness ... 298

Do-not-resuscitate order: a view throughout the world ... 299

Family Factors Affect Clinician Attitudes in Pediatric End-of-Life Decision Making: A Randomized Vignette Study ... 301

Withdrawal of care: A 10-year perspective at a Level I trauma center ... 303

Palliative Surgery in the Do-Not-Resuscitate Patient: Ethics and Practical Suggestions for Management ... 305

Law ethics and clinical judgment in end-of-life decisions—How do Norwegian doctors think? 306

Religio-ethical discussions on organ donation among Muslims in Europe: an example of transnational Islamic bioethics 308

Pediatric ventilation in a disaster: Clinical and ethical decision making 310

Use of the Medical Ethics Consultation Service in a Busy Level I Trauma Center: Impact on Decision-Making and Patient Care 312

Denying a Patient's Final Will: Public Safety vs. Medical Confidentiality and Patient Autonomy 315

End-of-Life Care Decisions: Importance of Reviewing Systems and Limitations After 2 Recent North American Cases 317

Attitudes Towards End-of-Life Decisions and the Subjective Concepts of Consciousness: An Empirical Analysis 319

The role of the principle of double effect in ethics education at US medical schools and its potential impact on pain management at the end of life 321

Death and legal fictions 323

The Ethics and Reality of Rationing in Medicine 326

Early Withdrawal of Life Support in Severe Burn Injury 328

Does Admission During Morning Rounds Increase the Mortality of Patients in the Medical ICU? 329

Refusal of Intensive Care Unit Admission Due to a Full Unit: Impact on Mortality 331

The Epidemiology of Intensive Care Unit Readmissions in the United States 332

A systematic review of silver-containing dressings and topical silver agents (used with dressings) for burn wounds 335

Pathogenic alteration in severe burn wounds 336

Chapter 12: Pharmacology/Sedation-Analgesia

Anticoagulation management around percutaneous bedside procedures: Is adjustment required? 339

Hydroxyethyl Starch or Saline for Fluid Resuscitation in Intensive Care 340

Early Intensive Care Sedation Predicts Long-Term Mortality in Ventilated Critically Ill Patients 342

Dexmedetomidine vs Midazolam or Propofol for Sedation During Prolonged Mechanical Ventilation: Two Randomized Controlled Trials 344

Author Index

A

Aboa-Eboulé C, 58
Aboumatar H, 99
Abu SF, 335
Agarwal HS, 107
Agarwal P, 200
Al-Mousawi AM, 296
Albertson TE, 137
Aldecoa C, 153
Aldous S, 20
Algra A, 198
Amiel J-B, 159
Amini A, 269
Andes DR, 79
Andriessen TMJC, 205
Aponte-Patel L, 105
Armada E, 13
Aronsky D, 64
Arvaniti K, 90
Aujesky D, 50
Aziz Z, 335

B

Bader T, 310
Bagiella E, 204
Bahus MK, 306
Baillargeon J, 80
Balogh ZJ, 275
Bandeali S, 26
Bart BA, 21
Barton CA, 339
Barton JR, 148
Bastero-Miñón P, 115
Baumgartner WA, 99
Bayer O, 17
Becker K, 140
Bednarik J, 207
Béjot Y, 58
Bellomo R, 226
Ben D, 336
Benson JJ, 317
Bentsen G, 210
Berardoni NE, 264
Bernard AC, 253
Bhaskar B, 183
Bhogal SK, 7
Biersteker HAR, 205
Bisbal M, 329
Bivard A, 206
Bize PE, 229
Blondon M, 50
Bloos F, 140

Böhling T, 288
Bouferrache K, 159
Bourbeau J, 7
Bowling WM, 216
Braune S, 141
Bressan S, 192
Brewster BD, 138
Brizzio ME, 182
Brown JB, 230, 232
Brown SES, 332
Brunkhorst FM, 86, 164
Bruno G, 83
Brusselaers N, 9
Buckley BA, 291
Burk A-M, 282
Burkle CM, 317
Butcher N, 275

C

Call M, 280
Canivet J-L, 81
Carbonara S, 83
Cardoso SO, 2
Carney N, 217
Carson JL, 185
Chan CM, 145
Chan KE, 68
Chandra MS, 55-56
Chesnut RM, 217
Chimot L, 159
Chiu S, 5, 6
Choi HA, 59
Chong NJ, 335
Christiani DC, 224
Chun B-C, 155-156
Ciaula GD, 83
Clabault K, 161, 163
Clement CM, 221
Clond MA, 247
Cloostermans MC, 191
Cohen MJ, 280
Collet J-P, 30
Corneille M, 272
Cotton BA, 251
Crook DW, 75
Cullen L, 20
Cuschieri J, 241

D

Dalmau J, 72
Dau N, 249

Davenport R, 257
Dawood FS, 77
De Backer D, 153
Dean NC, 64
De'Ath HD, 257
Dehmer GJ, 47
Den Hartog D, 60
Dente CJ, 262
Diaz EC, 237
Disseldorp LM, 131
Dobrowolsky A, 223
Dougherty PJ, 249
Dubose JJ, 278
Dulhunty J, 183
Dumas F, 23
Duran R, 229

E

Eastridge BJ, 255
Eertman CJ, 191
Eide PK, 210
Elman J, 4
Engel KG, 291
Eski M, 66
Esperatti M, 93

F

Farshadzadeh Z, 67
Ferraris VA, 253
Ferrer M, 93
Feudtner C, 301
Firat C, 66
Flierl MA, 282
Førde R, 306
Forth VE, 291
Frank AJ, 224
Franz RW, 259
Friedmann PD, 120
Friese RS, 269
Fu Y, 336
Fuller BM, 151
Fung C, 201
Funk LM, 128
Furlan AJ, 214

G

Gable MS, 72
Gaertner J, 315

Gainnier M, 329
Gajera M, 151
Galstyan GM, 172
Garvin JR, 305
Gates S, 16
Gerrard P, 132
Ghaly M, 308
Giacino JT, 204
Goldstein R, 132
Gordon AC, 45
Gottesman RF, 194
Goverman J, 119
Grega MA, 194
Greinwald R, 315
Grey B, 268
Griffin RL, 235
Gullo A, 299

H

Haanschoten MC, 43
Hacker S, 177
Hamilton N, 285
Hampton N, 168
Hamrahi VF, 119
Hardcastle J, 273
Harvin JA, 251
Havalad V, 105
Haydar SA, 170
Heard SO, 166, 174
Heenen S, 144
Hegarty C, 226
Helfenbein E, 14
Heltemes KJ, 219
Herndon DN, 178, 237,
  296
Hervieu M, 58
Hexem KR, 301
Higgins GL III, 170
Higgins R, 272
Hinder F, 140
Hodgman EI, 262
Hoerburger D, 177
Hoesch RE, 197
Hoffmann M, 248
Holbrook TL, 219
Holmes DR Jr, 47
Holmes HM, 80
Hopewell S, 187
Horn J, 205
Hoveizavi H, 67
Howells T, 211
Huang HD, 26
Humpl T, 115

Hussain A, 292
Hussain ON, 247
Hyde B, 253

I

Igonin AA, 172
Ikegami T, 188
Iuliano AD, 77

J

Jacobs F, 144
Jaenichen D, 164
Jairath V, 180
Jakob SM, 344
Jenkins DH, 239
Johnson LS, 312
Jones JP, 64
Joseph B, 269
Jule M, 142
Jung W, 119

K

Kahn JM, 332
Kallinen O, 288
Karakitsos D, 213
Katsahian S, 161, 163
Kaw R, 123
Kerby JD, 235
Khan N, 292
Khan S, 4
Kherad O, 180
Khosravi AD, 67
Kilic A, 110
Kim BD, 239
Kim HJ, 150
Kim P, 266
Kirkpatrick JN, 196
Kline JA, 135
Kluge S, 141
Ko S-B, 59
Koch CG, 182
Kohl M, 17
Kollef M, 168
Kollef MH, 63
Kopelman TR, 264
Kostalova M, 207
Kostousouv V, 251
Kraft R, 296

Kulik A, 101
Kumar M, 199
Kuo H-W, 70
Kwon S-S, 155-156

L

Lambermont B, 81
LaPar DJ, 96
Layios N, 81
Lee KH, 150
Lesandrini J, 312
Levine JM, 199
Lewén A, 211
Ley EJ, 247
Li H-L, 126
Liang CY, 293
Likosky DS, 103
Lin E, 197
Lin Y-L, 80
Lipsitz SR, 128
Logie D, 9
Lone NI, 298
Lopez-de-Sa E, 13
Lotto L, 319

M

Macauley R, 321
MacGregor AJ, 219
MacLennan P, 235
Madoff DC, 229
Maisniemi K, 288
Makris D, 213
Manetta JA, 2
Manfrinati A, 319
Manukyan MC, 138
Markert RJ, 55-56
Martin M, 282
Martin MU, 1
McArthur DL, 202
McGillivray D, 7
McKenna D, 74
McMillian WD, 339
Mees SMD, 198
Mega JL, 34
Mehta N, 26
Menger R, 266
Meskey T, 273
Micek S, 168
Michetti CP, 88
Miller FG, 323
Minei JP, 245

Mion T, 192
Mitasova A, 207
Mitchell AL, 145
Moerman T, 60
Monks T, 200
Montecalvo MA, 74
Moore EE, 243
Moore ET, 170
Morales J, 142
Morrison JJ, 278
Morse BC, 262
Mosier J, 6
Mosier JM, 5
Muckart DJJ, 268
Mullany DV, 183
Mullen MT, 166, 174
Murabit A, 10
Murek M, 201
Myburgh JA, 340
Myers J, 101

N

Nanchal R, 48
Nelson M, 280
Nguyen HV, 105
Nguyen MH, 71
Niederman MS, 63
Nierhaus A, 141
Nieuwenhuis MK, 131
Njimi H, 153
Nuis R-J, 116

O

Oddo M, 199
O'Neill PJ, 264
O'Neill R, 142
Ong GJ, 16
Osborne NH, 52
Osler T, 339
O'Toole RV, 273
Otto A, 328
Ozel L, 122
Ozer F, 66

P

Pannucci CJ, 52
Papa L, 221
Papanikolaou J, 213
Parikh G, 59
Park DW, 155-156

Parsons M, 206
Pasupuleti V, 123
Patel HDL, 285
Pattakos G, 182
Pauly V, 329
Perman SM, 196
Petrovic MA, 99
Pham TN, 328
Pickham D, 14
Pierrakos C, 136
Pitt M, 200
Porro LJ, 178
Presutti R, 209
Protsenko DN, 172
Puskarich MA, 135

R

Radford P, 285
Ranzani OT, 93
Rasmussen TE, 278
Rassen JA, 101
Ratcliffe SJ, 332
Raymondos K, 1
Redfearn S, 113
Reed C, 77
Reichley R, 84
Reinhart K, 17
Reitsma AM, 196
Restellini S, 180
Rey JR, 13
Righini M, 50
Rigoni D, 319
Ristagno G, 299
Robert R, 331
Roberts DM, 76
Rodés-Cabau J, 116
Rodriguez NA, 178, 237
Rodseth RN, 268
Romanato S, 192
Rosenberger LH, 96
Rosendahl J, 164
Rourke C, 257
Rozycki GS, 312
Ruppe MD, 301
Russell JL, 115
Russell T, 4

S

Sagi R, 310
Sakles JC, 6
Sakran JV, 88
Salhanick M, 272

Salinas J, 255
Santonocito C, 299
Saville BR, 107
Sawyer RG, 96
Sayharman SE, 122
Schaden E, 177
Scheunemann LP, 326
Schmid D, 70
Schmudlach T, 1
Schneider DF, 223
Schorr C, 151
Schortgen F, 161, 163
Scolletta S, 136
Scott TH, 305
Selchen D, 209
Selnes OA, 194
Semel ME, 128
Serpa Neto A, 2
Shah SK, 323
Shakir IA, 223
Shehabi Y, 342
Sheridan MJ, 88
Sheriff H, 72
Sherman D, 249
Shi Q, 209
Shields RK, 71
Shinn JA, 14
Shirabe K, 188
Shorr AF, 84, 145
Sibai BM, 148
Singh M, 47
Sinning J-M, 116
Sise CB, 303
Sise MJ, 303
Skinner H, 113
Sköld MK, 211
Skoyles J, 113
Slayton JM, 107
Smith JL, 16
Smith T, 60
Sorteberg AG, 210
Soto GJ, 224
Spratt N, 206
Stanworth S, 187
Steen PA, 306
Stein N, 202
Stiell IG, 221
Stolz U, 5
Stubbs BA, 23
Summers RL, 135

T

Tan W-H, 132
Tchorz KM, 55-56

Telford G, 266
Temkin N, 217
ter Woorst JF, 43
Thadhani RI, 68
Than M, 20
Thiele H, 38
Thomas S, 243
Thorndike JF, 303
Tran NK, 137
Tredget EE, 10
Trivedi A, 120
Truog RD, 323

U

Unal A, 122

V

Van Baar ME, 131
van Meulen FB, 191
van Straten AHM, 43
Vandertop WP, 198
Velissaris D, 136
Vent J, 315
Vespa P, 202

Vincent J-L, 144
Vogelaers D, 9

W

Wade CE, 255
Wahl WL, 52
Walker E, 123
Wallace DL, 292
Walley KR, 45
Walsh TS, 298
Wang D-X, 126
Wang HJ, 293
Wang N, 45
Wang W, 126
Wannemuehler TJ, 138
Warren HS, 68
Weiss ES, 110
Wenisch JM, 70
White DB, 326
White L, 23
Whyte J, 204
Willette PA, 259
Wisner DH, 137
Wissel MC, 71
Wohlauer MV, 243
Wood MJ, 259
Wu W-C, 120
Wunderink RG, 63

X

Xiao S-C, 294
Xie B, 294, 336

Y

Yang L, 187
Yao KP, 293
Yarrish R, 74
Yoshiya S, 188
Young M, 197
Young PJ, 216
Young SR, 328
Ytzhak A, 310
Yuh DD, 110
Yunos NM, 226

Z

Z'Graggen WJ, 201
Zhao H, 166, 174
Zhu S-H, 294
Zielinski MD, 239
Zilberberg MD, 84

Printed and bound by CPI Group (UK) Ltd, Croydon, CR0 4YY

08/05/2025

01864755-0011